Peter G. Douglas

$1.00

The BASIC *Neurosis*

The BASIC *Neurosis*

Oral Regression and Psychic Masochism

EDMUND BERGLER, M.D.

GRUNE & STRATTON, INC.
A SUBSIDIARY OF HARCOURT BRACE JOVANOVICH, PUBLISHERS

Grune & Stratton, Inc.
111 Fifth Avenue
New York, New York 10003

Library of Congress Catalog Card Number 49-9345
International Standard Book Number 0-8089-0054-4

Printed in the United States of America

TO MY WIFE, MARIANNE,

who, through her genius for real companionship and creation of a loving and contented home-atmosphere, has made my work possible and bearable.

Books by Dr. Edmund Bergler:

The Battle of the Conscience

Divorce Won't Help

Unhappy Marriage and Divorce

Psychic Impotence in Men

Frigidity in Women (in collaboration with E. Hitschmann)

Talleyrand—Napoleon—Stendhal—Grabbe

Contents

Preface

THE RIDDLE of the Sphinx in ancient Greece had this content: "What is that which is four-footed, three-footed and two-footed?" Young Oedipus of the saga guessed correctly that it was man; for the child crawls on hands and feet, the adult walks upright, and the old man supports his steps with a cane. Oedipus' smartness in solving the riddle did him very little good; he maneuvered himself into a great deal of trouble, but he achieved eternal fame thanks to the poet, Sophocles, and the scientist, Freud.

The riddle of modern times is not couched in symbolic language—it is simple, clear-cut and presented without circumlocution. Still, it is more difficult to answer than the ancient question and smartness alone does not do the trick—knowledge of the unconscious is necessary. Why do people have such an *insatiable unconscious craving for self-damage?*, does the question read. *The riddle of the Sphinx becomes the riddle of psychic masochism.*

Every new idea has an incubation time of at least a few generations. Yet this does not prove, as Schopenhauer scornfully assumed, "the miserable nature of mankind"; it is only natural, taking into consideration the inner obstacles preventing understanding and acceptance. Attempts at reducing these inner obstacles to the low level of intellectuality, are unjustified. Machiavelli's threefold division of heads, copied from Hesiod, is questionable:

> There are in the capacities of mankind three varieties: one man will understand a thing by itself; another so far it is explained to him; a third, neither of himself nor when it is clearly put before him.

Freud's discoveries of the dynamics of the unconscious shocked mankind. Freud himself acknowledged that humanity received three painful disappointments: Copernicus proved that our earth is not the center of the universe; Darwin, that man is not the unique crown of animal creation; and Freud, that man is not even master in his own house.

It took only one to two generations to acknowledge Freud's clinical discovery of the living reality of the unconscious, a fact which astounded the originator of psychoanalysis himself, though only after a long period of disappointment. The reason for the shortened incubation time was a coincidental factor: growing opposition to Victorian stuffiness and hypocrisy in matters sexual. True enough, what people understand of Freud's work is a rather silly simplification. But that "knowledge made simple," is also natural: mankind does not want to be bothered by new ideas in the first place, and even less with those which offend its narcissism. Thus, one can read even today the naive statement that "psychoanalysis is obsessed with sex," though Freud proved in the last third of his long scientific life that unconscious aggression is a full-fledged partner in the psychic household—the second partner being the previously discovered libidinous drives. All human actions and reactions invariably constitute a combination of *both* repressed tendencies.

It is in science as with grandmother's medical advice: it petrifies in a popular simplification the precepts of physicians of her mother's or grandmother's times. Newer discoveries are neglected and must wait for your children's granddaughter. Thus medical recipes become popular, though at the "wrong" time and when science is already miles ahead.

Psychologically interested readers are nowadays satiated with psychological half-knowledge. They still chew hopelessly on the early Freud of the nineties of the last century; and we are not to disturb that slow and painful process. Therefore, if an adherent of Freud comes out with some new explanations, the self-styled "psychologic connoisseurs" produce a supercilious "We-know-all-about-it" attitude. That mask of omniscience, though, has a Janus-face. On the one hand, every deviation from or "heresy" against Freud is gleefully accepted because it bolsters the old and deep-seated wish to reject analytic findings; the new fashion lasts approximately three to five years to slowly decline by segmentation. Or, if the contribution is genuinely Freudian and cannot be used for the purpose of bolstering inner resistances of the half-smart but fully neurotic set, it is ignored, or angrily rejected as complicating "unnecessarily" a complicated problem.

I am convinced that my contribution will be classed by more ignorant "connoisseurs" as belonging to the first, by more discerning ones to the second category. Foreseeing all this, the justified question arises: Why write the book in the first place?

The answer is simple: I am tired of constantly explaining my ideas on "orality" and psychic masochism, and hope to save myself time and fruitless effort in answering questions, by being able to refer to the book. I cannot be accused of harboring many other illusions about the present volume—for the moment.

Clinical work in psychoanalysis is unpredictable: you get a "simple" case into treatment, and find yourself on new and uncharted territory. That was, at least, what happened to me: even my first cases as candidate in training, sent to me by the Psychoanalytic Clinic in Vienna, were "complicated." I found myself—22 years ago—confronted with, or, I stumbled upon—as a malicious friend said—the deepest of all possible neuroses: "orally" regressed ones. Seemingly simple hysteriform cases turned out to be complicated ones in disguise. These cases had to be handled. They were, with the aid of first glimpses of a theory, gradually developed as "mechanism of orality," embodying the clinical fate of psychic masochism. I had at that time no idea of the universality and ramifications of the problem involved.

Even less did I suspect at that time that these studies would lead me to the conclusion that there exists but *one neurosis*, though one with many rescue-stations in later development, erected intrapsychically for the purpose of escaping the *deepest of all mortal dangers—psychic masochism.*

In a good portion of approximately 130 papers and 6 books, the bulk of which appeared in scientific journals and reviews in eleven countries, I gave an account of these experiences of two decades. Scientific journals are, unfortunately, a mass-grave, and not even a pompous one since it consists of paper walls. I have been constantly blamed that I "don't express precisely" what I mean, which, in general, is a polite word for reader's shifting the blame for not understanding the material presented—because of his own resistances—onto the innocent author. The same people have urged me to write a book on the topic, perhaps only to avoid reading (more precisely: seeing) my papers for some time in print.

I have been unfortunate enough to find "something" which every human being to a varying degree harbors unconsciously. Hence my statements were—unwillingly—"hitting below the belt." Neither that regrettable fact, nor my Cassandra-like warnings, to stop treating the great mass of orally regressed neurotics as hysterical ones, increased my popularity even in scientific circles.

In compiling my opinion about the "mechanism of orality," I absolve the reader beforehand from believing in the conclusions and results. An opinion is recorded—that is all. The inherent truth—or fallacy—will be tested and plagiarized a few generations hence.

I do not believe in Schopenhauer's slightly megalomaniacal self-consolation to the effect that the man with new ideas "buys centuries of fame by foregoing the applause of his contemporaries." I rather subscribe to Sir William Osler's candid statement: "In science the credit goes to the man who convinces the world, and not to the man to whom the idea first occurs." The implied advice to convince the world of your own ideas has a catch: you have to live a few generations after your own death. Since medical imperfection prevents that desirable state of affairs—at least in the meantime, as optimists believe—the pleasure of thinking up theories and making them work, is the scientist's only reward—past, present, and future.

EDMUND BERGLER

New York, February, 1949.

The author wishes to express his thanks to the editors of

Quarterly Review of Psychiatry and Neurology
The Psychiatric Quarterly
Diseases of the Nervous System
Bulletin of the Menninger Clinic
The Psychoanalytic Review
The Psychoanalytic Quarterly
Journal of Criminal Psychopathology
Medical Record
Quarterly Journal of Studies on Alcohol

for permission to reprint papers, or parts of them, previously published in these journals.

1

Symptoms and Signs of Oral Regression

FREUD started his discoveries of the dynamics of the unconscious on hysteric (phallic) neurotics and discovered first the libidinous drives which propelled these sick people: the Oedipus complex.

Viewing that fact from the aspect of "analytic geology," Freud first came across the most superficial layers of the unconscious, and, to complicate matters, focused his attention exclusively on libidinous drives. True, you cannot prescribe to a genius the sequence of his discoveries.

Imagine for a short moment the hypothetical possibility that Freud had discovered first the "geologically" deepest, and historically oldest, in the life of the individual, layers of the unconscious: those of oral regression. The result would have been the avoidance of a fantastically amorphous mass confusion. The "geologic" layers would have been presented in their "proper" order.

Things did not, of course, happen that way. The real development of the child starts with the oral level, and progresses to the "anal" and "phallic" phases. Freud discovered the phallic phase first, progressed later to the anal phase, and had very little to say about the oral phase.

Historic sequence of analytical *discovery*, and historic sequence of individual *development*, are thus reversed. Many people never clearly understood that confusing fact.

Not less tragic is the confusion in matters of libido and aggression. Once more, the sequence of discovery does not tally with the whole of clinical facts. All human actions are from the start a complicated mixture of both tendencies. Freud, however, discovered first the libidinous factors, and supplemented them only three decades later with aggressive components. Hence thinking in terms of libido *and* aggression, at the same time, at the same place, confronted with the same symptom, obviously overtaxes some heads. Clinical facts are seemingly not produced to make simplifying thinking more easy. Confronted with a boy's masturbation, for instance, we cannot simply say, as once upon a time, that the child satisfies his libidinous tendencies alone. He aggressively oversteps at the same time the educational command not to touch the penis, and this is clear even if one does not take into consideration his fantasies which either can have strong aggressive coloring or pertain to "forbidden" people.

Analytically, the journey into the past starts with the first phase in the child's development: the oral phase. The name, chosen by Freud, corresponds to the fact that the baby's main contact with reality is the mouth: eating, screaming, breathing, vomiting; he uses directly or indirectly, that passage.

What do we know about that phase? No direct reports are available, either at the critical time, or in later recollections. The grotesque fact is to be observed that the decisive first year-and-a-half of the life of the human being is not directly recorded—at least not in form of accessible memories. In direct contradiction to that lack, the unconscious wordless imprint, as deciphered through the later reactions of the child and the grown-up, is overwhelming. Philosophers may marvel at that dichotomy.

Clinically, there are good reasons for the assumption—expressed first by Freud and Ferenczi—that the child lives for some time in the fantasy of magic omnipotence. That means—to reduce it to a succinct term—on the basis of the "autarchic fantasy," as Jekels and myself named it. Autarchy denotes self-sufficiency, and we know, on the other hand, the complete dependence of the newborn. We, the adults, know it—imagine, however, the situation from the autarchic "angle." Then, not mother feeds the child—the child produces everything out of himself. Then, breast or bottle are not given to the child—these indispensable requisites of nutrition and pleasure are parts of the child's own body. Then, all wish fulfillments, so lavishly and automatically produced by mother, are the results of the child's own omnipotence. All that adds up to a pretty picture of magic misconception of reality.

The first rude shock is the child's gradual understanding that fantasy and reality do not coincide. That shock is rather a long and protracted series of disappointments, mostly connected in the child's first months with the feeding process. To exemplify: the child wakes up and wants "autarchic" milk. Mother is in the other room; even in the best regulated household there are delays. The half-minute the child cries, till mother comes with bottle or breast, is nutritionally and calorically completely unimportant. Quite correct—but as lesion of the fantasy of autarchic omnipotence, it may be decisive. Once more there is the crushing realization for the child that his fantasy does not correspond to facts. A deep narcissistic wound is inflicted—unavoidably inflicted—to the child.

Imagine a few thousand of these wounds and similar ones (pertaining later to all types of wishes), add to these the "tragedy"—once more unavoidable—of weaning, and you have in a nutshell the beginning of the most painful collapse of a grandiose fantasy—the fantasy of childlike omnipotence.

The gradual collapse of autarchic fantasies produces in the child important changes in the sphere of aggression: *every "refusal" produces fury.* That fury is out of proportion to the ability to express it, simply because of the *motoric helplessness* of the child. Later, three additional difficulties complicate the child's aggressive expressions: *punishment, moral reproach, guilt.* The objects of the child's anger are mother, later father—both people with a halo. Aggression against both is not only inhibited, a heavy moral argument is added: "How can you do that to your parents who sacrifice themselves for you?"

At that point the decisive dichotomy starts: one child takes the "triad of retribution" (punishment, moral reproach, guilt) in its stride, adapts himself more or less diplomatically to the environment, shifts manifestation of aggression to less holy subjects and objects. Another child persists in its original aims and subjects with the unavoidable external, later internal punishment in the form of guilt. These are frequently the children so enigmatic to educators: punishment is no deterrent to them.

This latter group of children becomes the material for "*psychic masochism.*" The term describes in *two words a life technique* of people who—despite conscious ignorance of so doing—are *unconsciously lovers of humiliation, defeat, refusal.* The question arises how such a monstrosity of feelings could develop in the first place.

The moment the aggression towards people with the halo is maintained, despite punishment, moral reproach and guilt, the problem for the child is one of libido-economy: how to maintain that position and still live on the basis of the pleasure principle, the foundation of childhood. That truly fantastic and seemingly unsolvable problem *is* solved by this type of child in an amazing way: pain, depression, punishment, guilt are changed into pleasure. *The only pleasure one can derive from displeasure is to make out of displeasure pleasure.* That is the astounding solution: by sugarcoating the painful situation with a layer of pleasure, derived from pain, punishment and guilt, the child gets libidinous satisfaction. A psychic masochist is in the making. Superfluous to state that the whole process is unconscious.

The moment the psychic masochist's aim is established in the oral stage, the mother of the pre-oedipal period is chosen as the great malefactor. Later, people from whom similar "pleasurable displeasure" can be obtained, are unconsciously identified with that "monster." [1]

Imagine a man standing before a candy-store, looking with hungry eyes at the display of candies. He has money in his pocket, he can buy the alluring "stuff." Nothing of the kind—he prefers to feel excluded, refused, rejected. For him—*unconsciously*—to act the refused child, is obviously more important than the wish to get the *consciously* desired candy.

For any understanding of the subject of psychic masochism, a precise differentiation is necessary between the *genetic* and *clinical* picture. The genetic picture comprises the sequence of early infancy: offense to megalomania incurred by a libidinous frustration, fury, motor helplessness, external, later internal, inhibition of aggression—boomeranging of aggression—libidinization of guilt. Here the *genetic* picture ends.

The *clinical* picture starts where the genetic picture ends. The clinical picture is based on the fact that the inner conscience (super-ego) objects to this peculiar type of infantile pleasure. The result is that the unconscious ego creates new secondary defenses. These secondary defenses comprise the "*triad of the mechanism of orality.*"

Oral neurotics are people who constantly provoke the situation of the following triad of the "mechanism of orality":

[1] These neurotics, too, try to rescue themselves to higher levels of libidinous-aggressive development (anal, phallic). They regress, however, after a few futile attempts. Baron Münchhausen, the famous liar, claimed that he rescued himself from drowning by holding on to his own pigtails. This technique does not work with oral neurotics.

(1) "I shall repeat the masochistic wish of being deprived by my mother, by creating or misusing situations in which some substitute of my pre-oedipal mother-image shall refuse my wishes."

(2) "I shall not be conscious of my wish to be refused and initial provocation of refusal, and shall see only that I am justified in self-defense, righteous indignation and pseudo-aggression because of the refusal."

(3) "Afterwards I shall pity myself because such an injustice 'can happen only to me,' and enjoy once more psychic masochistic pleasure."

This triad induces the ego-strengthening mirage of aggression, while in unconscious reality the wish to be refused, deprived and mistreated is foremost. Under the disguise of pseudo-aggression the oral neurotic enjoys masochistic self-pity and the pleasure of being refused.

Here are six clinical examples:

A patient in the thirties suffering from premature ejaculation, stated that all his plans for "happy marriage" miscarried. He always met with golddiggers or, at least, golddigging parents of his presumptive brides. He gave as an example his last experience. He "fell in love" with a girl of 18. When her parents made inquiries into his financial status, he represented his income as 80% lower than it really was. The purse-proud and money-conscious parents were horrified at his inability to support their daughter "in style" and prevented the match. Asked why he misrepresented his true income, the patient claimed that he wanted to "test" the bride. What he unconsciously really wanted was refusal and a good hitching post for his furious complaints covering masochistic enjoyment.

A woman in her forties had an affair with a man in the same age-group; respecting his "enormous drive for independence," she never talked of, but always counted on, marriage. Officially, she advised him to marry "later" a young girl. After some years, the man attached himself to an aggressive golddigger and was pushed by this calculating woman into marriage. "Terrible scenes" with my patient ensued, the man acting surprised: "You yourself always advised me to marry a young girl!" It took some time to convince the patient that she unconsciously committed a series of errors in the evaluation of the situation and provoked the éclat. First, she misunderstood and took at the face value "her friend's independence"; it represented his own defense against his latent masochistic danger. As his neurosis progressed, his wish to be kicked around, increased, hence he attached himself to an aggressive golddigger, being "bored" with the patient's kindness. Her second mistake consisted in treating a psychic masochist kindly. Her third mistake pertained to her hypocritical or self-sacrificial advice to marry someone else. "How was I to know that he would take me seriously?", asked the lady in despair.

An unsuccessful writer asked his wife, after the literary and financial failure of his latest book, to consent to live with the two children in the country on 100 dollars a month. He wanted to give up his 5000-dollar position in the city and devote himself entirely to writing. The 100 dollars monthly were provided by the remnants of his father's estate. His wife refused to give up the apartment in the city and the accustomed standard of living, pointing out very reasonably that such a proposition would be justified after a *successful* and not *unsuccessful* book. The man considered his wife a rather selfish person. It was obvious that he himself never believed that she would accept his proposition. And still he showed all the typical fury of the unjustly treated person and pitied himself extensively, depicting himself as "martyr" bearing a cross.

A young man had developed an amorous attachment for a girl outside his financial and social sphere, and was very conscious of the obstacles. He constantly reiterated the hopelessness of the situation and stated that the inevitable day must come when the family would convince the girl to give him up. One evening the girl told him that an old friend of her's was going to be in town shortly and asked him whether he would object to her seeing him. This trial balloon, testing his "notorious" jealousy, was immediately used by the young man for a violent scene, with which he unconsciously hastened the inevitable end.

How independent of reality factors these unconscious "prefabricated patterns" stemming from early childhood really are, is visible in the following example. A patient called me up on a Friday, told me the person who recommended him, and asked for an appointment. The appointment was arranged for the following Monday at 11 A.M. The following day, on a Saturday, the patient came at 11 A.M. and was informed by the doorman and, later, by the elevator man that he must have confused the day of appointment since "the doctor does not work on Saturdays and was not in the office." The patient waited, nevertheless, a full hour in the hall, assuming consciously that I had forgotten the appointment. After one hour, he left and complained bitterly to the person who recommended him to me that I had spoiled half of his day. An "injustice" was constructed—without his ever having seen me!

A young musician was confronted with the fact that his commercially minded family had no appreciation of his studies and refused to finance these any longer. His allowance was cut in a determined effort to force him to make his own way. Thereupon the schizoid young man fell into a state of excitement which finally convinced the family that he needed psychiatric help. It was possible for me to convince the family that the allowance should be restored, his musical studies financed, and his doctor's bills paid. After a short-lived period of gratitude "for achieving the impossible," the patient started to accuse me that I "sold him down the river." He suspected that I entered into a "secret deal" with his family to the effect that should the parents consent to his being treated psychiatrically, I should in return "make a good businessman" out of him. Despite the fact that the patient's fantastic accusation could be refuted by a statement of his mother who was present during the negotiations with his father, the young man continued for a long time to believe his fairy tale. Not even my argument that no power on earth could make a businessman out of him, was accepted as proof of his fallacy.

All these "*injustice collectors*" were not so foolish as their irrational actions would indicate. It was not wrong "testing," hypocritical advice, timing, forgetfulness, and hypersuspicion, respectively, which made the six patients described above act irrationally. They knew unconsciously very well what they were after. *First,* they unconsciously constructed or imagined a situation in which somebody was unjust and refusing. As *second* act they revelled in fury and anger from their arsenal of "righteous indignation," seemingly in self-defense. That they themselves constructed the imaginary injustice was fully repressed and therefore not conscious to them. As *third* and final act they pitied themselves, enjoying—once more without knowing it—psychic masochistic pleasure.

A great deal of confusion exists in our literature concerning this type which I have described in dozens of publications during the last 18 years. The main misunderstandings center around the following fallacies:

(1) The *original* oral-aggressive wish to get is confused with the *later neurotic* elaboration of that wish. The neurotic-masochistic elaboration leads to the strange but clinically observable fact that these neurotics do not want "to get" but—to "be refused." The historic sequence of events is this: wish to get—refusal or fantasy of refusal—fury and hatred—motoric helplessness—external, later internal, inhibition of aggression—turning of aggression against the own person because of guilt—masochization of guilt. Nobody denies that oral neurotics were, once upon a time, babies who wanted to get. As adult neurotics they reproduce the situation "Bad mother refuses." What they repress deeply is their masochistic enjoyment of that refusal.

(2) Constant confusion between the masochistic wish to be disappointed and the pseudo-aggressive defense. In other words, layers 1 and 2 of the "triad of orality" are confused.

This confusion is constantly made even by theoretically interested analysts. Even if the "mechanism of orality" is quoted, confounding layers 1 and 2 is maintained. Fenichel, in his last book "*The Psychoanalytic Theory of Neuroses*" (1946), manages to quote and misunderstand at the same time. He mentions some of my papers on aspermia under "Oral Character Traits" and says (pp. 489–490):

> . . . Other/oral/persons are completely ungenerous and never give others anything, an attitude tracing from an identification with a frustrating mother. Theirs is, indeed, an attitude of revenge. 'Because I was not given what I wanted, I shall not give other people what they want.' Bergler showed that some cases of ejaculation retardata are fashioned after this pattern. The penis represents the patient's breast, and the patients unconsciously refuse to feed their sexual partners.

This is a clear-cut confusion between the first and second layer of the "mechanism of orality," a term which Fenichel also avoids. What these oral aspermists in their refusal of sperm do, is but the pseudo-aggressive defense against the wish to be refused.[2]

[2] For details see "A Short Genetic Survey of Psychic Impotence." Psychiatric Quart., 19, Nos. 3 and 4, 1945.

(3) Incredulity that there should be people whose aim in life is being refused. This incredulity often is cloaked in the argument that it is improbable that the "life of oral people should start with suffering." Asked how they read this misconception into the "mechanism of orality," as sketched above, the answer is "Well, does not your formula start with the words 'I create unconsciously a situation in which I am refused . . .' ". This misunderstanding confuses once more the historic development ("genetic picture") with the neurotic-masochistic elaboration ("clinical picture"), as pointed out in misunderstanding No. 1.

(4) Confusion between pre-œdipal and œdipal mother is perpetuated. Though objectively one and the same person, psychologically two different entities are involved.

The *pre-œdipal mother* is unconsciously considered to be "cruel, malicious, refusing, devouring": the children-eating witch of Grimm's fairy tale "Hansel and Gretel" seems to be her prototype. The reason for that fantastic misconception of the child is, as the English school of analysis correctly pointed out, based on the projection of the child's own aggression onto the mother.

On the other hand, the *œdipal mother* is passive, weak, castrated—in the child's fantasy—completely under father's dominance.

Hence colleagues who have not digested this "dichotomy of mothers" —a late Freudian conception, to start with—cannot grasp the reason prompting the orally regressed neurotic to repeat disappointment with a "non-existent monster" of a mother. Naively, the objection is repeated: "But mothers are loving and sacrificing." Quite true, the mere existence of the oral neurotic proves it. Were the mother really so cruel, as her unconsciously enshrined picture in the neurotic's psyche is, the child would have died from hunger and exposure. Neurosis deals with fantasies—repressed fantasies—not with realities.

(5) That—long ago demoted—overevaluation of reality versus fantasy, plays other tricks with the believers in "reality factors", too. A hunt for the "bad" mother starts in analysis, and if her record is cleared, a question-mark remains, shifted secondarily onto the oedipal mother. A combination of confusion No. 4 starts all over again.

(6) The star argument against the "mechanism of orality" is the contention that no recollections can be produced in analysis proving its

existence. That is true: even the deepest analysis of an oral case cannot unearth recollections from the first eighteen months of life. But these objectors have either never heard, or do not believe in, Freud's contention that reconstructions and recollections have dynamically the same value in analysis.

That objection "No recollections—hence no value," thus conveniently overlooks the fact that human recollections never reach farther back than to the age of 1½. These objectors would either have to find a method of producing recollections beyond that age, or deny the fact that the child's first months of life have any influence at all. They do neither, of course, satisfied with sterile skepticism.

The whole overvaluation of recollections is also historically explainable. Since analysis started with hysterical and obsessional material, going back to the ages of 2½–5, where repressed recollections can be obtained in analysis (even then frequently incomplete, but that slight point marring the argument is conveniently forgotten), the yardstick of higher levels of development is applied to deeper ones.

(7) Another argument stresses the universality of the problem, not as a positive evaluation of the importance of the "mechanism of orality," but as devaluation. "You find that mechanism in writers, drinkers, homosexuals, pseudo-mental deficiency, and what not. Isn't that too general?"

The answer is simple: a universal problem is to be encountered universally. That part of the objection is rather an involuntary compliment, though intended as the opposite. It is like being surprised that every human being has an organ called the heart.

But that is not what our opponents mean. The objection claims that the same mechanism cannot produce so many different clinical pictures. That objection is based on—let us say—unprecise reading. Obviously, in every orally regressed case the "mechanism of orality" is to be found —provided one doesn't want to overlook it purposely. But to that *general* basis, a *specific* feature, characteristic for that particular subgroup must be added and distinguished. That *additional factor,* which I always stress specifically, is just overlooked: title-reading, as practiced in unprecise reading, results in unprecise understanding and criticism.

In Chapter VI the specificity of all oral (as far as now known) clinical pictures will be presented.

(8) Some colleagues, confronted with the "mechanism of orality" and the claim of universality in direct-, modified- and "retreat"-forms, simply get jumpy, as if the solid earth on which they feel secure, were withdrawn from under them. That "earthquake reaction" leads to not too intelligent objections, like: "Do you deny that hysteria or obsessional neurosis exist?" I don't. What I claim is, that higher developmental levels, on which these neuroses rest, are but rescue stations against the underlying "oral danger." More about it in the next chapter.

(9) A fundamental misunderstanding arises when a psychoanalyst does not clarify in his own thinking the basic fact that psychic masochism is neurotically displaced aggression. In some unclear way, many colleagues feel that psychic masochism is a libidinous problem. They forget or overlook the fact that Freud stated that the primary masochism (death-instinct) is directed against the individual himself, and is only secondarily directed against objects—by interaction with the life-instinct. Hence, in Freud's conception, psychic masochism is destrudo, secondarily libidinized.

What I call the *genetic* picture of psychic masochism, is identical with Freud's description. What is new, is the working out of the *clinical* picture and its interconnection with the oral phase—the "mechanism of orality."

Not less confusing is the fact that we never see clinically life- and death-instincts. What we see are not even the quantitative mixtures of both; only the third generation, namely derivatives of mixtures are observable. Simplified, we speak of libido and destrudo.

(10) The most amusing objection was reported to me in the form of a compliment. A colleague said to another: "You know, this man goes beyond the Oedipus complex and, that's the strangest thing, has clinical successes with it." The tone of voice was that of complete surprise—undigested variety.

"Beyond the Oedipus complex!" That is the sort of naive simplification, which I am fighting. What Freud always wanted to avoid in analysis—simplifying sterility—is petrified in this, I hope not too typical example.

I came to the conclusion that the best way of explaining *homo masochisticus* is to state what he is *not*. The *layman's* use of the *term* and *scientific* connotations are miles apart. The *scientific* "ten misunderstandings" quoted previously are paralleled by the *layman's* set of "ten misunderstandings." Here are some of those:

Misunderstanding No. 1: *Psychic* masochism is confused with *perversion* masochism. The latter denotes pathologic pleasure—consciously experienced pleasure—derived from being beaten, stabbed, tortured. It starts with a game-like attitude, to progress to more dangerous escapades. The direct *bodily* pain is perceived by these strange human beings as pleasurable. In *psychic* masochism pain is consciously rejected, hence consciously avoided.

Misunderstanding No. 2: Psychic masochism is confused with self-damage. True, every psychic masochistic action leads to self-damage, but self-damage may have entirely different reasons, e.g. inner guilt.

A very frequent misunderstanding of the "mechanism of orality" is based on the objection: "I did not *provoke* that specific situation; I am confronted with *real facts*." The objection overlooks gratuitously that "*provoking* a situation of being refused" and "*misusing* a given external situation for a masochistic fiesta," are in its effects identical. The "mechanism of orality" states specifically *both* types of masochistic misuse.

Misunderstanding No. 3: Psychic masochism is identified with feeling of guilt. Frequently, conscious guilt is alluded to which confuses the issue even more, if this is possible. Even if unconscious guilt is meant, the definition still does not make sense: psychic masochism means *unconscious* pleasure derived from self-punishment. Unconscious guilt plays a part in the pre-history of psychic masochism, but is by no means identical with it.

Misunderstanding No. 4: Psychic masochism is regarded as the result of a too severe conscience, and the advice given consists in "not being fooled by conscience." The whole conception is erroneous. First, the human being has no access to his inner conscience (superego), provided that the proponents of that misconception do not confuse conscious and unconscious parts of the conscience to boot. Moreover, psychic masochism is not the result of the punitive inner conscience, but just the opposite: *an unconscious act of outwitting the punishing conscience.* If a specific person makes pleasure out of punishment, he reduces the punitive authority to absurdity.

Misunderstanding No. 5: Psychic masochists are considered either *dumbbells or psychotics.* Wrong again: they are quite rational neurotics, with a normal I.Q., except in situations in which the allurement of their self-created and fantastic inner pleasure of self-torture is predominant.

Misunderstanding No. 6: Psychic masochism is viewed as "*inexperience*" which can be corrected by life-experience. That misconception overlooks the fact that experience has no access to the unconscious. Experience cannot change a psychic masochist. On the contrary, it is disregarded to achieve the neurotic aim. People then marvel at the naiveté of the psychic masochist, not understanding that he simply increases his self-damaging stakes in order to counteract the conscious "voice of experience."

Misunderstanding No. 7: Psychic masochists are believed to be victims of a "*biologic misfortune.*" Nothing of the kind: psychic masochism is an individually *self-created* unconscious attitude of defense in the "battle of conscience" raging from the cradle to the grave.

Misunderstanding No. 8: Frequently psychic masochists are credited with an unconscious *wish* to maneuver themselves right behind the eightball. Psychic masochism is not an unconscious wish but a complicated *inner defense mechanism,* created by the unconscious ego. It is, to quote a wit, "not an apple growing on a tree, but *synthetic* marmalade." The "producer" is the unconscious ego. Later, it is true, psychic masochism has the *power* of an unconscious wish, but it is only an unconscious defense-mechanism.

Misunderstanding No. 9: A never-ending chaos is produced by confusing the *genetic* and the *clinical* pictures: the questions "How does it start?" and "What is actually observable?" are confused with each other. Genetically, psychic masochism is an undigested *aggression;* that aggression is counteracted by *guilt,* and secondarily "*libidinized.*" Clinically, psychic masochists crave for a libidinous "pleasure" of refusal, humiliation, and defeat. Hence, clinically visible *libidinous* aim, and genetically deducible *aggressive* aim, are confounded.

Misunderstanding No. 10: Psychic masochists are frequently accused of being "aggressive." This misunderstanding arises from mistaking the *provocative technique* applied unconsciously to achieve the anticipated kick in the jaw, for the real aim. People underestimate the inner difficulties with which psychic masochists have to fight. The naive outer world has no inkling of the masochist's aim, which is his "daily dose of injustice." Hence the outer world has to be provoked to administer the defeat.

I conceive of the child's life as a running battle with passivity.

The winding road of the *battle line: passivity versus activity, starts in the cradle and ends in the coffin.* We have not to lose sight of the fact that the human child has been "spoiled" in tasting passivity by two biologic factors: protracted intra-uterine existence and protracted maturation. Nobody can "blame" the child for attempt at continuation of pre-natal and early post-natal paradisiacal existence. Reality, and to a lesser degree, inherent activity, force the child in another direction —very much *contre coeur.*

This is visible from the use the child makes of his "activity." The aggressive drive is "mobilized" in defense and fighting off "external intrusion" into the child's private life, allegedly magically regulated by his erroneous precepts of autarchy and megalomania. This anger and fury are immediately counteracted by his motoric helplessness, *later* by the "triad of retribution": punishment, moral reproach, guilt. All this diminishes the radius of activity and *reinforces passivity.*

To complicate this poor showing of activity, the child is confronted with bodily drives, forces and functions which are outside of his power: urination, defecation, even sleep. All these experiences, though banal and "natural," seen through the eyes of adults, are not only blows to the child's megalomania; they also push the newcomer in this unfriendly world even more into the passive situation. Once more: *passivity is reinforced.*

Add to this the fact that the child's aggression is quantitatively not less developed in the cradle (at least potentially) than that of an adult —and the conclusion is unavoidable that a ricochet of aggression, or— if you prefer fluid examples—a backward flowing of aggression against the child itself, is in the making. Inner conscience takes care of the "inflation money." [3]

The next development in the battle of passivity is a series of megalomaniacal-aggressive denials. The child denies:

[3] See Chapter IV.

(a) "It is not true that I want to be orally-*passively* penetrated by breast (or bottle), I don't want to take it into my mouth." This accounts for occasional vomiting, even refusal of nourishment, of unexplainable "hungerstrike," not due to intestinal troubles. Out of sheer consistency, the child would "autarchically" starve to death. This, however, is counteracted by the discovery of a new "libidinous pleasure" experienced during sucking. Still, there are reasons for the assumption (Freud) that the child conceives of the breast (bottle) as part of his own body, a modified continuation of the "autarchic fantasy."

(b) "It is not true that mother could refuse and withdraw breast (bottle), I have on my own body a similar organ producing fluid." In this anatomically, histologically, physiologically, chemically incorrect way of reasoning, penis and breast, milk and urine are identified. The anatomical, histological, physiological and chemical idiocies, underlying the identification, are laughable only to the adult: the child is neither informed nor impressed by them. True, a wit could reason that not even a megalomaniacal child could live on urine as milk-substitute. Quite correct. He overlooks, however, that the identification is performed after weaning when the child already learns to eat more solid food. Moreover, only a sham is performed—did you never hear of dethroned kings calling themselves Majesty long *after* being dethroned? Still, that compensatory identification with the purpose of negating dependence on a woman has decisive results for the whole masculine psychology.[4]

Not only does the male child negate his dependence on mother's nutritional apparatus (breast, bottle), he reverses the rôles. Using the "unconscious repetition compulsion" (Freud), meaning *active* repetition of *passively* endured experiences for *the purpose of restoring a lesion in narcissism, inflicted through passive submission*, the boy identifies penis and breast; milk, urine, and later sperm. Instead of being *passive* recipient of milk, he becomes *active* bestower of urine and, later, sperm. In coitus, the reversal is perfected: vagina = mouth, penis = breast, sperm = milk.[5] *The decisive point is eradication of a lesion inflicted to infantile megalomania.* That application of Freud's idea later proved fruitful for other mechanisms as well.

[4] See Chapter V, "Orality and the Myth of the Superior Male."

[5] See "The Breast Complex in the Male." (In collaboration with L. Eidelberg), Int. Z. f. Psa., 1933.

(c) "I don't want to be *passively* penetrated by urine, and especially feces. I produce these products myself, am proud of it and want to play with them." We see in children, later anally fixated, that the fight between "autarchically" produced feces and the wish to be internally-passively penetrated, goes on with a libidinous disguise: I want to be anally penetrated by *father's* penis (repetition of the breast-mouth experience with mother).

(d) The latter phase indicates already the shift from the "disappointing" and dangerous mother to the new power: father. This wish to be anally penetrated by father (negative Oedipus) has different tributaries:

1. old passivity from the oral stage is anally displaced;
2. rescue attempt from the pre-oedipal mother;
3. identification with the oedipal mother with added anal misconceptions of sex;
4. guilt reaction from the positive Oedipus: "castration" is accepted and identification with the "castrated" oedipal mother performed.

(e) The latest in these rescue attempts from and *denial of passivity* in the boy, is the famous *Oedipus Complex.* What it practically amounts to is borrowed strength from the father; the boy wants to act father's part and to demote the "dangerous" mother to a passive being; *at bottom to an image of his own self.* The *reversal of the rôles* is perfect: here *mother* is *passively penetrated* (as once the child was orally-anally penetrated); the active penetrating is done by the child. A perfect setting for an alibi!

What happens? *Passivity is triumphant once more.* The Oedipal push of activity via borrowed strength collapses: mother does not take the boy seriously, father threatens "castration" of the "active organ"—the end-effect is disappointment, bitterness, passivity. At best, these wishes are given up and de-sexualized (filial affection) and de-aggressionized (filial camaraderie).

A modern Aristophanes could well write a comedy of misunderstandings taking the Oedipus Complex as theme. How much indignation and irony has been heaped on the Oedipus Complex in the last fifty years! What appeared to be a morally terribly objectionable "fantasy" turns out to be (in my opinion) a desperate rescue attempt from desperate passivity!

One can, however, ask the question: Is everything taking place in the mouth-zone "oral"?

The analytic term "oral" has become a "weasel word," a generality with elastic qualities. According to Theodore Roosevelt a weasel-word denotes lack of content: "When a weasel sucks eggs the meat is sucked out of the egg; if you use a weasel-word after another there is nothing left of the other."

First of all, a distinction must be made between *neurotic* reactions called, in an abbreviated way, "oral," and physiologic and psychologic processes in the realm of practical *health.* By not making that distinction, a kiss or a drink, e.g., is subsumed under "oral tendencies" in the same way as is hysterical vomiting, or the oral stubbornness of the pseudo-mute, word-refusing husband.

To complicate matters further, there are "oral" cases in which the mouth *per se* is not directly involved. If we speak of certain complicated cases of premature ejaculation as being "orally regressed," we do not refer to the mucosa of the mouth. The same holds true of perversion homosexuality, erythrophobia, psychogenic oral aspermia, pseudo mental deficiency, etc.

Hence, not everything taking place in the mouth-zone, is analytically called oral, and, on the other hand, many results of oral regression do not manifest themselves in the mouth-zone directly: *hysterical vomiting, for example, is not oral but phallic in genesis; still it uses the "locality" of the mouth.*

What then does the analytic term on orality mean?

Historically, the term was first used by Freud in 1905 in *Three Contributions.* The term was descriptively applied as meaning "oral incorporation," hence the desire to get.

K. Abraham elaborated in his studies on oral personalities the identical connotation and worked out a series of personality traits, all fashioned after the principle "orality = I want to get."

Further clinical experience proved that the term as originally created and used, covered but the *historic* phase of orality. Yes, the baby wants to get; yes, the baby experiences oral pleasure in sucking. *But* —and that but is quite decisive—what we see later, in the *clinical* picture, is *not* a direct *continuation* of the "once upon a baby time," but a secondary *elaboration.* And that elaboration goes through masochistic channels, as sketched in its clinical end-results in the "mechan ism of orality."

Hence, people who parrot-like cling to the original meaning of the word and stubbornly refuse to yield an inch from their conservatism, remind one of an English humorist's definition of a conservative:

> A conservative is a man who will not look at the new moon, out of respect for that 'ancient institution,' the old one. (Douglas Jerrold)

True enough, it is easy to make fun of every innovation and quote that old reactionary, Dr. Samuel Johnson, as recorded by Boswell in "Dialogue with Rousseau":

> I told him Mr. Johnson's bon mot upon the innovators: that truth is a cow which will yield them no more milk, and so they are gone to milk the bull. Rousseau said, "He would detest me. He would say: 'Here is a corrupter, a man who comes here to milk the bull.' "

Still, all this witty talk does not change clinical facts. It is more advantageous to investigate the reasons as to why the idea of "I want to be refused," is so abhorrent. The answer is simple enough: psychic masochism, since present in every one, provokes immediately the superego reproach: "It's you!" The rebellion against that painful fact, has its reverberation in—rejection and disbelief.

Freud, who was a clear thinker, finally made the necessary step half-heartedly and described the pre-oedipal phase, though only in 1931. Many of his followers, however, did not have the psychic elasticity of Freud at the age of 75!

This "too little" of orality has its counterpart in "too much": some neurotic pictures have been erroneously connected with orality, though they have nothing to do with it. Fenichel, e.g., related boredom and jealousy to that stage, although he first misinterpreted the term and, secondly, applied it to clinical entities where it does not belong. Neither boredom nor jealousy have an oral substructure.[6]

In our whole deduction, the leading idea has been the following duality: The child's reactive *fear of passivity* and his desperate *narcis-*

[6] For a discussion see my studies "On the Disease Entity Boredom ("Alysosis") and its Psychopathology." The Psychiatric Quarterly, 1944. Furthermore: "Contributions to the Psychology of Jealousy." Int. Zeitschr. f. Psa. und Imago, 1939.

sistic rescue attempts to higher development levels, fleeing from the "dangerous mother" to father. What are the dangers, the child attaches to mother? Why is that kind and bountiful woman so "dangerous"?

The English school of analysis did good work on this problem and showed the infantile aggressive misconceptions of the child, frequently projectively shifted onto the mother. The furious opposition against these discoveries has two roots: the typical static thinking in science, and the exaggerations produced by the English school itself. In due time a selection of clinically confirmed facts and exaggerated superstructure will be made and the result will be beneficial.

My objection to the English findings is that—though the child's early aggression is admirably worked out—the masochistic elaboration is neglected. Fear of retaliation is directly connected with aggression —one gathers the impression that the psychic-masochistic phase is, if not overlooked, at least not properly centered. Still, on the day of scientific reckoning, the English contributions will find their proper and distinguished place in our science.

I believe that the child labors under a "*septet of baby fears*" [7] and lives through the following dreads:

Fear of being starved, devoured, poisoned, choked, chopped to pieces, drained, castrated.

These fears have little connection with reality factors. I personally believe that the whole development of the child hinges on the constant attempts of the child to maintain infantile megalomania and autarchy and ward off the constant blows directed against this noble aim by reality.

The trouble starts with the fact that the child wants to maintain its paradisiacal passive existence in utero where it had been spared even the effort of breathing and eating. Confronted with radically changed post-natal existence, it counters first with the illusion of omnipotence and sees even in nutrition an undesirable intrusion.[8] Normally, the newly discovered pleasure of oral intake prevails. Later, the "septet of baby fears" makes its dismal appearance.

Fear of starvation.

Mothers do not let babies starve—the fact that the later neurotic,

7 For elaboration see my book "The Book of Fears". The Linacre Press (at press).

8 See Chapter III.

harboring that fear in his unconscious, is alive, proves that conclusively. The "starvation" refers to megalomania: dependence upon and waiting for bottle (breast) even a few seconds is unconsciously magnified out of proportion.

In later years, the reproach of "starvation" is modified into that of being refused—whether love, kindness, gifts, attention, or what not. After *masochistic "stabilization on the rejection level,"* the game "cruel mother refuses the helpless child" is perpetuated on an unconsciously self-chosen and self-initiated basis.

Fear of being devoured.

That grotesque fear has been clarified by the English school as projection of the child's *own* aggressive designs upon nipple (bottle). The formula reads: "Not I want to bite, mother wants to devour me," Fairy tales and dreams, animal phobias and unconscious fantasies enshrine these early infantile conceptions.

Fear of being poisoned.

Even a child nourishing his "starvation grievance" cannot deny after some time that he is fed. Hence a shift is performed: "Mother feeds me, but harms me with poisonous food." Pathologic fear of impregnation, neurotic intestinal disturbances, hypochondriacal complaints centering around food, are in later life the remnants.

Fear of being choked.

Analysis of neurotics scared of "confined places," be it claustrophobia, elevators, subways, buses, proves that behind hysterical palimpsests repressed fantasies of being choked by mother's breast or body are hidden.[9] It has little to do with the disproportion of these organs and child's miniature mouth, nor with maladroitness of mothers' and nurses' pushing the nutritional instrument too forcefully into the baby's mouth.

The grotesque forms this fear can take is proved by an example of a patient who, after seeing an old horror movie in which a man in a mill was killed when valves holding back flour were opened, developed the fear of being choked by particles of the wall falling upon him during sleep. He protected himself in such attacks—with a gas mask! That "foolishness" finally convinced him that analysis was indicated.

Fear of being chopped to pieces.

That fear has a very banal basis: baby's misconception of mother's

[9] Contributaries of that fear are visible in the psychological aspects of asthma.

harmless designs during wash- and cleaning procedures. From the standpoint of the baby, a Procrustean bed fantasy is initiated. Once more, not the overforceful actions of the adult are responsible, the evil design is projected by the child.

Later, the cutting of meat, fish, foul, is adduced as proof positive of what a woman is "capable of."

An especially grotesque example, which I observed, was a man with a "masseur complex." He claimed that his fear developed after a "bad experience" with a masseur who nearly "disjointed" him. It turned out that behind the superficial, though also repressed homosexual layer, a deeper fear was hidden: that of being "chopped" to pieces by a woman. That could be proven in a strange "coincidence": the man had a hernia, was advised to undergo an operation, and refused stubbornly: "You know how these surgeons are, they just want to chop you to pieces." On a vacation tour, he inquired immediately (as he always did) into the surgical services of the nearest hospital, and found to his horror that the chief of the division was—in absence of the chief surgeon—a female doctor. Horrified, he thought: "My God, imagine falling into her hands!" He overexercised promptly on a mountain tour, his hernia became incarcerated, and had to be operated on—by the woman.

Later, these irrational fears are subsumed (as in the case mentioned) into fear of operations, and phallic castration fears.

Fear of being drained. The infantile prototype is the fact that the child is helpless against "propelling forces" in the elimination of urine and feces. The child feels "drained" against his wishes, retaliating secondarily with megalomaniacal and aggressive ideas connected with both products.[10]

In later life, one encounters that neurotic fear behind the façade of miserliness in money, sex, even words.

Fear of castration. This fear is the rationally disguised culmination of all previously described "ancestors," encountered in its clearest form during the Oedipal phase. The elaboration of phallic castration fear in later life is endless in its variations, ranging from impotence to any inhibition of function of any organ and mental act. Frequently, seemingly banal castration fear covers but the deeper repressed precursors and constituents of "baby fears."

[10] K. Abraham and later the English school collected extensive material on that score.

Not all children have actually been threatened with "castration." Still, all children manifest that fear, which fact has puzzled many analytic authors; today there is agreement, as visible in the literature, that a series of non-genital precursors is to blame for that fear. The sheltered existence in utero ended, the breast (bottle) was withdrawn; stool was "drained," milk-teeth fell out. Thus the basis is prepared for the idea that "pleasure leads to loss of the pleasure-giving organ."

The deepest reason is more complicated. It is identical with the fact that the "septet of baby fears" is very much alive, and shifted to successive phases and organs. Much which goes under the heading "phallic castration fear" is at bottom undigested oral fear, stemming from the "septet."

It is my contention that in every case in which the "mechanism of orality" is discernible in decisive situations in life—work, love, personality,—we are justified in classifying the neurotic as an orally regressed one, completely independent of what other symptoms and signs he shows.

The danger of not knowing, or not applying, this clinical experience, is eminent and imminent. Neurotics are prone to give up, or exchange, symptoms under pressure. But to renounce their basic conflicts, is an inner compromise they decline to the last moment of the analytic "battle."

What are the aims of the analytic patient? [11]

Every analytic patient enters analysis with, or develops, partly during analysis, five aims: one conscious and four unconscious ones. The conscious wish is self-evident: The patient suffers, is helpless and wants help. The second aim has been discussed repeatedly: [12] materialization of unconscious wishes.[13]

[11] First published under the title "Five Aims of the Psychoanalytic Patient." The Psychiatric Quarterly, 20:684-700, 1946.

[12] See Nunberg's "Über den Genesungswunsch" Int. Z. f. Psa., 11:179–193, 1925. Furthermore, the writer's contributions to the symposium on theory of analytic therapy. XIV. Int. Psycho. Convention, Marienbad, 1936. Published in Int. J. Psa., 18:146-160, London, 1937.

[13] Nunberg, *loc. cit.*, gives the example of an impotent man deeply in love with the wife of his friend, a mother of six children. He was impotent with that woman and interested exclusively in restoring his potency with that woman only. In other words, the man expected from analysis materialization of his repressed Oedipal wishes and nothing else.

This, the patient achieves in the transference-neurosis and he is rather indignant when the analyst uses the transference for exactly the opposite purpose: destruction of the infantile repetitiveness.

The third, fourth and fifth aims of the patient are seldom discussed. They are: The patient wants from analysis, unconsciously, not cure, in our meaning of the word, but *stabilization of his neurotic balance.* What disturbs him is only his inner feeling of guilt and its results. Therefore, his unconscious formula is: I want my infantile paradise without paying for it with the "hell within" (Milton). In other words, the unconscious aim of the patient is *continuation of neurosis* combined with *lessening or elimination of inner guilt.* Fortunately, such a possibility does not exist, otherwise neurosis would really mean what a naïve psychotherapist once expressed with the words "Be glad to be a neurotic." All analysts would starve and the neurotics would have advantages which normalcy cannot offer. The not *too* neurotic person, sometimes euphemistically called "normal," is inwardly forced to renounce materialization of infantile repressed wishes and gets the attenuated pleasures of normalcy. If neurosis would really mean preservation of the childhood paradise *without* paying with depression, pain and unhappiness, only a "fool" would choose to be—normal.

The free-floating inner feeling of guilt which can no longer be satiated in neurotic unhappiness alone, pushes the neurotic person into analysis. After having found out what analysis really endangers, the patient fights desperately *for preservation* of his neurotic balance with—subjectively desired—corrections. Whereas the analyst's aim is "*Your neurosis must be destroyed,*" the patient's third aim is "*My neurosis must be improved.*" This "improvement" pertains to two sets of facts: first, to his wish to diminish or even eliminate his inner guilt; second, to the *strengthening of his inner defense mechanisms,* which represent the patient's fourth aim. The majority of neurotic defense mechanisms are built upon the ironic formula: "I couldn't have killed the girl you accuse me of in Brooklyn, since I was stealing a watch in Manhattan at that time." In other words, the neurotic guilt is accepted and deposited but after the principle of the "lesser crime." Since every analysis tries to put the feeling of guilt at the place where it genetically belongs, the patient is furious.

The patient, caught in the "danger zone" of analysis, behaves, first, in a typically infantile-megalomanic way: He just does not believe that the danger could pertain to him, too. Naïvely, he clings unconsciously to his "neurosis-must-be-improved" theory. The more he finds out that there is real danger that his whole neurosis can be uprooted, he is as incredulous as the soldier who exclaims, full of surprise, during the first battle: "A guy can be killed here." It is precisely this inner incredulity which contributes to the fact that so many patients do not run away from analysis at that point. The combination of transference, the feeling of guilt, and partial intellectual understanding holds the patient back. In his desperation, he settles for the minimum compromise, the giving up of as little as he can. Thus the fifth—unconscious—aim of the patient develops in analysis: *maintenance of the neurosis* with the forced giving up of some trimmings.

The five aims of the patient are therefore:

1. (Conscious): "I am helpless, suffer, and want destruction of the neurosis."

2. (Unconscious): "I want living out and materialization of repressed wishes."

3. (Unconscious): "I want my neurosis improved: Feelings of guilt have to be eliminated through analysis."

4. "My unconscious defense mechanisms should be strengthened without endangering my attitude for taking the blame for the 'lesser crime' only."

5. (Unconscious, and developed during analysis): "I want my neurosis at least maintained and am willing to give up, under pressure, a few trimmings."

Let us start with a clinical example. Mr. A., a patient of 43, entered analysis because of depression, inability to work and fear of fire-escapes. Up to 42 and one-half, he had lived with his mother. Asked why he did not marry, he retorted that "somebody had to take care of the old mother." "Why exactly you and none of your five brothers and sisters?" "Well, they were married and had families of their own." Thus, confusing reasons with results, the patient remained at home with the domineering mother, clinging to his rationalization, which convinced him. His mother's heart failed—she was in the 80's; the patient did everything for her and lived for two years in a state of constant excitement. He provided day and night nurses, sacrificed his sleep, paid doctors who had to be at his call for 24 hours a day. When the mother died, she was deeply mourned by the patient who "nearly collapsed." Asked what kind of person his mother was, he declared her a "kind and loving person." It turned out soon that his mother had been, in reality, aggressive and tyrannic; the patient was under her complete dominance with occasional "attacks of suppressed fury." After his mother's death, he gave up the apartment because his sister's son-in-law wanted it. "Accustomed to sacrifices," he moved into a hotel room and here developed for the first time his symptom of fearing that "somebody" could enter the room through the fire escape when he himself was sleeping. This "somebody," more precisely, was a man, as the patient admitted after some time. In his consciousness, he developed fear of homosexuality, shifting unconsciously—after the principle of taking the blame for the "lesser crime"—his passivity toward his mother to the stranger. He left the hotel room, moved into another one, changed rooms again; the fear persisted. Finally, he took an apartment in the same building in which he had lived with his mother. His depression deepened, he more or less stopped working, covering up his inability with the thought that some of his millionaire-clients could eat "only one steak for dinner," an ability which he possessed, too. His "solution" was a vacation plan for six months. One of his brothers, horrified at the patient's change of personality, forced him indirectly into analysis.

In analysis, the patient was "deeply shocked" at his feminine identification and his wish to be overwhelmed by the aggressive mother. His psychic masochism was not less "shocking" to him. What convinced him was that his "girl friend" was not less domineering than mother. He had difficulties parting from his assumption that he was homosexual. The simple fact that he preferred to be guilty of that *imaginary* "crime," only to conceal his *real* "crime"—the passive wish of being overwhelmed by the mother—penetrated only slowly. He even started to coöperate in analysis and produced recollections going back to his early youth when he observed parental intimacies through the interstices of his crib. These interstices were later unconsciously identified with the fire escapes; the fear shifted from the inside to the outside.

After three months of analysis, the patient was a "changed man." He started to work, became more active in his profession and wanted to interrupt treatment "because analysis interfered with his work." It was possible to convince him of the spuriousness of his argument. He became aggressive and treated the analyst like a lawyer, "squeezing" the witness of the district attorney. It started with a harmless: "Let me ask you a question. . . and went on endlessly. This resistance, too, could be analyzed. The only thing which "still disturbed" the patient was his obsessional thinking concerning the damage he could have inflicted on one of his clients by "oversight." Then came my vacation (the patient was at that time eight months in analysis). On one of a few days before returning to work, I received from the patient the following letter:

August 21st, 1945.

Dear Dr. Bergler,

I am writing to express my thanks for your kind and efficient treatment and to advise you that I do not intend to take further treatment. I am well and planning a vacation in September.

Association with you left its indelible print for good upon me and broadened my views appreciably.

Hoping that you are enjoying a well-earned rest and vacation, and with kindest regards, I am,

Respectfully yours.

etc., etc.

I answered that I was glad to hear he felt well, suggested, however, that I see him once a week for some time. This letter was not answered, until—half a year later—February, 1946, when the patient called up and told me that he believed he should accept my proposition. I saw him once, and he reported that his situation was still "all right." The only thing which bothered him was "the usual torture" concerning "mistakes" which could endanger his clients. Asked whether he had gotten rid of his aggressive "girl friend," he answered: "This is impossible; she is still around." "Do you intend to marry her?" "Of course not. I am thinking of marriage, though. I never did previously." "Are you conscious of the fact that you are on the way to marrying her?" "I knew that you would tell me that. The only point confirming that suspicion is the fact that I don't look around for other girls. . ."

What was the patient's original aim in coming into analysis? He was completely "down" and could not help himself. His feeling of guilt because of the symbolic materialization of his neurotic wishes was so overwhelming that it could no longer be satisfied in his usual way. He had just lost his mother, the "legitimate" depository of his wish for "torture." His passivity—"homeless" after the loss of the accustomed depository—forced the creation of the new symptom (fear of fire escapes). The moment analysis showed him the reasons for, and the extent of, his neurosis, he feared that his original *unconscious* aim of enjoying his neurosis without paying the tribute of depression, pain and unhappiness, could not be materialized any more. He quickly gave up the most conspicuous and, at the same time, ridiculous symptom: his fear of fire escapes. Pressed in a corner—by the explanation of his passivity—he quickly established a *new* defense mechanism of pseudo-aggression which gave him the illusion of "cure;" he worked, coped with the difficulties of his profession, fought aggressively and efficiently his professional adversaries. He retained—of course—the main basis of his neurosis, now concentrated on the aggressive girl friend, and on his fears of damaging his clients through oversight. For both depositories, he had excellent rationalizations: The girl was not aggressive, *all* women are "bitches." Thinking about possible oversights gave him—so he claimed—excellent ideas. The moment I objected that his thinking was obsessional and not logical in character, especially since it came only *post facto,* he became disturbed. Not less "painful" was the analytic explanation that this theory was nonsense that "All women are bitches—therefore I cannot be blamed for choosing an aggressive girl." To avoid analysis of these two points, he left analysis.

This example shows how all five aims enumerated worked together:

1. The patient's conscious suffering was intolerable.

2. After the death of his mother he was unconsciously on the lookout for the *materialization and increase* [14] of his neurosis: Whereas his

[14] Very interesting was the fact that the patient, before he reached the *acute* stage of his neurosis (after the death of his mother), was a passionate reader of detective stories. At the climax of his sickness he lost interest in them. In a longer essay, "Mystery Fans and the Problem of 'Potential Murderers' ", (Am. J. Orthopsychiatry, *15*:2, 1945), I showed that the mystery fan enjoys a great deal of inner passivity in identifying with the *killed* victim. Mr. A. used that depository. His super-ego became—as he tried to *increase* the neurotic stakes—less tolerant, with the result that he could not use that outlet either.

mother previously had simply dominated him, after her death the "somebody" coming through the fire escape, raped him.

3. The patient unconsciously wanted his *neurosis improved*: He clamored for his inner passivity which he, by no means, wanted to renounce. He only wanted neurotic pleasure without paying for it with depression and guilt.

4. He wanted his *defense-mechanisms strengthened*, but for the purpose of maintaining his neuroses. Precisely because analysis tried to destroy his defenses, he ran away. The moment his two last depositories were attacked (girl friend, "torture" connected with perfectionism, the latter related to castration fears and their defensive counter-actions), he avoided analysis.

5. After realizing that there was real danger of losing his neurosis, he fooled himself with his newly established defenses against passivity (ability to work, aggressive approach in professional conflicts) and believed himself to be cured. He *gave up a few trimmings* (the minimum of the minimum) *to keep the basis of his neurosis.*

A witty patient once remarked that the definition of analysis as a therapy for neuroses, working with explanation and "working through" of transference and resistance, is much too complicated and should be simplified. He suggested such a simplification: "Why not simply state that analysis is an eternal fight between the couch and the door? The couch signifying analysis, the door the patient's tendency to run away. . . ."

The fight between "the couch and door" signifies but *one* of the phases in analysis. Running away is a rather crude method: Our patients use, in general, more refined techniques. These are numerous. To give only a few examples:

1. *Maintenance of the Feeling of Guilt on the Side-Track.* Mr. A., the aforementioned patient, clung for quite a long time to the assumption that his feeling of guilt pertained to the fact that he did not sacrifice enough for his mother. He recalled incidents in which he had been angry or impatient with her. Her physician took a vacation at the time of her gravest illness; perhaps if he had prevented *that*, his mother would still be alive, etc. In other words, he shifted the blame from his *real* crime (passivity) to the *imaginary* one (aggression). As stated before, every neurotic lives psychologically on the

basis of shifted guilt, the ironic formula being, "I couldn't have killed the girl you accuse me of in Brooklyn, since I was stealing a watch in Manhattan at that time." The blame is accepted, but always for the "crime" which was never committed. Mr. A. accused himself also of homosexual tendencies, a "crime" he was innocent of, only to disguise the—in his specific case—dynamically decisive "crime": feminine identification, with the wish to be raped by the mother. One could object that feminine identification could lead to homosexuality, an assumption proved to be completely wrong.[15] Mr. A.'s father was a passive person who did not play any important rôle in his life; Mr. A.'s mother was the real "boss." Furthermore, Mr. A. repeated in life the situation of being "mistreated" by a woman, as is seen in his relation to his tyrannical girl friend. The decisive objection to the assumption that Mr. A.'s suspicion could correspond to facts, is the clinical experience that what appears in consciousness is but the inner defense mechanism and never the unconscious wish.[16]

Mr. B., a dipsomaniac, entered analysis with the statement that he suspected "incestuous attachment to his mother." He was not guilty of that, his oral masochistic attachment to the *pre-Oedipal* mother was in the foreground.[17]

Mrs. C. entered treatment because of a neurotic triangle which she could not tolerate any longer. Her husband had maintained for the past twelve years a sexual relation to another woman and had asked both to consent to living together—all three of them. Said the patient: "I became so furious that I want to cut off my husband's genitalia. Do you believe I am a murderess?" As was to be expected, the patient repeated in life the situation of Cinderalla versus father-mother. Her Delilah-fantasies were only pseudo-aggressive defenses against her repressed masochistic attachment.

2. *Establishment of New Defense Mechanisms for the Purpose of Maintaining the Neurosis.* Mr. A. quickly established his ability to work and his activity in his profession—as defense against the analytic

15 See the writer's "Eight Prerequisites for the Psychoanalytic Treatment of Homosexuality." Psa. Rev., *31*:3, 1944. The paper also gives a cross-section of the extensive literature.

16 The Leading and Misleading Basic Identifications. Psa. Rev., *32*:4, 1945.

17 See: "Contributions to the Psychogenesis of Alcohol Addiction." Quart. J. Stud. on Alcohol, *5*:3, 1944.

mobilization of guilt pertaining to his passivity. This gave him the illusion of cure.

Mr. D., a neurotic dentist, full of undigested passivity and resulting fears, became, after he understood the main conflict in the first weeks of analysis, very overbearing toward his patients. Previously, he was afraid even to mention the fee; at once he was precise, demanding, meticulous in money matters. This, of course, gave him the illusion of being "cured."

3. *Worsening of Symptoms and Depressions.* The best "argument" the patient can provide—after exhausting his arsenal of "logic," irony and scorn—is the "objective" proof that analysis is "not only a fake but even dangerous." This is typically done when increases of depressions and symptoms follow. Here are two examples:

Mr. E., a man of 38, entered analysis because of a heart-neurosis. His symptom became so acute that he could not work, "or even live." This man, too, lived with his mother. He was having an affair with a girl who worked in his office. Just before aggravation of his heart complaints, this girl had tried to force him to marry her. To a great extent, he was uninterested in women, regarding intercourse as a disagreeable tribute demanded by "crazy women." He was interested only in the problem of motoring. Analysis revealed that his heart disease was chiefly the result of identification with his father's fatal illness, heart failure. His hysterical symptom was brought about by an unconscious feeling of guilt because of aggressive wishes toward his father and by the masochistic elaboration of this boomeranging aggression, complicated by the unconscious pleasure of being overwhelmed. His feminine identification also contributed to this sexualization of aggression directed against himself. In addition to his heart symptoms, disturbances of potency appeared. He was no longer capable of carrying out his former entirely pleasureless sort of intercourse; and he feared to die while performing the sexual act. That his hysterical heart complaints grew worse at the approach of marriage, was due to his unconscious identification of his fiancée with his mother. When analysis was beginning to disclose his attachment to his mother, he reacted with the typical resistance, which for him took the form of temporary aggravation of his heart complaints and the breaking off of his engagement. He then decided that his heart was "too weak" for both analysis and marriage.[18]

[18] "The Problem of Over-aged Bachelors." Medical Record, May, 1945.

Mr. F. was a "happy-go-lucky" whose false optimism did not prevent "slight troubles with his manliness." This euphemism covered a severe potency disturbance. The analysis of the pre-Oedipal components provoked a transitory depression which the patient blamed on analysis. The analysis of this depression contained a cross-section of all the typical seven [19] types of neurotic depression.

First: Our skill in therapy depends on our ability to trace the feeling of guilt to its proper source. Let's take a banal example: A patient feels deeply depressed because of his potency disturbance, and believes that his feeling of guilt is in connection with the injustice he does his wife in not being able to satisfy her sexually. We show him that this feeling of guilt because of aggression [20] is justified, but that it has reference to something else—unconscious identification of his wife with the mother of the Oedipal period. He satisfies in unconscious fantasy these incestuous wishes and at the same time disappoints the woman in reality. His feeling of guilt, therefore, belongs to his repressed libidinous and aggressive wishes stemming from early childhood and materialized in faint innuendos. His sense of depression is, therefore, the "fee" he pays to his superego for its permission to enjoy a part of the unconscious wish in a disguised form in his neurotic symptom. Remembering the witty expression coined by Freud, "unconscious currency," we can call this depression *"neurotic fee depression."*

Second: His depression is increased because the superego, having accepted the bribe of unhappiness for the symbolically-materialized part of the unconscious wish in the symptom, acts like a blackmailer who always makes veiled allusions to the fact that he has even more compromising material up his sleeve, only to prevent the victim from thinking of stopping payments. Since there is a "direct path between the id and the superego" (Alexander), the superego knows the whole extent of the id-wishes, which are only partly and in secondary defenses materialized in the neurotic symptom (*"preventive depression"*).

Third: The superego constantly shows the ego the self-created unconscious ego-ideal like a silent model, and every discrepancy between ego and ego-ideal manifests itself in a sense of depression and feeling of

19 See "Working Through." Psa. Rev., *32*:461–464, 1945.

20 That aggression is but pseudo-aggression, covering deeper repressed oral masochism, see chapter VI, section 2.

guilt. Dr. Jekels and I have described that mechanism in our paper, "Transference and Love" (Imago, 1934). One could call that type of depression a *depression because of discrepancy between ego and ego-ideal.*

Fourth: The id constantly claims, more and more, fulfillment of its wishes, as is demonstrated by the fact that untreated neuroses become more severe with age, and the part of the wishes which are not satisfied in innuendos and defenses, the "*nonfulfillment depression,*" appears in the unconscious ego as depression.

Fifth and sixth: The unconscious ego itself contributes two types of depression. The ego is constantly reproached by the superego, activated by the working-through process, on the accusation that the ego gives way to id-wishes and enjoys so doing. Since analysis, during the working-through process, continually points out that the pleasure-element and the superego take up the interpretation for their own purposes of torture, the patient must increase that *alibi-part of the depression.* Thus, we see why depression and unhappiness often deepen during analysis.

The sixth component of that sense of depression comes from the gradual realization that these wishes will be destroyed; we might call this a *regret-element* in the depression.

As a seventh and least important element, we might mention the fact that every person unable to fulfill his *conscious* ego-ideal-demands feels none too happy.

The differentiation and working-through in analysis of these seven elements of neurotic depression are of paramount importance. One could object to the breaking down of the massive depression of the patient into its constituents as superfluous miscroscopy. To that, I must answer that one has to recognize the specific meaning of the specific type of these transitory depressions. The unfortunate fact is that, only if one interprets the specific reason for, and type of, a specific depression, can one speed up its disappearance. General and vague interpretations simply don't work. On the other hand, as long as a patient takes his sense of depression at face value, without understanding and discounting it, he is a beginner in analysis, regardless of how many months or years he has paid his analytic bills.

4. *Danger of Losing the "Basic Fallacy."* Every neurotic dreads most

the loss of his "basic fallacy."[21] This fallacy which supports the whole edifice of the neurosis, consists of an erroneous assumption about, or mendacious misuse of, the real situation in childhood. The patient's "basic fallacy" assumed automatically that his neurosis is the *direct* result of environment. Every neurotic drags out his family skeleton, such as: "Father was cruel. Mother didn't love me; she preferred my brother. My sister hated me. The whole family was 'half-crazy.' Our neighbor's brother seduced me . . . etc., etc." One may be of different opinion as to how much influence "reality" really has on the child's development, whether the child sees everything through the spectacles of his own projection or only partly misconceives reality. One thing is clear: Without participation of the ego, the process of environmental influence is unintelligible. It is exactly the basic fallacy of the past which psychoanalytic therapy has to dispose of in every analysis. Assuming, for instance, that the mother in a specific case was really rejecting the boy, why should that child not create later in life a situation in which a woman loves him dearly? Without *masochistic elaboration*—a work done by the unconscious ego—the repetition of being unloved, created in later marriage, is not even conceivable.

By fighting for and clinging to the "basic fallacy," the patient can waste months and years in analysis.

5. *Dreams Embodying a Sense of Guilt in Connection with Recovery.* In the last stages of successful analyses, the unconscious sense of guilt is tremendously increased, for, in advanced stages of the treatment, the guilty feelings which were lodged in the symptoms, depressions, self-provoked punishments, ego-limitations, etc., are activated, thus transforming the *bound* unconscious sense of guilt into a *free-floating* one. When the analysis is far advanced, this sense of guilt, released from its former positions, temporarily increases the patient's sense of depression, his subjective uneasiness, and his aggressive impulses toward the analyst, although the symptoms have subsided. In its free-floating form, it now fastens with all of its force on the reproach leveled by the patient's conscience, "Why are you not well yet?" It is difficult to determine what part is played here by psychic-economic factors—the provision of a better outlet for the sense of guilt or indeed of any outlet at all. Of

[21] "The Danger Neurotics Dread Most: Loss of the Basic Fallacy." Psa. Rev., *33*:2, 1946.

course, that part of the unconscious sense of guilt which represents the patient's reaction to his sexual and aggressive pre-Oedipal and Oedipal wishes is resolved by the analysis; besides, analysis destroys these wishes.

This reproach of conscience, "Why are you not well yet," finds expression in typical dreams, in which the ego seeks to reject the superego's accusations. I have proposed that we should call dreams of this type "dreams embodying a sense of guilt in connection with recovery."[22]

I shall give one example: A young girl, suffering from agoraphobia and hypochondria, dreamed in a late stage of analysis in which her street-fear diminished to a negligible degree for a longer time: A person resembling the patient's sister declares during a quarrel that, if the patient does not get well, she will not feel bound any more to secrecy and will divulge the reason why the patient came to the city from her distant home-town. The patient curses the sister's child.

Consider the situation on the day preceding the dream: The patient did not feel happy at all at her improvement. She shifted the emphasis from the disappearing street-fear to the shape of her breasts. Even if analysis could completely eliminate her street-fear—so she argued—this alone would not help her, since the shape of her breasts was irreparable. The problem was thoroughly discussed in analysis, and it was proved to the patient that her pre-occupation with the breast was based on masculinity wishes. Her main objection to her breasts was their "softness" and smallness—she simply compared them inwardly with an erect penis. Neither the diagnostician nor the gynecologist could detect anything abnormal or even cosmetically objectionable in her normally-shaped breasts. During the last analytic appointment preceding the dream, she was shown how she sabotaged recovery, since she did not want health at all and clung to her masochistically-tinged complaints, covering materialization of infantile wishes. In the dream the sister takes over the rôle of the analyst and of her own superego, respectively, because the patient had consulted her sister about her breasts before entering treatment; her sister had declared that she was imagining things. She knew about the patient's "great secret," her analysis. The patient did not want to give any information to her sister; and the latter used

[22] First stated in the writer's contribution to the symposium in Marienbad, *loc. cit.*

the technique of taking a great oath of secrecy. Since both sisters were superstitious, the oath had the formulation: "I swear that my child shall die, should I divulge my sister's secret."

The dream could thus be interpreted:

Id wish: I want masochistic exhibitionism continued, want a penis and hate everybody who has a penis-substitute (child).

Superego Reproach: You don't want to change at all. First you centered your complaints around street-fear, now you are stressing the breasts. You don't want the cure at all, but indulgence in exhibitionism, masculinity and hatred, masochistically misused.

Ego-Compromise: It is not true that I don't want recovery, it is not true that I am jealous of my sister's child and what it represents. Quite the contrary! Not I am exhibitionistic! My sister is: She wants to misuse my secret for exhibiting at my expense. I, therefore, have the right to curse her child, since I am acting in self-defense. My complaints about my breasts are real enough! I am neither masochistic nor aggressive, I defend myself in self-defense.

The patient's dream satisfies both purposes: Fulfillment of unconscious wishes and rebuff of superego reproaches.[23]

The correct handling of the transference and of resistance, by "working through," activates the unconscious feeling of guilt and makes it a *vis a tergo* which pushes the patient out of his or her neurosis.

Freud once made, in an impatient mood, the remark that curing neurotics is like white-washing a colored man. Some neurotics, it is true, give this impression—fortunately not all. If we overlook, however, the obstacles to recovery, we must marvel, not at neurotics who don't want to be cured, who never enter analysis, or if they do, who run away after a few weeks. We should rather be surprised that there are neurotics who allow us to cure them. There are hundreds of thousands of neurotics in every great city and only a few hundreds of them are subject to our therapy. I exclude purposely matters of financial difficulties and ignorance of the existence of analysis. Experience with

[23] See Jekels-Bergler, "Dualism of Instincts in Dreams." Lecture presented before the XIIIth Int. Psa. Convention in Lucerne, 1934. Psa. Quart., 9:4, 1940. We claimed that every dream fulfills two aims: fulfillment of infantile wishes *and* refutation of super-ego reproaches.

patients of psychoanalytic clinics in Europe has proved conclusively that there are no differences in the basic structure of the neuroses of the millionaire and the poorest unemployed person.

Suppose a well-to-do patient with potency disturbance has ten wealthy friends. Suppose the patient is cured and tells all his friends about the way he achieved his potency. Suppose all his friends were impotent and had confidence in the cured friend. What would be the probable result? Of all these ten persons, perhaps one would enter analysis after five years.

There is *one more* prerequisite necessary besides neurotic illness, money, and knowledge of analysis, to make a workable patient. This indispensable prerequisite is an, at least potentially fluctuating, inner feeling of guilt.[24] I do not mean feeling of guilt *per se*, since every neurotic is full of it. The problem is the deposition of that guilt. As long as the balance of guilt and absorption of it in neurotic unhappiness is fair, the neurotic will not enter analysis—despite his suffering.

The fact that the unconscious aims of the patient in analysis and the objective fact of what that therapy has to offer, are so different, explains also why so few neurotics complete their analyses. At least fifty per cent of the analytic patients leave analysis after the model of Mr. A.'s "partial success," described above. Should the analyst mourn over these people? Not at all. The analyst should know what it is all about and take the results stoically. The neurotic idyll is the infantile paradise, paid for with unhappiness. Only the fact that the few persons who actually seek analytic help, engage us for precisely the destruction of this paradise, gives us the right to disturb it.

The theoretical knowledge of the five-cornered "aim" of the neurotic provides us with a compass to steer away from either therapeutic hyper-optimism or therapeutic nihilism.

That therapeutic skepticism is fostered by the fact that many analytically treated cases are not helped. True enough, there are incurable cases. One has, however, to distinguish between *unavoidable* and *avoidable* failures. I believe that the chronic disregard for the oral-masochistic regression is responsible for many avoidable therapeutic failures.

[24] See the writer's "Working Through." Psa. Rev., *loc. cit.*

2

One Neurosis—But Many Neurotic "Rescue Stations"

FREUDIAN psychoanalysis has existed for half a century and survived all death notices. The main body of our science has outlived attacks of enemies and even the "advice" of false friends who have been trying to reform, "advance," change and neo-"modernize" psychoanalysis. All these attempts have consisted in throwing overboard basic principles of psychoanalysis. It matters little in effect whether these attempts reflected personal inner conflicts of the reformers, or more conscious adaptations to prejudices and resistances of a "difficult" environment. Freud ironically called these split-off groups "Abfälle," a term which denotes in German secession and—refuse.

The attacks of enemies and pseudo-friends had, however, one deleterious effect: while defending analysis, analysts themselves became too engrossed in conservation and conservatism. The best example is the way Freud is quoted in analytic circles. I listened a few years ago to a lecture delivered by a colleague who "proved" with great learning and a multitude of quotations that Freud was biased on a specific topic. The curious thing was that the quotations stopped short before 1931, the year of introduction of the pre-oedipal phase, as if a heavy curtain were drawn, or Freud had died in that year. . . . To express it paradoxically: one quotation from Freud and another quotation from Freud are not the same thing. Freud may have believed one thing in 1908, and another in 1931. The technique of picking out whatever one chooses is—to say the least—misleading.

There are honest Freudian analysts who stopped in their psychic development at some time between 1900 and 1939, the year of Freud's death. They all quote Freud, and with good authority. The most typical example is one of Freud's oldest pupils who never overcame the shock of the introduction of the concept of the superego. His favorite question was: What's the difference between my—piles and the superego? The piles protrude from my rectum, the superego from my throat.[1]

Another mental obstacle is the fact that different types of neuroses stand around like primordial blocks without being interconnected. Hysteria and obsessional neuroses, e.g., are considered diametrically different diseases: connecting links are, though theoretically half-acknowledged, practically never made use of. The basis of obsessional neurosis is still considered "anal-*sadistic*," as in the good old days of 1908, when sadism and aggression were not at all, or inadequately, differentiated. Some of the younger generation of analysts in different countries are pitifully disoriented about anything which reaches beyond the most primitive principles of the "positive" Oedipus complex. Often these colleagues do not even know that a "negative" Oedipus exists, though Freud described it in 1908. Or if they have heard about it, they confuse it with homosexuality. And if you talk about the pre-oedipal phase, though discovered by Freud, they consider you a heretic with an "unorthodox" approach.

Psychoanalysis is still a science in the developmental stage. The history of *every* science proves with boring monotony that in these transitory periods there are people to be encountered who are content with the already known body of material, and others who continue to search for exactly the dark spots of *terra incognita*. Freud himself belonged to the second group; some of his adherents are emotionally drawn to the first category, fashioned after the principle "my learning days are over." There is no reason to marvel at that fact; there is, however, the necessity of stating the fact and its rather grotesque consequences.

Fully aware of the possibility of being misunderstood and berated, I would like to register *my conviction that there is only one basic neurosis and that neurosis is oral in genesis. All other nosologic groups, based on anal and phallic regression, are but rescue stations from the oral "danger."*

Nobody denies, of course, that hysteric and compulsive neuroses do exist *clinically*. So do a dozen other neurotic diseases. What is ques-

[1] "Wächst mir zum Hals heraus," untranslatable, because idiomatic; denotes something like: I am fed up.

tioned is not the undeniable clinical fact. *What is questioned is the correct application of the connecting links between oral, anal, and phallic phases.*

That those connections do exist, has been known for a long time to more discerning and less naïve analysts. These connections are even sometimes mentioned in the literature. Lip service, however, does not mean acceptance, nor understanding: to be "modern" you have to make a few concessions—best in a footnote.

What I claim is something different. *I claim that "remnants" from the oral phase are not carried around later in life like sentimental baggage, or a souvenir. I claim that that "later"—the anal and phallic phases and what follows in neurosis—is not understandable without taking cognizance of the fact that these phases are but rescue—and survival attempts from the oral danger.*

The "*story of the missing links*" is, as pointed out before, not new. It has been theoretically stressed by different authors. To quote a case history written in 1929, published in 1933: [2]

". . . The patient did, of course, reach in a token sense the later levels (anal-urethral-phallic); but he carried over to all these levels so many remnants from the 'breast complex' . . . to that he was always forced to regress. The complexity of the picture was comparable to the chaotic situation on the currency-market of a country in which five currencies are at the same time accepted (e.g., shillings, new Austrian crowns, old Austrian crowns, gulden and taler.) The population, however, has confidence exclusively in the oldest currency: the taler. Moreover, to continue the illustration: there exists also an exchange rate, according to which each of the different currencies is contained in the following one."

Twenty years ago, I did not suspect, when writing these words, that the attitude expressed in the monetary simile as "confidence," is in inner reality a desperate self-rescue action on the part of every neurotic.

One self-evident fact should be stressed, if only to avoid too senseless misundertandings. Biologically conditioned necessity forces the child to a cathexis of other organs, beside the mouth. What the con-

[2] Case II in "The Breast Complex In The Male" (in coll. with Dr. L. Eidelberg). Int. Zeitschr. f. Psa., *19*: 569, 1933.

tents of the cathexis is, and how much is carried over from the oral stage, is the problem.

I conceive of the child's life as a great intrapsychic escape from passivity. The real situation pushes the child constantly into that danger. That threat of passivity is counter-acted by defensive aggression. Neurosis or normalcy represent the result: if passivity wins out—neurosis is inevitable. Normalcy denotes the opposite outcome.

There exists in the child's life a long line of *enforced passivity stations.* To start with, the oral stage begins historically with the parasitic "gimme-attitude." That "gimme-attitude" is, however, vastly different from the parasitic attitude of an adult parasite. First, the fact that a person outside of his own ego is the dispenser, is not at all acknowledged by the child who lives on the basis of autarchic fantasies. Moreover, because of this megalomaniacal misconception, the *child perceives being given milk—paradoxically—as maternal aggression.* This is, perhaps, even more fantastic than the megalomaniacal idea of the child centered around its own supposed omnipotence. Still, it is a direct result of the latter. Since the child originally believes the breast (bottle) to be a part of its own body (Freud, Ferenczi), everything forced upon the child is conceived—for a transitory period—as coming from the outside, and therefore undesired; in the last resort, as *aggressive intrusion.*[3] The child feels *passively victimized.* This "aggressive intrusion" is counteracted by aggressive counteractions: biting the breast (bottle), refusal to take it, spitting, vomiting, crying. Normally, however, the libidinous contents of sucking prevail and the child gets, besides the necessary caloric contents, and oral pleasure as well.

The clinical material leading to the assumption of the child's misconception "milk as maternal aggression," came to my attention in the following way: My first observation pertained to a young man who acquired a potency disturbance after an attempt to strangle a girl who refused to masturbate him. The patient was at the time of his analysis twenty-one years of age. He met in an amusement park of the capital of his North European country, two years before entering treatment, a girl, a chambermaid, and tried to persuade her to have intercourse

[3] First stressed in "Three Tributaries to the Development of Ambivalence." The Psa. Quarterly, 1948, No. 2.

with him on the very evening they met. She refused, and he forced her to masturbate him in a dark street, threatening to choke her to death if she refused. The girl was frightened, and after a short time ran away. He caught up with her and started to strangle her. The girl freed herself and began to scream. A policeman arrested both. The young man pretended that she wanted to rob him; the girl told the true story with some exaggerations. The whole affair looked unfavorable for the young man, and only the girl's police record saved him. It seemed that a few weeks earlier she had been accused of stealing a ring from her female employer but had been freed on lack of definite proof of her guilt. The young man was from the "higher social circles": the family lawyer was able to convince the authorities that "such a well-bred person was incapable of committing a crime." No charges were pressed; after that "incident" the young man was sent abroad. He decided, after long peregrinations, to enter analysis.

The reasons for his criminotic action are unimportant in this connection.[4] For our purposes one incident which happened during the analysis of this orally regressed patient is pertinent. He had repetitive dreams of the following nature: An enormous ball (sometimes a stone) was pressed into his mouth. He was suspended in mid-air, face downward, his feet bound together on the ceiling, like a reversed fixture. These dreams could not be interpreted, as no associations were given. Having met similar dreams before, I suspected the connection with the breast without, of course, mentioning my suspicion to the patient. However, one day *he* mentioned an incident which seemed to have bearing on the accuracy of the suspicion. He had entered by chance, as he claimed, the room in which his landlady's daughter was nursing her baby. He withdrew with apologies and thought: "It looks as if she would choke the baby with her enormous breast." Since recollection from the baby-days are unobtainable in the deepest of analyses, only indirect conclusions are possible.

Years later, I analysed an inhibited radio actor who was afraid to face the microphone. He gave up his profession, worked in an underpaid position in some different field of endeavor and was indirectly forced by his wife to enter analysis. It turned out that the flight from

[4] See my "Suppositions About the Mechanism of Criminosis," Case 9, J. of Criminal Psychopathology, V: 215–246, 1943.

the microphone was preceded by the flight from the stage. The patient started his career as stage actor and "switched" because of neurotic and not realistic reasons, to radio. In the theatre he developed pathologic stage fright, was afraid of forgetting his lines; allegedly to avoid that danger, he entered the radio field where parts can be read. He dreaded the advent of television where that "advantage" would be lost. Many elements in his neurosis pointed—besides the obvious scopophiliac ones—in the direction of oral regression; these cannot be mentioned because of necessary discretion. For our purposes, two statements of the patient are important. The first was a recollection pertaining to the beginning of his stage fright, rather a flash of an "impression" as the patient called it, still important enough to be repressed. The thought was this: "It occurred to me one night, while on the stage and waiting my cue, that if one looks at the two galleries in the dark, they remind one of an open mouth ready to 'swallow you up'." The other statement, this time not repressed, was a description of learning a part during that phase of analysis in which he was able to take up his radio career once more. Said the patient: "While studying my part I had the impression that somebody wants to force down something into my throat and I resist violently." The patient did not connect that observation with the fact that "digesting" his part was his—"bread and butter," *forced* upon him by the "cruel" analyst in the transference repetition.

A well known writer, in analysis because of his writing-block lasting for years, showed all the typical reasons for writing-inhibition, as described in my previous publications.[5] He produced, however, one additional symptom when attempting to write: he vomited. The interesting feature in the patient's life history was that his father and stepfather were scholar and writer, respectively. His mother pushed him, first indirectly, later directly, into the writing profession, also because of her antagonism to the second husband who ironically denied that the "boy" had any literary chances at all. Full of glee she finally showed the skeptical husband the patient's first book, as if it were her

[5] "A Clinical Approach to the Psychoanalysis of Writers." The Psa. Rev., *1*:1944. "Psychoanalysis of Writers and Literary Productivity," In *Psa. and the Social Sciences*, ed. Dr. Roheim, Int. Univ. Press, New York, 1947. "Further Contributions to the Psychoanalysis of Writers," The Psa. Rev., *4*:1947 and *1*:1948.

personal triumph. The triumph increased with the success of that book.

The patient lived psychologically on the basis of his defense mechanism: "Not I want to be masochistically refused, *I* refuse aggressively." That defense corresponded to the second layer of the "mechanism of orality". Whereas the successful writer "eliminates" autarchically the "refusing" and "disappointing" mother by identifying unconsciously with the fantasy of the *giving* mother—he gives "out of himself" to himself "beautiful" words and ideas—, the blocked writer is incapable of that "self-cure." Under pressure of guilt, pertaining to his undigested psychic masochism, he is forced to maintain his pseudo-aggressive defense: *I* refuse. He thus furnishes his alibi, but, at the same time, his alibi makes him unproductive.

Hence the patient's vomiting represented unconsciously refusal of food allegedly forced upon him (science, writing milieu, "to suck on wisdom's breasts," Goethe's "Faust"). That intellectualized nutritional revolt of the patient was corroborated by a recollection of a statement of his deceased mother to the effect that he was a "strange child." He either refused the breast, *or* bit the nipple so forcefully that his father had to open his mouth to free the nipple. Later, the patient became an exquisite gourmet; most of his conflicts with his successive wives centered around food and culinary preparation of food.

In analysis, the patient behaved on the same defensive level. He had, for example, a dream:

"In a hospital patients are treated by a woman physician with a long rubber hose attached to the penis of the patient; a fluid is pumped in for the purpose of distending their stomachs."

The associations led immediately to recollections of fantastic stories, circulated at the beginning of the century, pertaining to the "water cure" applied to subdue rebellious Moris. The fact that breast and penis are unconsciously identified was known to the patient from previous dreams. That he mixed up his anatomy to such a degree (direct connection between penis and stomach) pointed to the infantile level and also to the reversal of the fact that he did not possess a breast—mother, however, did. Therefore he emphasized an organ which he had, and was missing in mother. The rubber hose represented the breast, the fluid milk. Thus the seemingly senseless use of anatomy becomes meaningful. Especially characteristic is the fact that the patient represented the solution of his inability to give words in writing by a maternal aggression in the transference: the analyst "forces" him to write.

The material in these and similar cases was convincing enough, still I doubted for years the child's misconception: milk = maternal aggression. What convinced me finally were two theoretical considerations based on clinical experience: cases of psychogenic oral aspermia and the psychic superstructure in intercourse.

There is a group of oral neurotics, which I have described elsewhere (see Chapter VI), who despite prolonged friction in intercourse never achieve an ejaculation. There is no organic disturbance present: these people ejaculate during masturbation and in wet-dreams. Analysis proves that unconsciously for these neurotics ejaculation is identified with bursting of an explosive charge, like a bomb. There is no infantile prototype for this fantasy, with exception of the milk-stream.

The second argument is the assumption made by a long series of analytic authors: that the psychic superstructure of intercourse corresponds to a reversal of the dual situation: suckling mother-sucking child. A short survey of our literature on that subject will elucidate this: First must be mentioned Stärcke's paper on the castration complex. He was the first to signalize the fact of oral castration through weaning. Ferenczi (in "Attempt at a genital theory") stressed that every human being, man or woman, is capable of acting the double role of child and mother with his own body. The act of sexual intercourse is characterized by a "maternal regressive trend" in which a threefold identification takes place: identification of the whole organism with the genitals, identification with the partner, and identification with the genital secretion. The rhythm of suction persists as an important part of every following erotic act, and great quantities of oral and anal eroticism are shifted toward the vagina. Here the vagina assumes in coitus, as H. Deutsch has asserted in "Psychoanalysis of Female Sexual Functions," in a shift from above to below, the passive role of the sucking mouth, the penis being identified with the breast. In this function coitus means for the woman a repetition of her first relation with the outer world, where the object was incorporated orally, a repetition of sucking on the mother's breast, an overcoming of the trauma of weaning. O. Rank, in his "Genesis of Genitality," has shown that the child finds in his own genitals a substitute for his mother's breast, and answers the question of how the "shabby remnant" of libido is shifted from the oral to the genital level by pointing to masturbation of the infant. In this transition—following a hint of Bernfeld—the hollow hand is substituted for the mouth, and later the penis is substituted for the breast and sperm for milk. The normal sex act is, in that conception, not only a substitute but also sadistic revenge for satisfaction denied by the breast. Eidelberg and I have stressed, in "The Breast Complex in the Male," the *active* repetition of the *passive* experience (contained in Freud's conception of the "unconscious repetition compulsion") as a means of overcoming the trauma of weaning. By means of this device the child restores his injured and mortified narcissism and megalomania, since, instead of passively receiving milk, he becomes the active dispenser of urine (later sperm) and thus denied the loss of the breast, identifying breast and penis. In this conception a mixture of erotic and thanatic impulses are directed at the penis. We stress the fact that the thanatic elements in the mixture of impulses are attenuated in coitus to such a degree that their satisfaction is possible without danger. In intercourse the man finally achieves, in identification with the phallic mother through active repetition of the passive experience, the overcoming of the trauma of weaning.

All six of the authors just mentioned assume, as we see, that the sex act is basically a repetition of the situation of sucking. In "Transference and Love,"[6] however, Jekels and I go one step further and postulate the basically *narcissistic character of intercourse.* The object-relationship, which is usually stressed, is not decisive at all, since through identification with the object the infant situation is found again. The logical conclusion from that is that the wish to be loved can be traced back to the wish *not to be separated from the "unending stream" which pours from the mother's breast.* However, that nostalgia does not apply to the mother's breast as such; it represents rather a narcissistic attempt at restitution, since it has the breast as object only insofar as that was *conceived as a part of one's own ego.* That grotesque mistake of the infant—assumption that the breast belongs to him—has far-reaching consequences in love. It leads directly to object-rela-

[6] Imago, *1*:1934.

tions in love with the purpose of helping to restore the lost narcissistic unity.

The problem of love cannot be understood without taking into account the role played by the superego. That that is necessary seems strange because it has never been attempted before, and at first glance the connection between the superego and love seems far-fetched. In our paper Jekels and I attempt to separate the insufficiently differentiated portions of the superego more clearly, making use of the Eros-Thanatos theory. We come to the following conclusion:

"Both portions of the same, ego-ideal ('Thou shalt') and 'Daimonion' ('Demon') ('Thou shalt not') [7] are various as to *instinctual psychology and genesis*. The ego-ideal has two roots: One of these consists in the attempt of the ego to put upon objects the aggression of the death-instinct directed against the ego itself. These objects thus become fear-inspiring, and thus an internal danger is merely exchanged for a projected external danger, an unsuccessful attempt. This achievement of the destructive instincts is parried by Eros by absorbing this object of fear into the ego, where it becomes the object of the individual's own narcissism. The second root of the ego-ideal formation is to be sought in a compromising attempt of the ego to maintain its supposed omnipotence. This fictitious omnipotence is severely shaken by the demands of the outer world (intervals between feedings, training to cleanliness, etc.). Because of his helplessness, the child has the choice of reacting in only two ways: either to give up his infantile megalomania or to take to himself the commands of the parents and then disguise this involuntary act as voluntary, in order to preserve his fictitious omnipotence, and invest the introjected commands with his own narcissism. But if Eros really succeeded in parrying Thanatos by setting up the ego-ideal by means of identification, then only love would be found there, which, in fact, is not the case. Thanatos parries this stroke of Eros [8] by desexualization, which is known to accompany every identification.

[7] The word "Demon" has here not the prevailing English meaning of "devil" but the sense of a malignant spirit akin to the "Daimonion" of Socrates. In the above presentation, Demon and Daimonion are synonymous, the latter with the modern connotation.

[8] It is clear, according to Freud's statements, that Eros and Thanatos never occur unmixed, that is, that only secondary *derivatives of mixtures in various proportions* can be studied analytically.

Thus, the ego-ideal is desexualized Eros, and corresponds to the indifferent narcissistic energy postulated by Freud in 'The Ego and the Id', which may at times be added to one of the two fundamental instincts and increase the total cathexis of the one or the other instinct. The ego-ideal thus becomes the real aim of the combat between these two gigantic forces. Like a neutral zone between two parties at war, it becomes the plaything chiefly of the Thanatos section of the super-ego ('Daimonion'). The formation of the 'Daimonion' is due to the unsuccessful attempt of Eros to divert to objects the aggressions of Thanatos originally directed against the individual's own ego by means of projection. The projection is unsuccessful to a quantitatively greater or lesser degree: first, because of the helplessness of the individual, as the little child is powerless against its environment, and hardly able to carry out aggressions to any extent; second, because the same objects against which the aggressions of the child are directed —the parents—have already been absorbed into the ego-ideal, and this results in a decrease of aggression or in aggression against himself. Both cause stasis and redirection of the aggression against the child's own ego. The ego, thus endangered, becomes fearful and gives the danger signal. The ego-ideal, the repository of desexualized Eros, is made use of by the ego-disturbing tendencies of the 'Daimonion' and causes the ego to experience feelings of guilt by constantly holding the ego-ideal up to the ego as a model, and pointing out the discrepancy between the ego and the ego-ideal. The ego-ideal, which was originally erected to bolster up the child's own threatened narcissism, thus becomes the most dangerous weapon of Thanatos against Eros. This holding up of the ego-ideal as a model by the 'Demon' is far from harmless; every deviation from the self-erected ego-ideal appears in the ego in the form of guilt. The remarkable thing about this procedure is that the suffering which the 'Daimonion' causes the ego always takes the route over the ego-ideal. It is as though an opponent of the regime in a dictator state stood before a special tribunal; the outcome of the trial is all decided upon beforehand, but the prisoner is condemned 'legally,' according to certain laws, etc. This comedy of justice is also carried out intrapsychically; a discrepancy between ego and ego-ideal must always be demonstrated before guilt and the desire for punishment arise in the ego. The destructive instinct beats the Eros with its own stick by making use of this desexualized Eros against the Eros itself. It should also be noted that the ego-ideal is an unhomogeneous formation, a not-at-all completely successful alloy of two substances of unequal value, the original unconquerable narcissism, with the introjection of the parents, to which cannot be attributed anywhere nearly equal resistance."

The authors believe, too, that love is partly the expression of the fight between erotic and thanatic tendencies. Here the purpose is to disarm the "Daimonion" by wresting from it the instrument of torture, the ego-ideal, and to add the indifferent energy of the ego-ideal to the erotic tendency. Love presupposes a *tension between ego and ego-ideal.* In his despair—to rid himself of the constant reproach of not having achieved the high-pitched demands of his own ego-ideal—*the lover first projects his ego-ideal on the beloved object.* Then he re-introjects the projected object, a procedure which implies that the object is tinged with narcissistic libido. Thus is explained the over-valuation of the beloved object; it is one's own narcissism which one admires so much. Basically, love has the purpose of restoring the narcissistic unity of the personality.[9]

The strange fact, not generally regarded as strange at all, that love pushes the afflicted person so imperatively to sexual unity and satisfaction is explicable from that point of view. "Tender" and "sensual" love have basically the same meaning; they both represent *narcissistic attempts at restitution of unity* under pressure of the repetition compulsion. The sexual act manifests bodily the same thing that tender love does psychologically. What comes to the fore in tender love, through re-introjection of the object that is substituted for one's own projected ego-ideal, also manifests itself in sensual love through the "Kontrektationstrieb" (Moll), that enigmatic wish of lovers to embrace each other as closely as possible, seemingly inseparably. Only the combination of both tendencies—the tender and the sensual—is the strongest negation of the feeling of separation, incompleteness, basically, of the lesion in narcissism.

[9] The difference between love and transference consists of the fact that in love *only* the ego-ideal is projected; in transference, the whole superego is projected—ego-ideal *and* Demon. The result is that the object of the transference is not only loved but also dreaded. For elaboration see "Divorce Won't Help" (Chapter V, "Neurotics Can't Love"), Harper, New York, 1948.

One point was, however, never stressed in all these assumptions: frictional movement. The prototype for this could only be the feeling of being pierced at the breast.

The penis is—as people observed millions of years ago—a strange organ: in a queer organic economy it serves urinary *and* sexual functions as well. It is *passive* passage way for urine, and *active* expeller of semen, preceded by active frictional movements (thrust). In neurotic regressions, it is even used for passive aims: bedwetting, nocturnal emissions, premature ejaculation when the "semen flows out like urine" (K. Abraham)—without erection and thrusts. The passive and active "use" of the penis perpetuates the old fight between passivity and activity in the male child. Small wonder that the passive use is considered abnormal. Nor should we forget the large group of men who basically want to be *passively* stimulated by a woman's handling of the penis, and have an abhorrence to all active movements in sex. Ironically, one could say that their *activity in sex is reducible to an "active dislike" of activity*. The latter is visible even if coitus is half-heartedly attempted; they fail or, at least, insist that the insertion should be performed by the woman.

The constant fight between *active-progressive*, and *passive-regressive* tendencies, explains also one of the hitherto unsolved mysteries in psychopathology: *the problem of ambivalence.*[10]

Bleuler's terminus technicus, "ambivalence," later accepted by Freud and made famous by the founder of psychoanalysis in his studies of obsessional neurosis, denotes the presence of *two* contradictory psychic tendencies toward the *same* person at the *same* time. As time went on, the term was applied to all neuroses and became typical in the description of practically all contradictory feelings. First it meant: conflict between love and hate, anal submission and aggression; then: conflict between masculine and feminine tendencies in the same person; to be a "bad" and a "good" boy at the same time, dirty and clean. Some analysts apply the term to the contradictory splitting off the "good" and "bad" mother in all its consequences; some to the rapid alteration of introjection and projection. Freud spoke in later years of ambivalence as result of the fight between life and death instincts.

[10] First published in a shortened version in "Three Tributaries to the Development of Ambivalence." The Psa. Quart., 2:1948.

Despite a great variety of explanations, Freud's final statement on the subject in 1926, to the effect that we do not know exactly why ambivalence plays such a decisive part in obsessional (compulsive) neurosis, still holds true. Since ambivalence in no other diseases is so pronounced as in obsessional neurosis, there is no hope of solving the problem except in the study of compulsion neurosis.

In my opinion the problem of ambivalence in obsessional neurosis can be explained only on the condition that we take into account the interconnections between the oral and anal levels of development. It has been repeatedly stressed, for instance by K. Abraham, that mouth and anus are psychologically and biologically very similar. It has, however—strangely enough—not been stressed at all that the child repeats in both zones, though not at the same time, similar passive experiences. Some children perceive the harmless act of getting milk from bottle or breast as maternal aggression. Being given the breast (bottle) means for these children something like being pierced.[11] Caloric kindness is perceived as maternal aggression.

The problem as to why the child forms this fantastic misconception is complicated. It has little to do with maladroitness of mothers and nurses who sometimes push the nipple or bottle too forcefully into the baby's mouth. In my opinion the reason for this misconception of "milk or maternal aggression" is due to a lesion of infantile omnipotence. Since the child originally believes that breast (bottle) is a part of its own body (Freud, Ferenczi), everything forced upon the child is conceived—for a transitory period—as coming from outside, therefore undesired in the last resort, and is perceived as *aggressive intrusion.* The child feels *passively victimized.* This "aggressive intrusion" is counteracted by aggressive counteractions: biting the breast, refusal to take it, spitting, vomiting, crying. Normally, the libidinous value of sucking prevails and the child gets besides the necessary caloric contents an oral pleasure as well.

Children who have perceived being fed in earliest childhood as maternal aggression, misconceive the passing of stool in no less fantastic ways. They feel "drained." "Something" most powerful, uncontrollable, and overwhelming is forcing them to expel a "part of the body." Once more, the child feels *passively victimized.*

[11] See p. 40 ff.

Here we meet the *connecting link* between the oral and anal phase: in both phases certain children feel *passively victimized.* First, the "piercing" fantasy of breast (bottle)—mouth; second, withdrawal of breast (oral castration—Staercke); third, being "pierced" against one's will by feces (anal castration—Freud), all this adds up to *passive* experiences.

Normally, the child overcomes passive experiences, offending his childlike fantasy of omnipotence, by an *active* repetition of the passive experience (Freud, "unconscious repetition compulsion"). The boy nullifies the withdrawal of the breast (culminated in weaning) by identifying his penis with the breast: instead of being *passive* recipient of milk, he becomes the *active* bestower of urine (later sperm). Through these channels narcissism is preserved, dangerous passivity in the male counteracted, as I have previously stressed (in collaboration with Eidelberg) in "The Breast Complex in the Male".

In the anal stage the fantasy of being *passively* pierced by feces leads—as inner defense—to *aggressive* fantasies in connection with anal functions. A classical example is the case of the child mentioned by K. Abraham [12] who threatened his governess in the following fashion: "If you annoy me, I shall shit you on the other side of the river." To which Abraham adds: "According to the thinking of the child, one gets rid of a person not loved any more through defecation."

Obsessional neurotics labor under specific conflicts which, in my opinion, are more complicated than usually assumed. The problem hinges on the question whether or not the aggression displayed by obsessional (compulsive) neurotics is original or defensive in nature. I have stressed the latter view in a series of previous publications.[13] There exists a strange contradiction in the attitude of many colleagues toward the fact that obsessional aggression is but pseudo-aggression. They "feel" that all analysts are familiar with the role of aggressive defense against passivity in compulsive neurotics because Freud described that defense—for paranoia. On the other hand, they cannot name *one* publication which brings that fact into prominence for obsessional neurosis. In scientific literature, feelings do not count, only

[12] "Versuch einer Entwicklungsgeschichte der Libido." Int. Psa. Verlag, 1924, p. 14.

[13] E.g., "Two Forms of Aggression in Obsessional Neurosis." The Psa. Rev., 1942.

publications do. Nobody denies that every analyst must have come across in his clinical experience the pseudo-aggression of obsessives. Still, as far as I can observe in the continuation of unfinished analyses, their aggression has been taken at face value. Obviously, the old formulation of the "anal-*sadistic*" regression in obsessives is being taken too literally. I have stressed in previous publications on that subject that I do not claim to have "invented" the pseudo-aggression of the obsessives; I do claim to have focused attention on something —let's say—neglected in our literature.

First: I do not believe that the aggression displayed by obsessional (compulsive) neurotics is real; it is instead, *pseudo-aggression.* I believe that male obsessional neurotics, after their symptoms and anomalies of character have been established, labor under a continuous unconscious reproach of conscience regarding their passivity. This passivity is *secondarily* warded off by the unconscious Ego in such a way as to prove: "I am not passive; on the contrary, I am extremely aggressive." Thirdly, this defensive is also warded off. Therefore, a *three-layer structure* is observable in obsessional neurotics. This observation has decisive therapeutic consequences: if in clinical analyses of obsessional neurotics one constantly points out only their aggressiveness and resultant feelings of guilt, one gives support (without wishing or meaning to) to their defense mechanism instead of destroying it. The poor therapeutic results with obsessional neurotics are—in my opinion—based on that misunderstanding of the three-layer structure.

Second: The wish to be anally penetrated by the father is not only the result of inverted oedipal wishes and the result of castration fear. These wishes resulting from the "negative" Oedipus in anal regression are also the *refuge from an oral conflict secondarily projected onto the father.* The child escapes into the normal *positive* Oedipus only to be driven back by his passivity into the *negative* Oedipus. Castration fear connected with the positive Oedipus speeds up this reversal. The reason why oedipal castration fear is so effective in these cases is due to the fact that the old allurement of passivity has paved the way by oral-anal *passive* experiences. What the anally regressed child expresses is the old *oral fantasy of being pierced* at a higher (oedipal) level.

Not enough attention has been given to the fact that the anal penis conception ("Kotstange") is but an autarchic attempt to negate the dependence on the breast, and later, as a substitute, on the paternal penis.[14]

This does not deny the importance of castration fear leading to the regression. The unconscious reasoning runs something like this: "It is not true that I want to be penetrated in feminine identification, *anally* by my father's *penis* (repetition of the mouth-breast conception of being pierced). The truth is that I am *autarchic,* have an anal penis myself and want to play with "autarchic feces." Later the anal ("dirty") penis conception is warded off, too, leading to reactive formations.

Third: I believe that the contents of anal repression is the wish to play with "autarchic feces" as defense mechanism against oral-anal passivity. The inverted oedipal wishes are a palimpsest of the oral masochistic fantasy of being pierced, projected onto a *later developmental level,* since the return of the repressed material cannot be forced back any more by the "autarchic defense."

Here, we find the *first* tributary to the stream of ambivalence: it is the *conflict between the "progressive" autarchic defense mechanism*: "I want to play autarchically with self-produced feces and not be orally (maternal breast) and anally (paternal penis) passively penetrated," and the *"regressive" passive wish of being orally-anally penetrated.* Since this fight never ends, ambivalence is perpetrated. We note further that the simple fact of not completely accepting oral-anal passive surrender but putting up some kind of pseudo-fight, in itself suggests the attempt to ward off those passive tendencies with aggressive though ineffective means. Secondarily, ambivalence, too, is used for passive purposes: the obsessional neurotic, for example, uses it for self-torturing purposes.

The second tributary to ambivalence is also to be found in a pseudo-aggressive attempt to ward off passivity. Feces have a strange fate in the child's education. In the first 10–15 months they are over-valuated, mother and nurses being highly interested because of nutritional reasons in their amount, color, odor; the child being coaxed into defecating at specific times and places. Later the same anal products become taboo: It is bad manners to even mention anal functions. The obses-

14 See the writer's "The Leading and Misleading Basic Identifications." The Psa. Rev., 1945.

sional child, constantly on the look-out for an aggresive palimpsest to disguise his oral-anal passivity, uses feces as such alibi. By holding up the old *over-valuated* interest in fecal matter at a time when the same products are already educationally classified as "dirty," therefore, *deprecated,* the child uses it as weapon against its own superego. By constantly reiterating the real contradiction in the educational evaluation of feces, the child tries to prove the hypocrisy [15] and inconsistency of the later internalized educators. In other words, the autarchic attempt at playing with self-produced feces, as stressed in Point 1, complements the pseudo-aggressive defense against oral-anal surrender.

The *third* tributary to ambivalence is to be found in a frantic attempt of obsessional neurotics to utilize pseudo-aggression against oral-anal surrender via "*narcissistic gratification.*" In a paper published thirteen years ago [16] I have pointed out that obsessional neurotics use four unconscious mechanisms for "teasing" their superego:

1. *Mechanism of the inner contradiction of all "compulsive rules."*

Federn showed in his "Frohngesetze," [17] that practically every one of these "compulsive rules" contradicts the others: exactness of content, successful insulation, undivided affect, and the rule of the participation of the entire ego, are mutually irreconcilable, from which much of the insolubility of the compulsions is to be explained. I supplemented this with proofs that the fact that the several rules of compulsion are a mass of contradictions is by no means a matter of chance, nor is it to be fully explained by ambivalence, but by a narcissistic gratification to the ego in reducing the superego *ad absurdum* as well. By way of illustration I referred to an assertion of, Alexander,[18] who pointed out that the obsessional neurotic constantly tends to reduce the demands of the superego *ad absurdum.* "The ego fears the superego, but attempts to abrogate its own dependence upon it. This independence is attained by means of arousing the superego to unjust demands, thus enabling the ego to break off its moral dependence on the superego.

[15] "Hypocrisy." J. Clin. Psychopathology, 1944.

[16] "Notes on an Obsessional Neurosis in Ultimis: Four Mechanisms of Narcissistic Gratification in Obsessional Neurosis." Int. Z. f. Psa., *2*: 1936. Partial English translation in "Two Forms of Aggression in Obsessional Neurosis," *loc. cit.*

[17] Int. Zeitschr. f. Psa., *19*: 1933.

[18] Alexander: "Psychoanalysis of the Total Personality." Nerv. & Ment. Dis. Monograph, No. 52.

At that same time the ego, because of unjust punishments, achieves complete justification for giving way to the forbidden tendencies of the Id."

One of Alexander's patients, "who had been incapable of any sort of work for a long time, suddenly, while he was being analyzed, entered upon an extraordinary activity. Son of an academically educated man, and himself preparing for a professional career, he took a beginner's job at some manual labor. Completely idle up to this time, he now got up at six o'clock and worked in overalls for eight hours, came to his analytic hour every day, dead tired, and even took a daily lesson afterwards. He overworked in the most incredible fashion; instead of accomplishing work, he was working out a compulsion. The point of this distortion is clear: he was making a mockery of his analysis, which made the same demands as his superego (to give up his idleness), and he reduced it *ad absurdum,* in order to feel fully justified in abandoning all activity."

One of my patients, a young lawyer, behaved in a similar manner. Among other things he had the compulsion to read all foreign legal journals. He managed to borrow these, and worked at them compulsively until he was exhausted, for he "supplemented" his professional work with these senseless studies until he fell asleep from exhaustion. By about the tenth of the month, when he saw with despair that because of the mass of material and the language difficulties he would not "get through" with his reading, he gave up, and resolved to read "thoroughly" only the subsequent numbers of these periodicals, which appeared on the first of each month. Thus, after he had reduced the demands of his superego *ad absurdum,* he could permit himself to indulge in sexual fantasies during precisely the time which before he had been spending in compulsive reading.

Now this *reductio ad absurdum* of the superego is generally regarded as a sort of defense against a too strict superego. Another motive, however, is the great narcissistic gratification which the obsessional neurotic attains by means of this obsessional check-mating of the superego. Thus the "mechanism of an inner contradiction of all compulsive rules" is not only an expression of ambivalence in the obsessional neurotic and his tendency to reduce the superego *ad absurdum*, but also a really extreme narcissistic gratification. To be sure, this sort of gratification puts one in mind of the peasant woman who quarreled with her husband about the best method of cutting garden flowers. She insisted upon scissors, and he preferred a knife. In the end the man drowns his wife in a near-by stream, and she, in the very act of drowning, makes a triumphant, scissors-like gesture with her fingers.

2. *The mechanism of direct disparagement of the superego.*

It is well known that obsessional neurotics maintain a sort of "slave"—officially, master; that is, "they manage to acquire an authority beside themselves who can free them from obsessive doubt and obsessive panic. Whenever possible, this role is transferred to the analyst by the patient." (Federn). That the obsessional neurotic is incapable of coming to a decision because he is harried back and forth by his own ambivalence, that he would place the responsibility of a decision upon anyone rather than upon himself—these are Freudian axioms. I have noticed, however, that the obsessional neurotic regards his "slaves" contemptuously as being far beneath him. That in spite of this attitude, he invests them with the authority to make decisions, is an *aggression against his own superego,* somewhat according to the formulation, "What a miserable superego, that can be replaced by every Tom, Dick and Harry!" Thus it may be seen that when the obsessional neurotic attempts to force the analyst into this role, he is merely making use of him as a means of aggression against the superego. Therefore, the old analytic rule, not to give advice to the obsessional neurotic, but only to examine the motives that lead him to ask this advice, should be extended to require the analysis of the aggression and disparagement of the analyst (superego) which underlie the demand for advice.

3. *The mechanism of relative crudity in the compulsion.*

It is generally known that the obsessional neurotic arrives at strange compromises between the divergent commands and prohibitions of his superego (insulation, undoing). In spite of their complexity there is a childish and primitive quality in these compromises. At the same time they contain a boundless aggression against the ego-ideal. Almost every obsessional neurotic confronts himself with "obsessional alternatives," such as Freud has described in the "Rat Man."

I submit an example from the analysis of a patient of mine, who had set up the following "obsessional alternative" before taking a language test which he had been putting off for months. "Either I must cheat at the examination (using a dictionary or a 'pony') or my analysis will prove a failure." The connection with the analysis he established as follows: it was true that the analyst would give him no advice since this was against the rules of analytic technique. But *if* the analyst were to give advice, he would advise against cheating, saying it was a device of the patient to harm himself, and would prophesy *failure* of the cheating. Since the patient might not be caught by the professor, and might pass the examination *just because* of the cheating against which he had been advised, the prophecy of the analyst might be false. This would be proof that the rest of the analyst's assertions were incorrect, and therefore the analysis would be doomed to failure. . . .

The entire argument of the "obsessional alternative" is based on a *false premise*, the "prophecy" of failure. This is characteristic of the childish efforts of the unconscious portion of the ego to swindle the superego, which can only be resolved by tracing them back to the ambivalence conflict and infantile material. In fact, one might well assert that the relative crudity with which the superego is reduced *ad absurdum* is typical of the compulsions. The cruder the trap into which the superego falls, the greater the gratification of the unconscious portion of the ego.

4. *The mechanism of "guided miracles."*

It is known that things are always happening to obsessional neurotics which seem to confirm their omnipotence of thought. I have named these occurrences "guided miracles."

A patient had occupied himself for some time with the project of a school of agricultural fertilizers. Although he knew nothing of this speciality, and in his proposal was unconsciously trying to sublimate anal tendencies, he attempted with some astuteness to interest various agricultural authorities. After months of effort, he succeeded in drumming up a meeting of several interested people in a provincial town. On the way to the meeting (naturally the journey itself was beset by evil omens), the patient, in high spirits, decided to indulge himself by buying a better cigar than his usual brand at four cents a piece. To buy a more expensive cigar, however, would be tempting the fates, whose protection at the impending meeting he badly needed. So after long hesitation he decided on a compromise, and bought two cigars at four cents and one cigar at five cents. When he came to pay, he was completely prostrated when the clerk stated the total: thirteen cents!

Such a "miracle" is to be explained by ambivalence. Since ambivalence functions continuously, the defensive, negative striving is also constantly on hand; the more so, as these "blows of fate" are secondarily sexualized, and are looked forward to with unconscious enjoyment. One might add that the unconscious portion of the ego knows that the obsessional neurotic himself is the manager of these miracles. It is thus the product of his own omnipotence that appears to be enacted by an external fate. That fate constantly plays the role of observer, and the fact that it is so noticeably preoccupied with the obsessional neurotic, is a further proof that he is beloved by fate, and therefore has power over it.

These mechanisms provide narcissistic gratification and *are at the same time part of the chronic truly frantic attempts* of these sick people to utilize *pseudo-aggression as a means of defense against oral-anal surrender.*

Expressed differently: by teasing the superego and deriving thus narcissistic pleasure, the obsessional neurotic "proves" to himself that he is *not* passive. This spurious face-saving device is visible in ambivalence, too. The formula runs something like this: "I doubt whether I should do this or that. . . ." The emphasis is on "*I*". In inner reality, something beyond his control *makes* him doubt. By changing the role of the passively victimized into that of the active bearer of a doubt—some "activity"!—narcissism is autarchically "preserved."

Ambivalence denotes chronic presence of *two* contradictory feelings toward the *same* person at the *same* time. Three not hitherto described tributaries to that mechanism are worked out with the common denominator of being drawn towards inner passivity and fighting against it with "autarchic" fantasies. The original feeling of childlike omnipotence in the child is constantly hurt by reality. Some children perceive suckling as maternal aggression, misconstruing that harmless act as being passively pierced. Loss of stools is also later misconstrued as internally being pierced. Against these passive misconceptions aggressive and libidinous counter-devices are normally set in motion. Where these counter-measures do not suffice, ambivalence develops—especially in children regressing to the "anal" stage. Ambivalence is the outward manifestation of a *desperate inner struggle between the wish to be orally and anally pierced and denial of this dangerous wish by pretending aggressively that autarchy is preserved.* The whole struggle is fully excluded from consciousness.

I recently received a confirmation of my assumptions of the oral basis of ambivalence from a distinguished colleague for whose opinions I always had respect—prior indeed to his latest utterance. Dr. Henry Alden Bunker, President of the New York Psychoanalytic Society, published a few weeks after appearance of my study on ambivalence the following case: [19]

"The day after I read Dr. Bergler's paper, 'Three Tributaries to the Development of Ambivalence,' a male patient, a fairly severe compulsive character, reported a dream which seemed to me to confirm directly one of the constructions set forth in Bergler's paper. In this, it will be recalled, Dr. Bergler states *inter alia* that the anal regression evidenced in the wish to be anally penetrated by the father is an expression not only (as is well known) of the escape from the threat of castration connected with the positive oedipus into the passivity of the negative oedipus, but also of 'the old fantasy of being orally penetrated' by the mother's breast—nursing, Bergler has concluded, having been experienced by some persons as an act of maternal aggression: 'some children perceive breast or bottle feeding as acts of maternal aggression—for some children, at least, something like being pierced.' My patient's dream is noteworthy because it expresses the fantasy of anal penetration as including at the same time the fantasy of being orally penetrated, as though these two were the same and indistinguishable from each other.

> I was riding as a passenger in what used to be called the tonneau of an automobile, when a dickybird flew in the rear window. It then began to sing in two parts. Its name was Amelia.

"Passing over as self-evident the dreamer's passive rôle as a passenger to say nothing of the rather gratuitious introduction of a French word in this connection, it may be remarked that while the symbolism of a bird is familiar enough in psychoanalysis, the dreamer's own associa-

19 "Note on an 'Ambivalent' Dream." The Psa. Quart., XVII, pp. 389–390, 1948.

tions arrived at the same result: 'Dickeybird, dickey, (isn't that a slang word for penis?) prick, penis . . . In two parts /the patient is a musicologist/: an impossibility, of course—you can't sing in two parts any more than you can play a chord on a flute; being both masculine and feminine at the same time; I'd love to be able to do it; but we have a lot of collateral evidence also that "two" may refer to the breasts.' 'Amelia: a meal,' was his instant association; to which he added, 'the bird comes in and it's a meal.'

"In the light of Bergler's designation of ambivalence as the presence of two contradictory feelings toward the same object at the same time, and as 'the outward manifestation of a desperate unconscious struggle between the wish to be orally and anally penetrated, and an anxious denial of this dangerous wish', it was rather arresting to hear my patient then go on to say, 'This begins to suggest to me my wanting a thing and not wanting it at the same time. When a thing is forced on me,' he continued, 'then I feel I must rebel, even though I am attracted to or want the thing. You remember Miss Y., the aggressive woman with big breasts who forced the piano on me; and what did I do? I didn't practice, and I couldn't practice and I can't play the piano.' "

The allurement of, and fight against, passivity continues on the phallic (*oedipal*) level, too. We know from Freud that there exists a "positive" and "negative" (inverted) Oedipus. In the former, the boy wants to usurp father's place and do all the "forbidden" things father does in the child's imagination with mother; he "hates" the father as competitor and "loves" the mother. In the latter, the boy identifies (also under pressure of castration fear) with the mother, wants to replace her in father's affection and be sexually "mistreated" by him, as he imagines mother is; he "hates" mother as competitor, and "loves" the father.

Both phases of the Oedipus relation are correctly observed. *What is missing, is the connection with the oral-anal phases. Is not the passivity of the "negative" Oedipus but the continuation of the old oral passivity? And is not the activity of the "positive" Oedipus one of the desperate attempts to rescue oneself from that passivity via the tour de force of enhanced aggression?*

Viewed from that viewpoint we can state that man's whole psychic life is a desperate attempt to *escape from passivity*. That passivity was biologically, because of the helplessness of the child, most pronounced in the first months of life—on the oral stage. Hence my conviction that there is only *one* neurosis, the oral one, but many rescue stations. These different rescue stations correspond to the many nosologic groups subsumed as results of regression to anal and phallic phases. So long as these groups are not genetically interconnected with the start, the oral level—we are missing both understanding and continuity. We are fighting on the outskirts and not in the center of the enemy's stronghold.

The higher developmental levels (anal, urethral, phallic) remind one in neurotics of a man hanging above an abyss, holding on to the edge with his naked fingers. If he regresses to orality, his grip loosens and he plunges back. Crawling forward or falling back, seems to be the modern neurotic equivalent of Hamlet's "to be or not to be" problem.

Table 1 schematizes the fight between regressive-oral-passive tendencies, and progressive pseudo aggressive defenses in the male:

TABLE 1. *Conflict Between Regressive-Oral-Passive Tendencies, and Progressive Pseudo Aggressive Defenses in the Male.*

Psychic level	*Passive wish to be penetrated*	*Pseudo-aggressive autarchic defense*
Oral	Fantasy of being pierced by breast (bottle)	Grasping breast (bottle), crying, spitting, vomiting
Anal	Fantasy of being passively pierced by feces, shifted to paternal penis	Fantasy of aggressive and autarchic use of feces
Phallic	Feminine identification (negative Oedipus)	Masculine identification (positive Oedipus)

If we ask: is neurosis the result of undigested libidinous OR *aggressive tendencies, the answer is simple:* OF BOTH. Only the interconnection of both explains the complicated mechanism.

It is senseless to ask whether libido or aggression are "more importand." Both are constantly interwoven, both are constantly used as defense against reproaches of conscience. The real problem is not to find a priority scale between two partners of *equal* importance, but to follow their complicated interconnections in the specific case.

The psychic development of the girl—a much neglected chapter—acquires some additional clarification by applying ideas expressed in the "Breast Complex." The girl is incapable of using fully the compensatory fantasy: penis = breast. She tries, though, the "solution," hence the clitoris is considered by the girl *her* penis. The full impact of "being castrated," in the phallic phase, has an oral substructure. That inability of overcoming the trauma of weaning with penis-fantasies, pushes the girl finally into acceptance of femininity and passivity—at least, in matters sexual. The social penalities for passivity as in the case of the man do not exist for her, quite the contrary. In the end, the child she bears is, as Freud proved, the last and full compensation for lack of the penis.

A wit once asked what would happen if the girl would develop breasts before puberty. Well, she does not and that settles the question. The girl's breasts develop too late to compensate.

One can adduce an additional argument for the amazingly high percentage of *vaginal* frigidity among woman (80–90%),[20] an argument based on the incessant fight between activity and passivity. In puberty, as Freud proved, a "push of passivity" shifts the active cathexis of the clitoris to the passive cathexis of the vagina. If this does not occur, vaginal frigidity results. If the balance sheet is overdrawn, i.e., fear of masochism is too extensive, every passivity—even a normal one—is identified (unconsciously, of course) with masochism—hence avoided. The contents of these masochistic fears is not just "self-damage" and corresponding fear. This fear of "damage" is drawn from the arsenal of the "septet of baby fears."

[20] See the monograph (in collaboration with E. Hitschmann) "Frigidity in Women" Nervous & Mental Disease Monographs, 1936.

3

The Nine-Point Basis of Every Neurosis

EVERY neurosis, in my opinion, rests on the following basis:

(1) The conflict is unconscious and repetitive.

(2) The end-result of the infantile conflict in neurosis is always oral-masochistic.

(3) Every neurosis represents a rescue-attempt from the oral danger.

(4) Every neurotic symptom has a three-layer structure: only the defense against the repressed wish becomes visible.

(5) Every neurotic aggression is but pseudo aggression.

(6) The differentiation between "leading" and "misleading" unconscious identification gives the clue to the resultant neurotic personality.

(7) In every neurosis fear is predominant.

(8) Every neurosis is regulated by the mechanism of acceptance of inner guilt for the "lesser crime."

(9) Neurosis is a progressive and not self-limiting disease.

(1) *The neurotic conflict is unconscious and repetitive.*

These Freudian axioms are nowadays seldom questioned even outside of psychoanalytic circles. They contain in a nutshell Freud's basic contribution to psychopathology. Freud changed the nebulous philosophical term "unconscious" into a *clinically* provable, *dynamically* effective and *therapeutically* accessible fact.

Not less epoch-making has been Freud's discovery that neurotics are unconsciously repetition machines. Patterns acquired and undigested in early childhood, are repeated in later life on innocent bystanders. This "*transference*"-addiction is a characteristic of neurotics; small wonder that they do that same thing in analysis, too. The latter fact is of prime importance in therapy—provided the emotional repetition is correctly explained.

(2) *The end-result of the infantile conflict in neurosis is always oral-masochistic.*

I have believed for many years that the most dangerous pitfall in psychoanalysis is the *confusion between unconscious wish and unconscious defense.* The underlying fallacy can be reduced to the belief that unconscious wishes come to the surface in direct form. Many an analysis fails on exactly that point.

Here is an example showing the importance of being able to make this differentiation.

A young man consulted a physician, stating that after seeing a movie he became impotent with his wife. The situation persisted for months, his depression and despondency were marked. The movie was entitled "The Human Beast," a dramatization of Emile Zola's novel. In it the hero shrinks from having intercourse because he fears that in his sexual frenzy he might strangle the girl. This attitude is erroneously attributed by Zola to "hereditary alcoholism." The young man could not forget that central scene, applied the situation to himself and feared that he too would commit such a crime. He became completely impotent, and felt close to a "nervous breakdown." The physician who was interested in analysis, sent the patient to me, stating: "The man identifies himself with the murderer; his guilt makes him impotent." I questioned that assumption immediately, because, if this had been his real conflict, the patient would not have become aware of it. I suspected that behind the facade of aggression, deep passivity was hidden. Analysis of the patient confirmed that suspicion; the symptom was removed after some time on the basis of that interpretation, given through the transference repetition. It is obvious that an interpretation of his "aggression," taken at face value, would never have induced any change in the patient. It would merely have strengthened his neurotic defense-mechanism and not destroyed it.

I see now that the pitfall of confusing wish and defense, is *matched by an even greater danger: overlooking the differentiation between historic-genetic development and the clinical picture.*

Genetically speaking, we are confronted with a three-layer structure:

(1) Infantile libidinous wishes, frustration, offence against megalomania, resultant fury.

(2) Stabilization, called "end-result of the infantile conflict."

(3) Exchangeable defenses against the "end-result of the infantile conflict."

The "end-result of the infantile conflict" in neurotic cases is in my opinion always and without exception—masochistic stabilization on the rejection level. It preserves, as it were, the solution of an undigested *aggressive* conflict, aroused by refusal of libidinous wishes of different caliber. One should never lose sight of the fact that the child lives on the basis of megalomania. Hence every "refusal," be it real or fantasied, unavoidable or not, is counteracted by aggression. *The further handling of that helpless aggression determines the future of the individual.*

Now, there is only one inner defense against an "aggressive" conflict: using the opposite, namely libido. That is exactly what happens in neurosis. Libidinous wishes seem to predominate. I use the word "seem" purposely, because these libidinous wishes—*though historically they begin the conflict*—are later, in the *clinical picture, used as a defense.*[1]

In other words, the unconscious ego admits to a punishable crime, but to a lesser one. Pleadingly, it says to the superego: "Punish me, I am guilty. But I am guilty of a different crime than that you accuse me of."

That "*mechanism of admission of the lesser crime*" is of paramount importance in understanding of neurotic actions and reactions. Reduced to absurdity, the neurotic formula reads: "I could not have killed the girl in Brooklyn you accuse me of, since exactly at that time I was stealing a watch in Manhattan." *Clinically, we can state that the "great crime" of every neurotic is his masochistic solution of the undigested aggressive conflict. The lesser crime he unconsciously admits to is—libidinous wishes.*

That formulation is, of course, not complete without mentioning the fact that inner defenses end only with the death of the neurotic: *secondarily*, the libidinous wishes are contradicted too, with the result that pseudo-aggression is used once more as defense.

The question now arises as to why exactly masochistic wishes are so high on the priority list of the punishing conscience. The explanation is very likely connected with the fact that psychic masochism includes teasing and reducing to absurdity of the punishing conscience. Nothing enrages a sadistic dictator more than when his enemies get

[1] The silly question "What is more important—libido or aggression," is easily answered: both are 50 per cent partners!

pleasure out of intended punishment. And that is what happens to the superego when the unconscious ego "enjoys" punishment meted out by the superego. The psychic-masochistic solution corresponds to an outwitting of the superego. The inmate of a concentration camp ironizes and outwits the jailer.

On the other hand, one could ask why the jailer is so easily taken in by this indirect slave revolt under hypocritical disguise. The reason is that the superego basically wants to torture the ego. And the masochistic ego tortures itself to a high degree. That appeases the inner conscience which is perhaps even fooled for a long time. The same holds true for seizing upon substitute-crimes which the unconscious ego presents as punishable material. The pleasure of torturing blinds the jailer.

To repeat, there exists an amazing degree of confusion surrounding the problem of psychic masochism. The fact remains that many colleagues are surprised when confronted with the bland statement that psychic masochism goes back to a conflict connected with aggression. Somehow they consider psychic masochism a libidinous problem. This it is, but only in the end effect. The sequence of unconscious events is: *aggression, guilt, libidinization of guilt.* That *triad* is unchangeable in its repertoire; there is no other way in which psychic masochism is formed.

Psychic masochism is further confused either with inner guilt or punishment. Were psychic masochism and inner guilt identical, we could cure practically every neurotic—an ideal state of affairs which, as we all know, does not exist. We have only to resolve the inner guilt—a task easily performed. Only afterwards are we confronted with the morass of the pleasure of suffering. It is exactly that admixture which makes the greatest obstacle to cure.

The decisive element in psychic masochism is the tendency to outwit the punishing superego. The latter imposes punishment for the purpose of torture. The unconscious ego performs the most amazing act known in psychopathology: it makes pleasure out of it.

We have furthermore to admit that the dichotomy between children giving up their pre-oedipal and oedipal wishes and aggressions and those who do not is by no means clarified. We can play around with words like "strong" and "weak" ego; there is freedom of phrases guaranteed in science. Words *per se* are meaningless; the simple fact remains that *the X making a specific person a psychic masochist is unclarified*, although the steps leading technically to masochization are already understood and therapeutically accessible.

Judging from the amount of confusion surrounding the problem of psychic masochism, one cannot repeat frequently enough the steps in its genesis. It starts with the fact that every child's megalomania is offended by refusal of libidinous wishes. The result is fury and *anger* in the child. That anger and hatred is directed against people with a halo: mother, later father. Not only is that aggression inhibited because of the motoric helplessness of the child, but the weak attemps to express it, are curbed, prohibited, punished, first externally, later internally by the inner conscience. Heavy moral retribution sets in as is visible in education: aggressions directed against people with a halo are punished also with implanted guilt: "How can you do that to your mother (father) who sacrifices herself for you?" After some time every aggression directed against the bearer of the halo associates itself with the feeling of guilt, It is exactly that triad of punishment, moral reproof, and guilt, which drives the normal child out of the untenable position: the penalty is too heavy ("it does not pay"), hence aggressions against the halo-group is given up, shifted and modified, now directed against less holy people. The opposite happens with candidates for psychic masochism: the aggression is maintained *despite* punishment and guilt. Practiced for any length of time the situation becomes untenable, simply because every human being, including psychic masochists, lives on the basis of the pleasure-principle. *The only pleasure one can derive from displeasure is—to make a pleasure out of displeasure.* That is exactly what the psychic masochist does *unconsciously:* by sugarcoating the painful situation with a libidinized layer of pleasure, he gets some kind of satisfaction.

The classical *clinical picture* of psychic masochism is the "*mechanism of orality*". That mechanism consists of the following triad:

(1) "I shall repeat the masochistic wish of being deprived by my mother, by creating or misusing situations in which some substitute of my mother-image shall refuse my wishes."

(2) "I shall not be conscious of my wish to be refused and denied,

nor of my initial provocation of refusal. I shall see only that I am justified in righteous indignation to fight in self-defense the meanness of my self-created adversary."

(3) "Afterwards I shall pity myself because such an injustice can happen only to poor little me, and enjoy once more psychic masochistic pleasure."

This mechanism is constantly misunderstood in our literature. It contains in a nutshell the "end-result of the infantile conflict" stemming from the "*genetic* picture" and the following defensive "*clinical* picture."

The strangest thing is that the oral-libidinous wish to get, and its alleged frustration, started the conflict, and was originally real enough, with no strings attached. After establishing the "end-result," however, the identical wish to get is used intrapsychically as—defense. Hence the main confusion: the majority of my colleagues believe that an orally regressed person is "greedy" and grasping. The tragedy is that if one explains to an oral neurotic his "*wish to get*," he accepts it readily. But if his "*wish to be refused*" is stressed, he objects violently. The analyst who misunderstands the masochistic substructure of oral cases, in his ignorance strengthens the patient's neurosis!

The same holds true of the oral neurotic's "aggression." *Everybody lives intrapsychically on the basis of his pet defense mechanism.* And that pet defense in oral cases happens to be pseudo-aggression, mobilized to deny the wish to be masochistically refused. This is visible in premature ejaculation and psychogenic aspermia: the two main types of potency disturbances on the oral level. In both, milk (sperm) is refused: the milk is spilled before it can reach the mouth (in the oral identification of penis-breast, vagina-mouth, sperm-milk), or the milk is refused altogether.[2]

If one interprets to the man with premature ejaculation or aspermia, only the aggressive refusal, one confuses the wish with the defense, hence plays the strengthener of the patient's defense, instead of destroying it. Therapeutic failures are the result.

Every aggression in neurotic cases is but pseudo-aggression, covering the deeper repressed masochistic "end-result of the infantile conflict."

[2] See Chapter VI, *2* and *3*.

And the latter is without exception—stabilization on the masochistic rejection level.

It is—historically—easy to understand why and how the confusion about the inter-connection of libidinous and aggressive tendencies started. Freud discovered the repressed libidinous wishes first, the aggressive ones, however, much later. You cannot prescribe to a genius the sequence of his discoveries. Freud himself stressed the interconnection of both tendencies in later years, as his Eros-Thanatos-theory proves. Many analysts had difficulties in adapting themselves to that duality. To quote from a previous paper:

> "If a boy plays with his penis, he not only satisfies his libidinous wishes but also transgresses an educational rule not to touch his penis. He is therefore also aggressive. We simply must learn to think in terms of libido-destrudo."[3]

The simple fact is that the majority of analysts have not yet learned to think in these terms.

Another difficulty in adapting oneself to these newer conceptions, is also historically explainable. Freud discovered first the Oedipus complex. In other words, he started his epoch-shaking discoveries from the superficial and historically latest levels of the unconscious, only to progress later to deeper ones, for instance, the anal. The deepest regression, the oral, was little stressed. That inverse geology confuses many colleagues; they have difficulty in thinking in the reverse order. The bare fact of the sequence: oral-anal-phallic, is theoretically acknowledged; but in actual practice they think in the order of their discovery.

Every attempt at genetic development must, however, go the opposite way: from the deepest to the highest levels. Hence the confusion.

Biologic facts force the child to invest libidinous-aggressive tendencies—after the great oral experience—in other organs as well. Schematized: urethra, anus, phallus, eye. *The oral experience remains—and that is decisive—paradigmatic for the child. In other words, oral experiences are expressed in subsequent depositions in an urethral, anal, phallic, scopophiliac "language."*

[3] "On a Five-Layer Structure in Sublimation." The Psychoanalytic Quarterly *14*:91, 1945.

Once more, that thought is difficult to assimilate, if one thinks in different disease entities, without asking the question how they are interconnected. If one does so, one has pigeonholed hysteria, obsessional neurosis, hypochondria, agoraphobia, and so on, without any connecting links. Confusion is the inevitable result.

There are colleagues who find theoretical considerations "boring" and rather superfluous. Unfortunately, clinical practice depends on theoretical knowledge. If one confuses, for instance, an orally regressed case with a phallic one, lack of theoretical knowledge leads to therapeutic failures.

A malicious colleague years ago uttered the dictum that it is unfair to demand of every analyst an interest in theory: do we ask that every operator of an electrically propelled train be also a member of a society for experimental physics? The fallacy of the comparison lies in the subject-matter: you can teach the driver a few empirical rules, the "mechanized" analyst, however, is out of necessity a poor therapist.

(3) *Every neurosis represents a rescue-attempt from the oral danger.* Little is to be added to the deduction of Section II.

(4) *Every neurotic symptom has a three-layer structure.*

The original analytic formulation of neurotic symptoms and signs assumed a *two-layer structure:* compromise between repressed wish and repressed inhibition. The "substitute gratification" thus achieved, was considered the masterpiece of the neurosis.

Later experiences proved to me that the neurotic masterpiece is even more complicated. To make a long story short: *an unconscious wish never appears in consciousness directly, only the unconscious defense against the repressed wish is visible.* Hence a *three-layer structure* in every neurotic sympton and sign is discernable: wish—inhibition—defense against the inhibition. Only the third layer appears as neurotic symptom and sign.

What is the advantage of piling layer over layer in explanations, producing a skyscraper structure? No, personal architectonic predilections are not involved; rather clinical observations are being translated and expressed. Confronted, e.g., with a case of street fear (agoraphobia) in which exhibitionistic repressed wishes are predominent, the old *two-layer* structure explains: repressed wish: *exhibitionism;* inner prohibition: veto; result: street fear, combining both elements. Every time the patient thinks of going out, he exhibits unconsciously, appeasing his inner conscience with suffering.

The *three-layer* explanation is: repressed wish: *voyeurism;* inner prohibition: veto; result: the unconscious ego is forced to produce a defense, that defense consists of changing voyeurism into the opposite, in exhibitionism. The exhibitionistic defense—not wish—is the basis of the symptom.[4]

The advantage for the unconscious ego seems to consist in *forcing the whole "battle of the conscience" to be fought on a spurious front—"mechanism of admission of the lesser crime."*

How did the discovery of the three-layer structure occur? In investigating cases of depersonalization,[5] I found—in collaboration with L. Eidelberg—that these neurotics are warding off an *anal-exhibitionistic wish.* To counteract the veto of the superego, the exhibitionistic wish was changed into *voyeurism.* That, too, is vetoed by conscience and the *pleasure* of peeping is changed into the *punitive* variety; these neurotics are constantly *observing* their symptoms—mournfully and painfully.

At that time, I believed that the three-layer structure has some special connection with the scopophiliac tendency involved. The suspicion was bolstered by the fact that I found in pathologic blushing (erythrophobia)—also a scopophiliac disease—a three-layer structure, too. (See Chapter VI, Section 6)

Only later did I become convinced that the *three-layer structure in neurotic symptoms is an universal neurotic manifestation.* What convinced me were cases of obsessional neuroses.[6]

Every analyst is familiar with Freud's frequently cited statement in "Inhibition, Symptom and Anxiety" that the problem of the obsessional neurosis remains unsurmounted. Most of us in reading this sentence must have felt that this is not so, and that the creator of psychoanalysis, who wrote it, himself made the greatest contribution to the under-

[4] Secondary identifications occur, of course. Every voyeur also identifies with the exhibitionist, and vice versa (Freud). The decisive point is the analytic emphasis on wish or defense. "This also occurs . . ." does not suffice in the interpretation.

[5] "The Mechanism of Depersonalization." Int. Ztschr. f. Psa. 1935.

[6] First published in "Two Forms of Aggression in Obsessional Neurosis." The Psa. Rev., *29*:188–196, 1942.

standing of this mysterious ailment. Whoever has read Freud's work on the obsessional neurosis, must recognize with awe and admiration that with his "shot in the dark" Freud hit the mark very successfully in precisely this field.

I assume that this very recognition has cramped many of Freud's followers. It is remarkable how little analysts—with exception of Jones and Abraham—have added to knowledge of the obsessional neurosis since Freud's basic discoveries. A further reason, among others, is probably the complexity of the phenomenon.

If an analyst who has had the necessary experience with obsessional neurotics is asked whether they are "aggressive," he will say "yes," and at the same time emphatically confirm the unconscious tendency of these patients to harm themselves. The usual analytic explanation of the connection between these two unconsciously determined tendencies is that these injuries, or constant unconscious guilt feelings, are a reaction against abundant aggression. Regarded genetically, the aggression is turned against the ego under pressure of castration fears, or of the stern superego.

All this is part of the fundamental knowledge of the obsessional neurosis laid down by Freud, Jones and Abraham, which has been tested and substantiated analytically a thousand times. I believe, however, that it is necessary to distinguish between *two forms of aggression to be found in obsessional neurotics:* between the *original,* which can only be understood genetically, and one nearer the surface, but also unconscious, which is used as a *defense mechanism.*

I shall select a clinical example to demonstrate this thesis. An obsessional neurotic whose unconscious passivity to his father had been pointed out in the transference and in his general behavior, came laughing one day into my office. When he was asked what made him so gay, he pointed to a vase of flowers in the room, saying, "Please look at the color of the water in that glass vase. It is all yellow. Your maid can't have very much respect for you, if she dares to treat you like *that.*" The usual interpretation would be that the patient has identified himself with the aggressive servant, and enjoys her suppossed aggression against the analyst (father). Laughter results, because the psychic energy which has been expended in holding down aggression has now become superfluous: it is not himself, but the servant who is aggressive. In short the patient behaves as if the aggressive action of the maid were a joke to which he can listen with enjoyment, free of guilt feelings. According to this interpretation, then, the patient is aggressive; [7] and the aggression seems to be tapped from the apparently inexhaustible reservoir of obsessional neurotic aggressiveness.

I believe that this interpretation should at least be amplified. It seems to me that at bottom the patient identifies himself, *not at all with the aggressive servant*, but with the servant *deserving punishment*. The patient believes that the analyst will be angered by the oversight and negligence of the girl, and will "blow her up." It is with this girl, who is to be scolded and humiliated, that the patient has identified himself.[8]

In my opinion, both interpretations are correct, but at *different* levels. It may be said that the *passive anal wish* of the patient appears in the deeper identification with the abused servant, and is *warded off by means of aggression*, which leads to a more superficial identification with the supposedly aggressive girl.

How shall we construct this process? I believe that male obsessional neurotics, after their symptoms and anomalies of character have been established, labor under a continuous unconscious reproach of conscience regarding their passivity. This passivity is *secondarily* warded off by the unconscious ego in such a way as to prove: I am not passive; on the contrary, I am extremely aggressive. Thirdly, this defensive aggressiveness is also warded off. We know from our everyday analytic experience how long it takes to show our obsessional neurotic patients their repressed aggressiveness. We can accordingly establish a *three story structure*, from which emerges a *conclusion which is of prime therapeutic importance. If in our analyses of obsessional neurotic*

[7] One might perhaps add that mixed with the aggressiveness of the patient is the expectation of punishment: he believes the analyst will be angry at him, and will "pay him back"—the obsessional neurotic vicious circle of unconscious aggression and unconscious self-punishment.

[8] For the sake of argument, I have simplified the facts. It is clear that in this example not only these two identifications are present, but a whole bundle of identifications seen in one cross-section. Thus, for example, the patient identifies himself with the "aggressive" employer who scolds the girl. Further, he identifies himself with the "kind, forgiving" employer, who shows by means of a sort of "magic gesture," how the patient himself would like to be treated. The patient furthermore identifies himself with the employer because the latter has been offered anal pleasure in a sort of symbolic representation ("yellow water"), and anal pleasure contributes much to the satisfaction of the patient, etc.

patients we constantly point out only their aggressiveness, we indirectly give support (without wishing or meaning to) *to their defense mechanism, instead of destroying it.* What we should interpret to them with the greatest emphasis, is their unconscious passivity, and the secondary use of aggression as a defense mechanism.

"According to this," you will comment ironically, "obsessional neurotics are not 'really' aggressive!" Of course they are. The very fact that they make use of aggression as a defense mechanism, that this fund of aggression is readily at their disposal, proves its presence in these patients.

The conception outlined above is at variance neither with Freud's conception of the obsessional neurosis, nor with the experience of other analysts. We have learned from Freud that the conflict of obsessional neurotics lies in the pathological elaboration of their aggression and anality in relation to their father. When I said above that male obsessional neurotics suffered under continuous unconscious pressure of conscience regarding their passivity *after* the formation of their symptoms and character anomalies, the emphasis falls on the word *after*. Otherwise expressed, before the sickness develops, the wild, uncontrolled aggressiveness of these children is outstanding. Consider Freud's patient so often referred to, whose father, dumbfounded by his fits of rage and hate, remarked that the child would grow up into either a great man or a criminal. Freud adds ironically that the man forgot the third possibility—neurosis.

Nor does the stressing of aggression as a defense mechanism in obsessional neurotics contradict the experience of other colleagues. Every one of us has occasionally shown our obessional neurotic patients perhaps in other words, that their exaggerated aggressiveness conceals the very opposite attitude. I only claim to have presented a point of view more sharply, and to have advanced its theoretic and practical application.

This *pseudo-aggressiveness*, as I would designate the use of aggressiveness as a defense against the inner passivity of these patients, also leads to a better understanding of the curious phenomenon of "narcissistic gratification" in the obsessional neurosis. In an earlier work entitled "Notes on an Obsessional Neurosis *in ultimis;* four mechanisms of narcissistic gratification in the obsessional neurosis," I described four mechanisms [9] in connection with an "obsessional

[9] See pp. 94–99.

delirium" that persisted increasingly and varyingly through half a century.

1. *Mechanism of the inner contradiction of all "compulsive rules."*
2. *The mechanism of direct disparagement of the superego.*
3. *The mechanism of relative crudity in the compulsion.*
4. *The mechanism of "guided miracles."*

The tendencies of the four mechanisms of "narcissistic gratification" with its accompanying pleasurable aggression outlined here are not, as I now see, to be regarded separately. The obsessional "narcissistic gratification" should be included with the chronic *truly frantic attempts of these patients to utilize aggression as a means of defense against anal-passive surrender.* The apparently unappeasible longing for ever new aggressions is explained only in part by the natural aggressive endowment of these people. It is probably also a constant denial of passivity.

When we consider obsessional aggressiveness from this point of view, we understand why *pseudo-hate* and *pseudo-aggression* appear on the surface, precisely where the opposite, a strong passive tendency, has been repressed, and is trying to force its way through. An obsessional patient fell into inexplicable fits of rage against his brother, for whom he had a passive-feminine attachment. It was possible to prove that these rages were a defense against his passivity, in the sense of disproving it in the manner I have described. His dreams were an indication. Whenever he dreamed passive-feminine dreams at night, he would be particularly aggressive toward his brother in the morning. A similar process naturally took place in the transference.

From these representations but one conclusion can be drawn for the therapist. If we show these patients only their aggressiveness, they at first object angrily, but soon accept the interpretation, and *actually look flattered and smile* when we draw their attention to a *new aggression.* When, however, we show them the *passivity behind the mask of aggressiveness,* the picture is quite a different one. The patient becomes angry and depressed, or represses the interpretation to an astonishing extent. The whole battle then centers around the exposing of this pseudo-aggressiveness.

In a series of cases that have been passed on to me by colleagues, I have found that these apparently "hopeless" and "incurable" cases of obsessional neurosis had gone up a blind alley for this reason. The analyst had always shown the patient his inner aggressiveness and accompanying guilt feelings, and traced both back to the infantile situation. After extensive working through of this material, the result was the cynical acknowledgment of the patient: "So I'm an aggressive pig and ought to be destroyed." Thus the technical error lay in mistaking a defensive for a primary aggressiveness.

From this emerges a general technical rule: *when obsessional neurotics show aggression, we must always find out against what oral-anal-passive wish they are trying to defend themselves by means of aggression.*

I am far from maintaining that with this knowledge the obsessional neurosis becomes 100 per cent curable. This is out of the question. We all know cases which break down every therapy because of the *quantitative* factor. But in cases where the neurosis has not yet consumed the patient, hair and hide, where a relatively intact sector of the ego is available for analytic co-operation, the prognosis for the obsessional neurosis is by no means as discouraging as is generally supposed.

What happens if we explain neurotic symptoms and signs to the patient on a two-layer basis? We are bolstering—without knowing, or wanting to—the patient's inner defenses, instead of destroying those. We—involuntarily—strengthen his neurotic defenses.

I believe that the history of great psychological discoveries is along the lines of inner defense mechanisms. I pointed out in my study of Stendhal [10] who presented in his autobiography two generations before Freud, a correct description of his individual Oedipus complex, that he could become aware of the latter, only in order to cover up defensively (and, of course, unconsciously) his deeper regression. Moreover, I stated in *The Battle of Conscience* that the enigma as to how Sophocles could have consciously expressed the universality of the Oedipus situation, is only solvable when we consider that the ancient Greek culture of the intelligentsia in Sophocles' times was a homosexual one. Since homosexuality is an oral neurosis,[11] one could imagine that as inner defense the Oedipus situation could become conscious.

5. *Every neurotic aggression is but pseudo-aggression.*

I am of the opinion that normal aggression *never* enters the neu-

[10] "Talleyrand-Napoleon-Stendhal-Grabbe." Int. Psa. Verlag, Vienna, 1935.

[11] See Chapter VI, *12.*

rotically diseased part of the personality.[12] I have seen numerous analyses fail due to exactly this analytic oversight: the *pseudo-aggression of the patient was considered real aggression.* Instead of interpreting that the neurotic aggression covered but deeper repressed psychic masochism, the aggression was taken at face value and the guilt pertaining to repressed masochism, secondarily unconsciously shifted to defensive aggression, was connected with the aggression. That "little mistake" kills an analysis.

The differentiation between "normal" and neurotic aggression is of paramount importance.[13]

Psychiatric-psychoanalytic experience proves that there is but a quantitative distinction between a normal and a neurotic person. For practical purposes we have to draw a dividing line; theoretically, people of both types struggle with the same inner problems. Their solutions are different; their unconscious technics preceding the unraveling of the Gordian knot are also different. Basically, normal men and women are not the opposites of neurotic ones; they are all "brothers and sisters under the skin," to use Kipling's phrase in another sense. In other words, a "not too neurotic person" can be *euphemistically* called normal. Everyone has neurotic tendencies, but not in everyone are they increased to such a degree that a neurosis results. It is a problem of quantity, not quality, though there is a point where "quantity changes into quality" (Hegel).

The decisive difference between a normal and a neurotic person is that the former has overcome to a greater degree his infantile conflicts and is capable of having a relatively more objective outlook on reality, whereas the latter misuses reality for the unconscious repetition of his infantile conflicts.

Every neurotic can be compared to a person carrying around constantly one phonograph record and continually on the lookout for a phonograph on which to play his only tune. In this simile the one and only record represents the basic unconscious neurotic tendency; the phonograph stands for the other person with whom the neurotic pattern can be repeated. Expressed differently, Freudian psychoanalysis has

[12] That some parts of the personality of neurotics react normally is not excluded. I am referring exclusively to the neurotic sector.

[13] First established in "Differential Diagnosis Between 'Normal' and 'Neurotic' Aggression." Quarterly Review of Psychiatry and Neurology, I. *1*: 1946.

proved in fifty years of clinical experience that certain unconscious behavior patterns acquired in early childhood become petrified, and under the pressure of the "unconscious repetition" (Freud) are repeated throughout the remainder of life with eternal monotony—and completely without conscious awareness of that repetition. Thus, the unconscious "repetition machine" reels off the unconscious behavior pattern.

Neurotic people are constantly in conflict with their environment. They are fighting their unconscious battles on two fronts: inside, as visible in their symptoms, signs, and personality difficulties, and outside in their quarrels, obstinacy, provocativeness. Hence the necessity arises to use a yardstick for distinguishing whether specific conflicts with the outer world are normal or neurotic. The differentiation is even more necessary, since a "normal" person can have, in a specific instance, a "neurotic" conflict, and a neurotic person a "normal" conflict.

The following tabulation makes a quick distinction possible:

Normal Aggression	*Neurotic Aggression ("Pseudo-Aggression")*
1. Used only in self-defense.	1. Used indiscriminately when an infantile pattern is repeated with an innocent bystander.
2. Object of aggression is a "real" enemy.	2. Object of aggression is a "fantasied" or artificially created enemy.
3. No accompanying unconscious feeling of guilt.	3. Feeling of guilt always present.
4. Dosis: Amount of aggression discharged corresponds to provocation.	4. Dosis: Slightest provocation—greatest aggression.
5. Aggression always used to harm enemy.	5. Pseudo-aggression often used to provoke "masochistic pleasure" expected from enemy's retaliation.
6. Timing: Ability to wait until enemy is vulnerable.	6. Timing: Inability to wait, since pseudo-aggression used as defense mechanism against inner reproach of psychic masochism.
7. Not easily provoked.	7. Easily provoked.
8. Element of infantile game absent; no combination with masochistic-sadistic tendencies; feeling that a necessary though disagreeable job has to be performed.	8. Element of infantile game present, combined with masochistic-sadistic excitement, usually repressed.
9. Success expected.	9. Defeat unconsciously expected.

I shall discuss now the specific points on the basis of a clinical example:

A patient of mine, a physician, called me one evening to inform me that his friend Dr. X, also a physician, wanted him to arrange an appointment for him to consult me because of his "personality difficulties," the nature of which was not specified in the telephone conversation. The appointment was made for the next day. At the appointed time the prospective patient appeared, and after introductions, started to shout in the waiting room: "I haven't the slightest confidence in you." I answered smilingly, "Well, this will be a short visit. Do you want to leave now?" The patient smiled, too: "No, let's have a talk." An observer would have classified the man's behavior as both irrational and aggressive: irrational because no one forced him to consult me without a minimum of confidence; aggressive because, being a physician himself, he was very sensitive to the upbraidings which physicians receive from patients. Asked why he had no confidence in me, he replied that the preceding evening he had had a theoretical discussion with the physician who recommended him to me, in which they could not agree on a specific type of anesthesia. "Well, if an analyzed man talks such nonsense, his analysis can't have been a good one—though I'll admit that my friend has changed for the better in other respects." The senselessness of his argument was augmented when I asked him: "Was your little speech prepared?" The man admitted that it was; in other words, his resistance was impersonal and rather unfair, because he didn't give me even a chance. "What would you have done to a patient who entered your office shouting in such a manner?" I asked. "I'd throw him out," was the prompt reply. "That was exactly what you wanted," was my conclusion. In other words, the man used pseudo-aggression to achieve masochistic pleasure. The naïve observer would diagnose his behavior as aggression, the analyst, as psychic masochism covered by pseudo-aggression. The whole life of this patient was based on that technic.

We see in this example all of the nine points enumerated in the Table:

1. *Self-defense or pre-fabricated pattern?* No self-defense was involved for the patient since the simplest way of defending his precious neurosis was to call off the appointment. His later analysis proved that he acquired the pattern of provoking conflicts in early childhood and

repeated it later like a parrot. His technic was always the same: First he unconsciously provoked a conflict. Not being conscious that he himself provoked the conflict, he saw only the aggressive reaction of the person attacked, who, of course, fought back. With righteous indignation the patient fought back on his side, seemingly in self-defense. As the final act, he pitied himself, reflecting, "Such a thing can happen only to me." In this final self-pity he was, of course, unaware that he was enjoying the "psychic masochistic pleasure" of being mistreated.

2. *Real or self-created enemy?* In our example there was no real enemy involved, since the man wanted help from a physician, and by no stretch of the imagination could the helping physician be construed as an enemy. Therefore the man merely used a harmless outsider for his unconscious repetition-repertoire.

3. *Presence or absence of feeling of guilt?* Neurotic aggression is always accompanied by unconscious guilt. The reason for this is that the original persons against whom the libidinous and aggressive wishes in childhood were directed were mother and father. For the more normal person this attachment is practically resolved; therefore no guilt appears in "real" aggression, since the enemy is never identified with images from one's own childhood. Moreover, the normal person does not pick a fight *per se;* he defends himself when attacked thus having the best of inner alibis. The patient described, on the other hand, immediately identified me unconsciously with a person in his childhood, as he revealed in his admission that his speech was prepared; therefore, the attack was "impersonal." As a result he suffered feelings of guilt, visible in the quick collapse of his aggression when, not playing his neurotic game, I refused to let myself be provoked.

4. *Discrepancy between provocation and counter-aggression?* Normally one doesn't shoot sparrows with machine guns. Where a normal person teases or uses repartee, a neurotic one strikes. True, he strikes only to be struck back (and harder, for that matter).

5. *Harm the enemy or oneself?* The normal person, if he fights, wants one thing only: to victimize the aggressor. What he abhors most is pain, depression, guilt. For him that trio is painful and disagreeable. He has no unconscious strings attached to it: pain is pain. But for the neurotic, the situation is different. He craves "psychic masochistic pleasure." In other words, he makes pleasure out of pain. Without knowledge of this fantastic fact, neurosis is incomprehensible.

To give an example from the analysis of a perverted masochist: A patient's masturbation consisted of striking his penis forcefully on the edge of the table and the more painful the procedure was, the more pleasurable it was. He brushed aside the objection that to a normal person pain and pleasure were exclusive of each other, and considered the analyst's statement that his way of achieving sexual pleasure might be a punishment in a concentration camp, simply as the expression of "jealousy."

Imagine the same pleasure, consciously rejected but unconsciously approved, and we have a clue to the behavior of the physician of our example. He "hated" being mistreated, played the part of the "he man," but because of his unconscious provocation, was constantly "mistreated." In other words, he was a "psychic masochist" and not a "perverted masochist." Psychic masochism and perversion masochism are different entities.

6. *Waiting for the propitious moment possible or impossible?* There is a clear-cut distinction in the timing of aggressive actions. The normal person more often uses the right, the neurotic person the wrong, moment. The reason is that the normal person wants victory, the neurotic unconsciously wants defeat. The normal person strives after the current aim, the neurotic person after the current defense mechanism.[14] Therefore, to furnish his inner alibi, the neurotic cannot wait.

7. *Easy or difficult to provoke?* The normal person has a fair-sized narcissism which protects him from outside criticism; the neurotic is "touchy" to the nth degree. Since the normal person does not start fights for the sake of fighting, but fights only in self-defense, he is relatively difficult to provoke. On the contrary, neurotics see an offense even where a normal person does not. In our example the patient felt provoked because of a divergence of opinions on narcosis.

8. *Presence or absence of masochistic-sadistic excitement?* The normal person feels, in acting out his aggression in self-defense, that a necessary though disagreeable job has to be performed, nothing else. The situation is quite different for the neurotic person. He feels a queer excitement, often in the genital region. That feeling is often unclear to him—it is a combination of infantile masochistic and sadistic remnants. The element of infantile game is discernible, whereas

[14] See the writer's "On the Psychoanalysis of the Ability to Wait and of Impatience," Psa. Rev., *26*:11–32 Jan. 1939.

it is completely absent in such situations in normal people. To be sure, the feeling of neurotic-sexual excitement (pain, tension, shrinking of penis or erection, infrequently even involuntary ejaculation) is more or less repressed; the defense against masochistic tendencies with pseudo-aggression is often the only surface reverberation. A patient, for instance, related a newspaper report of rape by colonial soldiers in a captured city, as if it were some amusing game. His logic told him that his feeling was shameful, but it was there. Analysis could prove that he identified with the raped women and secondarily warded off his identification with queer pseudo-aggression in thoughts. The element of infantile game was very pronounced in this case. In the evening he felt a strong sexual urge and had intercourse twice with fantasies centering around the rape. Consciously he identified with the raping soldiers, unconsciously with the victims. This can serve as a typical example of the warding off of unconscious feminine-masochistic wishes with pseudo-aggression, intercourse being misused for that alibi.

9. *Success or defeat sought?* The normal person wants consciously and unconsciously victory if he is forced to fight. The neurotic person unconsciously seeks external defeat, which feeds his unconscious masochism though consciously he wants victory. His *real* victory is achievement of masochistic pleasure. These self-constructed defeats are brought about by using arguments which boomerang—for instance, the illogical behavior of the patient in our example.

Neurotics fight their battles only to lose them. The consequences are far-reaching if one takes into consideration their lack of success, which includes also inability to enjoy even transitory success. Those neurotics who are of the criminal variety make use of courts of justice to administer to them their required portion of masochism. The literature on that subject is too extensive to be reported here; it has been dealt with elsewhere.[15] In my opinion the criminal is the embodiment, not of aggression, but of exactly the opposite, passivity.

Knowledege of the differential diagnosis between normal and neurotic aggression is of decisive importance in the understanding of neurotic

[15] "Suppositions About the 'Mechanism of Criminosis,'" J. Crim. Psychopath., 5:215–246, Oct. 1943. See also "Psychopathology of Impostors." J. Crim. Psychopath., 5:695–714. April 1944.

actions. If one confuses in psychotherapy the superficial pseudo-aggression of a neurotic with real aggression, and interprets to the patient only his "hostility" and "bellicosity," one cannot achieve therapeutic success.

6. *Clue to the neurotic personality: differentiation between "leading" and "misleading" unconscious identifications.*

The great amount of misunderstandings rampant on the problem of unconscious identification, is reducible to a simplification which assumes that identifications are the reasons for human actions and reactions. The conflict preceding the identification is mostly overlooked.

Freud himself never intended to be misunderstood in this way. The best studied identification, described by him, is the identification of the boy with the oedipal father, laying the finishing touches to the formation of the superego. Freud pointed out that castration fear shatters the oedipal wishes; the boy introjects the image of the stern father into the superego and *avoids thus the danger of overwhelming drives*—corresponding to libidinous wishes toward the mother and aggressive wishes toward the father. Hence that type of identification is—*a defense.*

In other words, the situation preceding the identification is the decisive problem. The identification is but the result. Compare the complicated conflict with the simplifying headline: "Boy identifies with Father," and the difference is clear.

The next difficulty arises when one assumes—as I do—that an unconscious drive *never* comes to the surface in its original state. This excludes the theory of "Triebdurchbruch," that is, volcanic eruption of deepest unconscious drives in *direct* form. That idea was the result of the original assumptions about perversions: the latter were considered "negatives of neurosis." That means that the covering cloak which is used in neurosis, was assumed missing in perversions. That idea was later modified and restricted, partial repression and defense conceded. Finally, the conception became fully untenable after I proved in collaboration with Eidelberg, in 1933, in our paper "Breast Complex of the Male" that even in the perversion homosexuality such a volcanic eruption does not take place.

After long and circuitous clinical trials and tribulations I concluded that every neurotic symptom has a three-layer structure. Hence, the amount of "portable" unconscious identifications of every person must be greater than originally assumed. *The decisive point seems to be that identifications are performed for the purpose of acquiring a crutch in the fight against superego reproaches: the other fellow does the forbidden thing, too.*

Every identification presupposes an *inner readiness* for it. It is erroneous to conclude that certain actions are the result of certain identifications. Quite the contrary; genetically the *ground is fertile* for such an identification, and *therefore* the identification is accomplished. Often the person used for the identification serves simply *as a tool* to solve an inner conflict.

The employment of identification-tools increases the moment every changing defense is "covered up" with an introjected "sinner" as inner alibi.

Moreover, a very specific distinction must be made between "*leading*" and "*misleading*" *identifications.*

I stated previously that the "*end-result of the infantile conflict*" is in neurotic children without exception—stabilization on the *masochistic rejection level.* This represents *Defense I.*

Then follows a series of neurotic rescue actions: flight into higher developmental levels. The neurotic child either becomes fixated on one of these levels, or regresses to the starting point. In any case, a stabilization on the *second* auxiliary rescue level takes place. That leads to an unchangeable.[16] identification—"*leading*" *identification.* That is *Defense II.*

Because the superego objects against that defense, too, a *third* layer of varying denseness must be established, leading to exchangeable identifications—"*misleading*" *identifications.* That is *Defense III.*

Table 2[17] lists schematically the differences between the two types of identification.

If we ask ourselves what is different in this approach, we find that it is the revival and partial reformulation of the following facts:

1. An inner drive, whatever its contents, can never come to the psychic surface in its pure state. It is always modified by a covering

[16] That means: unexchangeable by the person himself. Only analysis can reverse the process.

[17] First published in "The 'Leading' and 'Misleading' Basic Identifications." The Psa. Rev., *32*:263–295, 1945.

defense mechanism. This excludes the old theory of "Triebdurchbruch," that is, volcanic eruption of deepest unconscious drives in *direct* form.

TABLE 2. *Two Types of Identification*

Type of identification:	*"Leading"*	*"Misleading"*
Time of establishment:	2–4 years of age.	Exchangeable throughout life.
Psychic level:	Established by unconscious ego as attempt at compromise between id and superego.	Established by unconscious ego under pressure of superego exclusively.
Status:	Unchangeable	Exchangeable as defense-mechanism wears out.
Genesis:	End result of infantile conflict.	Defense mechanism against end result of infantile conflict.
Sequence of events:	1. Solution of infantile conflict. 2. Adoption of identification as alibi.	1. Establishment of identification as end result of infantile conflict. 2. Adoption of exchangeable identifications to cover up first line of defense.

2. Identifications per se are not the reasons for human actions. Quite the contrary, they are adopted to serve the purpose of already-established neurotic or "normal" solutions of an inner conflict.

3. The terms "leading identification" and "misleading identification" are rather antiquated terminology, since they represent a compromise with the old form of thinking in our science, which assumed, on the basis of simplification, that identifications in themselves did explain something. There is no objection to this compromise in terminology, provided one bears in mind the actual genesis of identifications.

4. The problem often discussed in our literature, of whether or not new decisive identifications can take place in *adulthood* (the most outspoken proponent of this theory being P. Schilder, who stated: ". . . during the whole life identifications take place which basically never end"), is based on a slight misunderstanding. We are obviously dis-

cussing at cross purposes if we deny obvious facts and stick to misunderstanding of theory. The truth is that the *psychic* elasticity of the human being is exhausted after the age of five—as absurd as this may sound. On the other hand, it is also true that Schilder's observation is clinically correct. How can we reconcile both facts? Very simply, by differentiating between leading and misleading identifications. What Schilder described pertains only to the secondary defense mechanism, that is, the *misleading* identifications. The basic *leading* identifications, once established, become petrified and are unchangeable during the lifetime (except by psychoanalysis). But the inner defense mechanisms against them are time bound; time wears them out. Therefore *new types of defense and inner alibi must be furnished*, and they are via new identifications. These identifications are the new defenses used to cover the basic, old, leading identifications. To put it precisely: Only the secondary defense mechanisms change after the age of five.

5. The search for the "disjecta membra" of different identifications often occupies too great a place in clinical analysis. Not that finding out whom the patient "copies" unconsciously is not a legitimate part of analysis; but the decisive factor in understanding the psychic mosaic is *the reason leading to the specific partial identification and the differentiation between wish and defense.* The moment greater attention is placed on the hunt for the original image, we find that the patient co-operates too willingly once he understands what it is all about. In some kind of masochistic self-denunciation, he will even bring forward minute details proving whom he plagiarizes unconsciously in tone, posture, opinions, behavior, prejudices, etc. On the other hand, the moment the emphasis is placed on the genetic reasons for this identification, he offers very little cooperation, indeed, a distinct reluctance, in following this path. I once analyzed a patient who had previously spent one year being analyzed by a beginner. The other analyst had tried to solve the puzzle of the patient's complex personality by hunting down mechanically every trait copied from someone else; he made a mistake typical to beginners. He did not even discuss the dynamically-effective reasons for the patient's choice of such identifications. The patient, once he understood the difference in procedure in his second analysis, remarked ironically: "I see now; the psyche is more than a collection of plagiarisms and missing persons bureau."

6. The greatest danger in therapy is the possibility of confusing the original drive with the covering defense mechanism.[18] This confusion is responsible for numerous failures in therapy, since it does not break down the neurotic symptom but, on the contrary, bolsters the unconscious defense mechanism. In a typical process of displacement, such a therapist does not see his own shortcomings but accuses the patient of hopeless resistance.

(7) *In every neurosis fear is predominant.*

Neurotic anxiety is viewed analytically as an anticipatory action of the unconscious ego which "rings the bell" when inner tension surpasses the safety mark. This formulation is based on Freud's book "The Problem of Anxiety" and has been interpreted by R. Waelder [19] as follows:

> In our earlier theory we assumed that anxiety bursts forth from the id, as a direct result of the tension produced by overwhelming, unsatisfied cravings, and that the ego is helpless before its attack. Now, however, we have modified our views to this effect: we hold that in a situation of danger, i.e., when threatened with such tension, the ego may forestall it by experiencing anxiety. At the same time, this is the signal to the organism to get ready to deal with the danger. whether by taking flight or by preparing appropriate measures of defense, so that the signal serves a biological purpose. Naturally, in this work Freud did not intend the newer conception to cancel or supplant the older, nor did he mean that anxiety originates sometimes in the one way and sometimes in the other. Undoubtedly he meant only to indicate that, in actual life, the two theories—that of the irruption of anxiety into the ego and that of the fashioning of the anxiety-signal with a biological purpose, by the ego—represent two aspects of a real process, the phenomenon of anxiety being, as it were, described now from the standpoint of the id and now from that of the ego.

In the older theory—that of direct transformation of libidinous repressed tendencies into anxiety—the libidinous wish has always been considered the—malefactor. Much later, aggression was added as 50% partner in unconscious tendencies, hence aggression, too, was

[18] For a typical example, see the writer's "A New Approach to the Therapy of Erythrophobia," paper read at the XVth Internat. Psychoan. Convention, Paris, 1938. Published in Psa. Quart., Vol. XIII, No. 1, 1944.

[19] "Das Prinzip der mehrfachen Funktion", Internat. Zeitschrift für Psychoanalyse, 1930, XVI, p. 285.

considered as having identical power in the production of anxiety. We hear frequently of interpretations to the effect that the patient experiences deep anxiety because of his overdimensional repressed aggression. It seems that in this dualistic approach, libido and aggression—both repressed—are considered equals—as far as being potentially the cause of, and material for, developing anxiety.

Freud himself tried to solve the contradiction by suggesting in "Civilization and its Discontents" that every time a drive is repressed, "*the libidinous components change into symptoms, and the aggressive components into feeling of guilt.*"[20] This suggestion is forgotten—it is, as far as I can observe, practically ignored.

I submit the thesis that *every neurotic fear pertains exclusively to repressed psychic masochism* and shows a three-layer structure:

(1) *Stage of libidinized inner passivity* (psychic masochism) and narcissistic offense to infantile megalomania.

(2) *Stage of pseudo-aggressive defense* and narcissistic restitution, using: (a) change of contents: by accepting the punishment of the superego, but for the "lesser crime" (mirage of aggression), thus "sidetracking" the guilt and "restoring" by "activity" the lesion in narcissism; (b) change of locality: an inner fear is projected outwards.[21]

(3) *Stage of "hostages":* the superego, being interested exclusively in torturing the ego, accepts the pseudo-aggressive "hostage", especially since the ego increases *artificially* its guilt to "keep the inner tormentor occupied." The ego, having overdone its own defensive pseudo-aggressive efforts, gets "scared" of its own courage, and gives preventively the anxiety signal.

The suggested "triad of anxiety" presupposes that fear pertains to libidinized inner passivity, and is only secondarily shifted to an aggressive "crime" for which the blame is accepted. Hence fear seems to be attached secondarily to the inner defense and not to the real "crime." My supposition claims also that the amount of fear does *not* correspond to the amount of repressed wishes to be discharged. It is increased out of proportion—artificially—to hoodwink the inner conscience, and is attached to the defense. The whole "*battle of anxiety*" is fought on

[20] Ges. Schr. XII, p. 107.

[21] In phobic and paranoic cases; in hypochondria an organ is chosen as malefector.

a spurious front representing the ego's triumph which is *Pyrrhic victory.*

The statement "every neurotic fear pertains exclusively to repressed psychic masochism", requires for its understanding a precise distinction between the *genetic* and *clinical* picture.

To repeat: Genetically psychic masochism is misplaced and undigested aggression, and has a three-layer structure. Every offense against infantile megalomania—provoked by a libidinous frustration—results in mobilization of aggression in the child. That aggression is motorically helpless and counteracted by the "triad of retribution": punishment, moral reproach, later inner guilt. Under normal conditions, the process stops right here; the child finds out that it "does not pay" to be aggressive toward people with a halo (parents); hence aggression is shifted to less holy people, redirected, partly sublimated. Under neurotic conditions, the story reads differently: the aggression is perpetuated—despite the triad of retribution. Continued for any length of time, the situation becomes untenable: even the future candidate for psychic masochism lives on the basis of the pleasure principle. *And the only pleasure one can derive from displeasure is to make the displeasure a pleasure.* That is exactly what the psychic masochist does: by libidinizing the guilt and punishment he extracts pleasure from guilt and punishment.

At this point, the genetic picture is completed.

The *clinical picture* starts, where the genetic picture ends. Once established as *modus vivendi* of the unconscious ego, the psychic masochist has to fight his never ending "Battle of the Conscience." [22] One cannot do business with the corrupt neurotic superego without establishing inner defenses and paying the penalties of the "inner bribe" in form of depression, dissatisfaction, self-damage. The clinical picture—repeatedly described by me as "*mechanism of orality*"—comprises the following triad: *First,* the psychic masochist manoeuvres himself unconsciously into a self-damaging situation, either by unconscious provocation or by misuse of reality factors; he does not rest content till someone (the representative of the pre-oedipal mother) denies, refuses, inhibits his "wishes."

Second, not being aware that he himself provoked his pitiable situa-

[22] "The Battle of the Conscience," Washington Institute of Medicine, 1948.

tion behind the eight ball, he fights with great energy—seemingly in self-defense and with righteous indignation—against the other fellow's meanness, thus establishing the defense mechanism of "pseudo-aggression."

Third, he pities himself extensively and consciously as the innocent victim of human malice, and—at the same time—enjoys unconsciously in outwitting his inner conscience psychic masochistic pleasure.

The question arises: why does the superego tolerate this strange pleasure? The answer has something to do with the cruelty of that restricting and punishing department. The inner conscience has but one aim: to torture the victim. The psychic masochist does this extensively. Why should the cruel jailer overlook the pleasure derived? Imagine a Nazi jailer, observing with glee how a prisoner bangs his head against the wall. He will call him a model prisoner and feel that the prisoner's folly saves him the effort of torture. . . . The situation is similar with the superego: blinded by its lust for cruelty, it is for long times the dupe of the psychic masochist. Only much later—after many years—does the inner conscience catch on; then the real trouble starts. Nothing is more pitiful than an overaged psychic masochist: he increases his stakes, his defeats and depressions lengthen. Clinical experience proves that every neurosis increases as years pass by.

Where does anxiety enter this dismal picture?

Anxiety seems to me an auxiliary defense of the unconscious ego, used in situations in which

(a) a dramatic demonstration is required to convince the superego of "good intentions"; hence depression precedes anxiety. Only if the latter is insufficient as an alibi is anxiety produced.[23]

(b) the amount of narcissism (or the narcissistic "type" of the personality) makes it intolerable to endure the passive situation of being constantly reproached by the superego and pushed by masochistic-passive aims; hence *active* repetition of the *passive* situation is installed by admitting to an "aggressive" aim (application of Freud's unconscious repetition compulsion).

[23] There is only one exception to the observable fact that depression precedes anxiety: traumatic neurosis. Freud explained convincingly that anxiety has in these cases some kind of curative effect post facto, since ante facto the protective veneer of "*fear as cushion*" could not be applied.

(c) the defensive pseudo-aggression to which the unconscious ego admits as "lesser crime" surpasses the safety mark; the ego is caught between both horns of the dilemma: to produce defensive pseudo-aggression *and* to maintain the desired "low pressure." In such situations, the older mechanism of maintaining low tension seemingly wins out, and the nearly automatic signal of anxiety is given.[24]

Before going further into theory, I present sketches from clinical material.

Case I: Mrs. H., a woman of 26, entered analysis because of constant conflicts with her partner in a manufacturing outfit. The man having acquired in devious ways some knowledge of analysis, recommended treatment, "hoping against hope" that his life would become easier. He described the woman's behavior as "tense and leech-like": "She wants constant attention, admiration, love. If I give it to her, she is insatiable and dissatisfied; if I work, she feels excluded and a Pariah." Confrontation of both partners resulted in a series of accusations and counter-accusations. They both acted the neurotic game of "pulling a nobody-loves-me", hence the previously described "mechanism of orality."

The patient informed me that she suffered from a series of fears: "I know they are irrational, still I'm scared stiff. I'm practically afraid of everything—of fainting, collapsing, being exposed as fake, and what not." Asked where her fears came from, she claimed that "my sadistic mother implanted in me a chronic insecurity by always criticizing and reprimanding." The father was described as a weakling, long deceased, who never stood up against the mother. Asked how she felt about mother, the lady claimed that she had "detached" herself completely.

Analysis of her case showed first superficially repressed hatred toward mother. This accounted for her fainting spells in which, in unconscious identification with mother, she killed mother via a heart-attack and as penance—herself. After working out that material, a

24 The pseudo aggressive defense against deeper repressed psychic masochism seems to me confirmed in cases of suicide: the alleged killing of the introjected disappointer is in my opinion but the defense against overdimensional masochism. One could say that the suicide must convince himself, even in death, that he is capable of aggression. See the writer's "Problems of Suicide," The Psychiatric Quarterly Supplement, *20*:261–75, Part 2, 1946.

slight improvement took place, only to revert very soon to the previous state.

In the transference, the patient repeated first the positive Oedipus, always intermingled with "injustice collecting" and "aggressive" complaining toward the analyst. That attitude pointed in the direction of masochistic attachment toward the pre-oedipal mother. This—and the mother transference—were interpreted to the patient who soon understood: her fears pertained basically to her gluttony for libidinized punishment. That deepest masochistic layer was warded off with pseudo-aggression as palimpsest, the fear, now secondarily shifted to the aggressive thoughts toward her mother. That fear was artificially—though also unconsciously—exaggerated, to cover the real conflict—masochistic attachment.

The patient was cured. I doubt whether by exposing the aggression towards mother this could have been achieved especially since she was well aware—even consciously—of her antagonism toward mother, though she had no idea of the extent and depth of her hatred.

Case II: Mrs. I., aged 28, was, as she claimed, "obsessed with fear." She was afraid of everything: from elevators to subways, from leaving the home to visiting friends, from street fear to worries over health. She lived and dressed "for the emergency." For a long time she never took off her coat or fur in winter—in her own apartment. "I must be ready to leave at a moment's notice." Asked what she was afraid of, she claimed that her heart might fail and "then I must run to the physician." Asked whether in such an emergency (her heart was, by the way, completely normal) calling in a specialist would not be preferable, she said that she had three telephones installed—"just in case"—, but could not trust mechanical devices. Interrogated whether her belief in physicians was not exaggerated, she stated that she was well aware of the "stupidity of her fears." "Still," she said, "here they are."

Refusal to undress became so intolerable, that having slept one night fully dressed in her mink coat (!), she decided to enter treatment.

The case was practically identical with that of Mrs. H. Her "heart attack" represented unconscious identification with her mother, performed out of inner guilt. That aggression covered but thinly the deeper layer of masochism. The only difference was that Mrs. I. had also to cope with strong exhibitionistic wishes, covering voyeuristic tendencies.

Case III: Mr. J., a writer of 30, suffered from innumerable hypochondriacal fears. At the time he consulted me, he became "stabilized" for some time on—cancer of the tongue. He lived in panic; he constantly pressed and rubbed his tongue against his teeth and the small abrasions were taken as proof positive of cancer. Specialists denied any pathology, the patient remained unconvinced.

Analysis of his writing block does not concern us here.[25] As far as the substructure of the cancer fear was concerned, it was part and parcel of his oral regression. He acted in every respect the frantic "injustice collector," pushing his mother in the rôle of the refusing monster, he himself being the "innocent victim". The unconscious aim of gaining masochistic pleasure was, of course, repressed. In previous years he had been still capable of building up inner defenses, at least in his writing. He produced a few mystery stories in which a lawyer—his father's profession—had been regularly killed. This defense (based on pseudo-aggression) collapsed—he became literally sterile. His cancer of the tongue phobia pertained to mother's breast "forced" upon him. His "aggression" toward his innocent tongue pertained to mother, that aggression was, however, but pseudo-aggression covering masochistic attachment. (See previously discussed difference between clinical and genetic picture in orality). After working through the fact that "*his* tongue was but *his* tongue," the fear disappeared, to go through a series of other shifts and variations, before being given up.

The sequence of events leading to the cancer phobia was this: his infantile conflict had been solved with masochistic submission toward mother. That submission was warded off with pseudo-aggression—he damaged symbolically mother's breast. That defensive aggression was contradicted by the superego and had to be warded off, too,—with fear. The latter was, of course, secondarily libidinized ("Angstlust," pleasure of anxiety.)

An interesting detail was the fact that the patient "loved" to suck his mother's and wife's arm—but only if it was "cold." This strange predilection was complicated by an even more peculiar condition of

25 See f.i., "Psychoanalysis of Writers and Literary Productivity" in Psychoanalysis and the Social Sciences, ed. Dr. Róheim, Int. Univ. Press, New York, 1947.

coldness of the arm. Asked in a jest what he did in summer, whether he put both women into the frigidaire—he answered seriously, that during these months he was forced to dispense with that pleasure. What it practically amounted to was an unconscious "proof" that he did not want to be refused; on the contrary, he wanted to get. But—to prove being victimized and unjustly treated—the arm was "cold," like mother's emotions. This—self-provoked—alibi bolstered his "basic" fallacy.[26] He fortified himself, so to speak, with a new dose of mother's "coldness" and rejection.

Case IV: Mrs. K., a woman of 45, suffering from innumerable fears (mainly of "losing her mind") attached herself three times to husbands who "mistreated and exploited" her. She "suffered" and did not do anything about it until "thrown out by these ungrateful dogs." In her—otherwise cultured—vocabulary the word "dog" had a strange priority. Even in her dreams, dogs were predominant. It turned out that there was in her childhood a real dog—the prototype of her "personality." That dog was dearly loved by the child who felt "completely rejected" by the rather disagreeable and nagging mother and the "impersonal" and detached father. That dog was extremely submissive and docile. Still he ended his career with an "aggressive" action: he bit the patient's sister, and as punishment was given away by the mother. The dog became the reincarnation of the girl's inner conflict: she was masochistically submissive, and as inner alibi (defense) pseudo-aggressive.

The patient's fears belonged to her overdimensional masochistic submission; the fear was secondarily shifted to her alleged aggression. She was afraid that one day she would harm "in some cruel way" one of her husbands.[27] In her dreams, she frequently "watched" over the dog's "ready-to-bite" attitude. In other words, she, too, shifted her guilt to a side track in her self-appointed role of preventing a cruel action. She, too, accepted the blame for the "lesser crime."

[26] See the paper "The Danger Neurotics Dread Most: Loss of the Basic Fallacy." The Psa. Rev. 1945.

[27] See a similar case of a woman who—despite fantastic submission to her husband—produced the fear of cutting her husband's genitalia during his sleep. Her Delilah-fantasy was but a defense against masochism. Described as Case B. in "Divorce Won't Help" (Chapter I), New York, Harper, 1948.

Case V: Mrs. L., aged 31, came into analysis because of pathologic fears connected with her son of eight. She was constantly on the lookout for some sickness in the child. She took his temperature twenty times a day, every cough was interpreted as incipient pneumonia. If the child was in school, the mother worried whether or not he was warmly enough dressed, only to revert a few minutes later to the opposite fear, dreading the thought that the boy was too warmly dressed. During the night she could not decide whether the window in the child's room should be closed or remain open. She changed her mind constantly and acted according to the last doubt, only to reverse her decision shortly afterwards.

The case looked at first like a typical example of repressed aggressive attitude, her ambivalence [28] having an obsessional basis. Not the slightest change was achieved by working out that material, till it became clear that the whole conflict had no connection at all with the child and that the woman had chosen the innocent child as battle ground for realing off an unconscious conflict of masochistic variety—with her own mother.

She acted out a "magic gesture" [29] with the child. A magic gesture of this type has a complicated three-layer structure. The deepest layer is masochistic whining; under pressure of the superego a defense is installed: I hate mother (father). That defense, too, is vetoed by the conscience with the result that a new defense appears: "I'm neither masochistic nor aggressive towards mother and father; I just show them how I really wanted to be treated: kindly and lovingly." That defense appears as "magic gesture."

That problem was worked out with satisfactory results. One day, Mrs. L. enlarged the list of her symptoms, confessing to a "new-old fear." She was "scared to death" of her approaching vacation tour in Canada. That fear consisted of leaving home, and made its appearance on the condition that the absence was protracted for a series of days. Said the patient: "Why I should be frightened, is not understandable to

[28] See "Three Tributaries to the Development of Ambivalence." The Psa. Quart., 1948, No. 2. For details see: "Fear of Leaving the Apartment," *Samiksa*, J. of the Indian Psa. Soc., *1*:281–84, 1947.

[29] "The Problem of Magic Gestures." The Psychiatric Quart., *19*:295–310, 1945. Also Ch. VI "The Injustice Collector" of "The Battle of the Conscience."

me. I hate staying in New York. The boy is in camp, my husband and I both need and want that vacation. By the way, it was always so: every vacation, more, every little excursion involving leaving home for a few days, produces automatically that fear."

Since the connection with the child could be fully excluded (this specific fear made its appearance whether or not the child accompanied her) the attention was directed to her main problem: the masochistic attachment to the image of the "cruel" mother. It turned out that the patient lived "by chance" in the same building as did mother. That chance was unconsciously meaningful.

Seen in slow motion, Mrs. L.'s fear of leaving home had these layers:

Layer I (end-result of the infantile conflict): "I want to be masochistically rejected and tortured by mother; I want to stay home to be object of her wrath."

Layer II (first superego reproach): "You have no right to enjoy masochism."

Layer III (first defense created by the unconscious ego): "I'm not masochistically attached to mother, quite the contrary, I hate her; I want to stay home to protect her from *my* wrath."

Layer IV (second superego reproach): "You have no right to be aggressive either."

Layer V (second defense of the unconscious ego): "I'm neither masochistic nor aggresive toward mother. I love mother, want her protection."

The patient's fear pertains to layer I and is secondarily shifted to layer III.

All five examples have the following features in common:

(1) Unconscious wishes do not enter the symptom in direct form; only the defense against the unconscious wish is visible in the symptom. The problem hinges on the question whether a neurotic symptom has a two or three-layer structure.[30]

(2) The unconscious ego sidetracks the guilt from the dynamically decisive masochistic "crime" to the "lesser crime" of pseudo-aggression.

(3) Clinically, anxiety always pertains to the defense; lack of dif-

[30] For a theoretical discussion of the problem see Chapter III of "The Battle of the Conscience," *loc. cit.*

ferentiation between genetic and clinical picture leads the observer to erroneous conclusions.

(4) In confusing pseudo-aggression of neurotics with the underlying psychic masochism the therapist bolsters involuntarily the patient's inner defenses, which in turn leads to therapeutic failures.

Freud's formulation: "If a drive is repressed, the libidinous components change into neurotic symptoms, the aggressive components into feeling of guilt," is thus confirmed by clinical material. The formulation needs, however, two amplifications:

1. The aggression changed into guilt and fear is but pseudo-aggression, covering psychic masochism.

2. The libidinous wishes do not constitute the material for symptoms directly, only the defense against the repressed wish is used.

(8) *Mechanism of acceptance of inner guilt for the "lesser crime."*

Every neurotic operates intrapsychically on the basis of acceptance of guilt for the lesser crime. That means that the *role of the inner conscience (superego) is of prime importance for the neurotic structure. The whole neurosis rests on constant "appeasement" of inner conscience.*

The man with premature ejaculation accuses himself of cruelty toward his poor wife, though the guilt pertains *re vera* to the masochistic substructure, secondarily shifted to the pseudo-aggression of denying sexual satisfaction. And so on.

The fact is to be recorded that the moral code of the unconscious ego is—to put it mildly—slightly paradoxical: it does *not* correspond at all to the accepted standards of the specific society.

Every society establishes a penal code according to which the "punishment fits the crime." For instance, parking one's own car in a restricted area is considered a smaller offense than stealing a car; and stealing a car is "small fry" compared with killing a man who does not want to part from his car.

The grotesque fact is to be analytically observed that the moral code of the *unconscious* ego is not at all in conformity with the accepted priority list of crimes of the *conscious* ego. Crimes that are "*greater*" from the conscious viewpoint can be used as defense and alibis for "*smaller*" ones. The reason is not too difficult to detect: the unconscious ego, violently accused by the superego of a *specific* "forbidden wish"—the crime of the unconscious—defends itself, first by denying any guilt at all, and secondly, when forced into a corner, with the admission of being guilty but of a different offense from the one the indictment claims.

Expressed paradoxically: the unconscious ego first claims "I don't know from nothin'," only to change the defense according to the formula "I couldn't have raped the girl in Brooklyn as you say I did, because at that moment I was killing a man in Manhattan."

Thus, the crime admitted may be viewed from the penal code of reality a greater offense than the crime intrapsychically admitted.

The purpose of this procedure is simply to refute a specific accusation of the inner conscience. The plan is: "Punish me thus, but for something else."

To exemplify: A patient entered analysis after reading a paper of mine on potency disturbances. He had tried analysis four times in the last twenty years with four different colleagues in three different countries. His main symptom—premature ejaculation—remained unchanged. He finally lost confidence in his analysts and decided to make some research of his own, hoping that "something new" had been discovered in that specific field.[31] He started to study analytic publications and came across one of my papers dealing with premature ejaculation. He claimed that he did not understand the article (inability to understand was one of his symptoms), he was acting pseudo-mental deficiency, too, admitted however, that he gathered that I put stress on orality of which he had never heard. What the term meant, he claimed not to understand.

In his first dreams he confessed to practically every possible infantile "crime": masturbation, aggression, homosexuality, passive phallic castration; he had even a refutation dream proving that if his nagging mother would have been as nice and understanding as his father really was, no harm would have come to him.

The mechanism of admission of the lesser crime is a happy hunting ground for therapeutic errors. If the analyst falls for the wrong clue —neurosis is victorious.

[31] E. Stengel claimed that two types of patients existed: one believes in science and disrespects the doctors, hence never accepts incurability. The other is fatalistic and believes more in physicians, being skeptical of science. That patient was obviously of the first type.

(9) *Neurosis is a progressive and not self-limiting disease.*[32]

Neurosis, as Freud proved fifty years ago, is an illness of the unconscious. In unraveling the Gordian knot of neurosis we find with greatest regularity an unconscious wish, an unconscious inhibition and an unconscious defense mechanism. The neurotic end-results are deposited either in neurotic signs and symptoms or in "personality-difficulties."

The question arises as to the fate of untreated neuroses. What happens to them? Do they burn themselves out automatically? Are spontaneous "cures" effected? Is neurosis basically a progressive or self-limiting disease?

Clinical experience proves that neurosis is, unfortunately, a progressive illness. An untreated neurosis deteriorates as the years pass by. Symptoms may change and be shifted from one organ to another; depressions and worries attach themselves to different rationalizations but the neurotic basis remains. Not only does it remain, but the ability of the personality to absorb like a sponge libidinous-aggressive conflicts, decreases and the general picture worsens.

Every neurosis contains a quantitatively different amount of self-damaging tendencies. This psychic masochism can, as life goes on, be placed at different points. Confronted with either self-created or purely external painful or unhappy situations, the neurotic spends his wish to suffer, with the result that he has, temporarily, less symptoms and feels better. He might be compared to a drunkard who needs a specific dosage of alcohol every day; at what bar he gets it, is unimportant. Freud mentions apparently incurable cases of severe obsessional neurosis who lost their symptoms subsequent to organic disease, loss of money, or after other external unhappy events occurred.

If we do not take into account the exchangeability of neurotic manifestations and overlook the static basis of neuroses we may be led to erroneous conclusions. Specialization of medical science bolsters this fallacy. A girl of eighteen may develop a "nervous stomach" and after treatment by a gastroenterologist be helped. Two years later she may suffer from migraine-like headaches and a neurologist is consulted. In the meantime she has married and divorced two husbands. After her return from Reno she has severe abdominal pains; appendi-

[32] First published under the title "Neurosis—A Progressive or Self-Limiting Disease?" Diseases of the Nervous System, VII, 6, 46.

citis is suspected; a laparatomy is performed but the appendix proves to be normal. A few months later the headaches set in again. She consults another neurologist. Later the patient complains about all sorts of hypochondriacal ills, and consults in rapid succession a gynecologist, an internist and a sinus specialist. All her life she remains a patient of "universal medical science," a non-diagnosed and not improving neurotic.

In determining whether or not a neurosis deteriorates, one has to take into account the development of this illness. Neurosis is the petrification of an infantile conflict which is repressed. The infantile conflict itself, without psychiatric help, is indestructible. Every neurosis, which is latently present from early childhood, manifests itself first in form of depressions and fears. That does not mean that these are genetically the first depositions; they are merely the first visible ones. The "personality" *per se* absorbs the conflict first. Only after this "sponge is saturated," do symptoms and signs appear which the conscious ego treats like a foreign body. In other words, the "queer" personality precedes the "queer" neurotic symptoms.

Deterioration of a neurosis is difficult for the patient and the non-specialized physician to trace because there are years in the life of a neurotic when, seemingly, everything is "all right." The process of deterioration reveals itself only if one takes into account an overall picture of the personality. Then, and then only, does it become apparent that the neurosis of the thirties is worse than in the twenties, and so on in direct progression. If one meets a man with severe neurotic symptoms today, loses sight of him, to encounter him two years hence, and at that specific time the person has "shed" all his neurotic difficulties, a fallacy is possible in the judgment that the man "overcame" his neurosis. In probing deeper, however, one finds, for instance: that in the meantime the man had gone through an unhappy marriage and divorce which, since unconsciously self-created, consumed unconsciously, for the time being, his psychic masochism and therefore he feels "fine."

It is amazing to what degree the progress of an untreated neurosis is independent of reality, or more precisely, how reality is just used as a tool for the neurosis. A tragic example of this fantastic tendency is the following:

Many years ago, I was requested by the family of a compulsive neurotic to treat this man who spent all his time washing his hands (wash-compulsion). Of course, I wanted to see the patient first but he declared himself an enemy of psychoanalysis and refused even to see me. A few years later, the patient, a Viennese, was summarily arrested during a Nazi pogrom and placed in a concentration camp. There he behaved most strangely; the same man who had washed himself all day stopped washing altogether. At that time the Nazis were still in their beating-torturing stage; the outright killing and extermination came later. One day the S.S. guards decided to "teach" the man cleanliness; on an extremely cold winter day they stripped him in the open yard and kept pouring buckets of water over him for several hours. A few days later the victim died of pneumonia.

The reasons which prompted this man to give up washing can only be vaguely surmised. Clinical experience with analysed cases of compulsive washing proved that these neurotics constantly repress the wish to play with feces as end-result of their infantile conflict. The wish, having for these people a "sexual" connotation, is counteracted by a severe reproach of the inner conscience, with the result that in consciousness the opposite tendency appears; namely: Compulsive hypercleanliness. Since both, unconscious conflict and unconscious reproach never end because of inner ambivalence, the wash-compulsion is perpetuated. In the concentration camp the man obviously appeased his severe inner conscience with the objectively unhappy situation, with the result of "acquiring" the inner permission to indulge in his dirt-mania. At the same time he shifted the punitive factor of his inner conscience to the Nazis. There is reason to assume that he would have survived had he behaved differently. At that early stage the Nazis released non-political prisoners who could produce a visa to a foreign country, which his parents were able to secure.

A third example I present is the case of a young lawyer whom I treated for a few months, fifteen years ago. The patient entered analysis because of psychogenic impotence based on hysteria. After a relatively short time he was able to perform intercourse successfully for the first time in his life. Immediately afterwards he stopped treatment declaring himself "cured." I protested in vain, pointing out that he fooled himself completely about the depth of his neurosis. I advised him to continue treatment lest he suffer a predictable relapse. The man could not be influenced even so far as to discuss my experiences with similar cases. He felt cured and "that was that." Some months later I received his marriage announcement. Shortly after he consulted me in great excitement informing me that his wife suffered from vaginismus and had been treated surgically. The patient was aware that this condition was the manifestation of a neurosis and tried to convince his wife to enter psychoanalysis. Surgical treatment of vaginismus was, as could be expected, without effect. His wife refused to be analysed and took her condition fatalistically. The patient, too, accepted the situation with remarkable stoicism. What it really amounted to was that neither of them wanted genital sex. Every attempt at explaining this to the patient failed, though he admitted that even before marriage he had had the "vague feeling" that his wife was "sexually not too interested." What he did not admit was that this impression was precisely the reason for his choice. Fourteen and a half years later I met this man on the street. He was still married to his wife. She remained virgin because of her neurosis but still refused to be treated. He accepted her dictum without complaint and was still "faithful" to her. His external circumstances were poor, his wife earned more than he did. He often remembered my advice to continue treatment. Perhaps, he remarked hopefully, he would even do so—one day. . . .

Neurosis is a dangerous and progressive disease. Symptoms may be exchanged, but the condition advances; the masochistic stakes increase; the overall picture deteriorates. To hope for spontaneous cure in neurosis is as senseless as to expect the Niagara Falls to flow in the opposite direction.

4

The Underestimated Superego

THE MOST cruel and consistent enemy of human happiness—the inner, selfcreated Frankenstein, called superego—had analytically for decades an inconspicuous existence. Compare the "censor" of the "Interpretation of Dreams", with "the accumulation of death instinct" in the later presentation of the superego in Freud's works and you will see the superego has had a spectacular scientific career.

The reason for that long continued underestimation of the unconscious part of conscience, has once more to be found in the exclusive focusing of attention on libidinous drives, characteristic for the first three decades of analysis.

Even after discovery of the importance of the inner conscience, by Freud, analysis could not even find a word in the language to express what that inner demon really meant. The popular ideas of conscience current and expressed in every language, understand it as a benevolent though stern institution, easily appeasable by being a good boy. The ideas of reward and punishment, meted out in an ideal nursery, are naïvely projected upon the inner conscience. Add to that fact the surprise occasioned by the discovery of the existence of an *unconscious* part of conscience and you have the reason why the outerworld never understood or digested, what that strange analytic "invention"—called superego—really denotes.

To complicate matters, there is no uniformity of views on the problem in analytic circles, either. Shifting the center of attention to the decisive role of conscience in neurosis—as I have tried to do—surprises and makes many colleagues feel uncomfortable.

In a long book, "The Battle of Conscience," I have summarized my opinions on that topic. My deductions are based on Freud's Eros-Thanatos-theory, which has remained in the opinion of many people merely a philosophical conception. Applied with strict consistency, it leads to the *clinical* assumption that our whole life is but a fight between the *pleasure-principle* and the *torture-principle*. The latter is, it must be admitted, difficult to accept.

Different approaches have been tried to explain the conundrum of conscience.[1]

1. The *religious* approach assumes a manifestation of God as the basis of conscience. Scientifically that statement can neither be proved nor disproved clinically and therefore is outside the realm of science. If a religious man of any denomination asserts to the scientist that without the preordained will of God, education and intrapsychic mechanisms could not have built up the phenomenon called conscience, the discussion stops at that point. Religious beliefs are the most private affairs in a man's life. Science is neither competent nor willing to argue outside its own circumscribed zone. Hence, respect for the convictions of others—as well as the knowledge of having little to contribute to the emotional experience of the religion accepted in his specific society—debars the scientist from further argument. Science and religious beliefs work on entirely different psychic levels, and should stay in their respective domains, as far as scientific and religious polemics go. The two approaches do not contradict each other, as is shown by the fact that there are scientists who are deeply religious.

2. The next approach may be labeled: *conscious identifications with the specific environment.* Here stress is put on consciously performed imitation. Parents and educators provide a set of rules for the child, implemented by good examples. The difficulty here is based on clinical observation that in many cases, though constantly confronted by "good examples," the child behaves contrariwise. It remains unclear why one child accomplishes the identification, the other not; why one child comes under "bad" influence, whereas the other remains immune under identical conditions. Moreover, it remains more than doubtful whether the identifications, if accomplished, are of the conscious type. Every child is confronted with good and bad examples alike, not all "take" to them.

3. *Early psychoanalytic theories* connected the development of conscience with the normal overcoming of the Oedipus complex. Freud assumed that every child goes through a period in which it attaches libidinous wishes to the parent of the opposite sex, and aggressive-competitive tendencies to the parent of the same sex. These wishes are

[1] See "Crime and Punishment—Why Punishment Fails to Prevent Crime." The Psychiatric Quarterly Suppl. 21, 2, 1947.

detached after the age of five; they are shattered on the castration complex. To take the example of the boy: He is afraid of his father's retribution and prefers the intactness of his bodily integrity to the not-realizable wishes directed toward the mother. The result of that conflict is that the maternally-directed wishes are de-sexualized, deprived of the previous libidinous content,[2] and the father's prohibitions are internalized; and thus the inner conscience is established.[3]

4. *Later psychoanalytic theories* stressed the fact that the child does not perceive reality as it really is, but through the spectacles of "projection." [4] Projection denotes unconscious shift of a person's inner problem to the outside, without awareness of so doing. If, for instance, the boy experiences great aggression toward his father, he may shift that aggression projectively on the father and now feel that the father is "cruel." If the boy later introjects and incorporates the father's prohibition, the severity of the inner conscience so formed is in direct proportion to his *own*, and not to the father's aggression.

Other theories stressed the assumption that the child shows signs of the existence of the superego long before the age of five, that the superego antedates the development of the Oedipus complex, and is, thus, brought into connection with the mother.

The decisive element in the structure of the superego has been more and more understood to be its fantastic severity. To quote a late statement of Freud: "The superego seems to have made a one-sided selection and to have chosen only the harshness and severity of the parents, their preventive and punishing functions, while their loving care is not taken up and continued by it."

Freud finally came to the conclusion that every bit of aggression which—under cultural conditions—cannot be placed externally, is taken over by the inner conscience.

5. *Freud's Eros-Thanatos theory* assumes that there are two basic instincts operative in every human being. Our whole life consists of a constant fight between two giants: the "life-instinct" (Eros) and the

[2] The child has, of course, different misconceptions of what parental sexual activity consists of. These misconceptions have little to do with adult intercourse.

[3] *Mutatis mutandis,* the same process was assumed to take place in the girl, although the severity of feminine conscience never reached that of its masculine counterpart, according to that conception.

[4] Especially emphasized by the English school of analysis.

"death-instinct" (Thanatos). Eros attempts to discharge upon objects in the outer world the destructive tendencies of Thanatos, originally turned upon the individual himself. What is apparent as an instinct of destruction is genetically the original death-instinct, forced into a changed direction by the life-instinct. Guided by Eros, the destructive instinct rages outwardly, instead of inwardly.

Imagine two giants fighting each other; the first wants to kill the second. The second tries to divert the destructive energy of the first toward a third party. Imagine further both giants operative as instincts in one personality, and you have in a nutshell the Eros-Thanatos theory. These drives never appear "unmixed." They are combined in quantitatively varying degrees at different times. There is also an "indifferent narcissistic energy" which can be added to one drive or another, thus increasing its cathexis. Of course, what we see clinically is never life-instinct or death-instinct *per se*, or even their original mixtures, but only the derivatives of these mixtures. In this sense we can speak of "libido" and "destrudo" (aggression), assuming that each contains admixtures of both drive, libido more of the derivatives of Eros, destrudo more of the Thanatic elements.

Freud himself did not apply this theory to the development of the superego. This was done by two of his pupils.

6. *The Bergler-Jekels theory* represents an application of Freud's dualistic Eros-Thanatos theory to the development and working of the superego.

Freud's original conception of inner conscience was based on a compromise between the original megalomania of the child, confronted with a stronger reality, represented by the parents. The child solved that conflict by a face-saving device: He identified himself with the commands of these educators, sugar-coating the defeat by an illusion. That illusion is: Nobody forces me, I'm good of my free decision. The amalgam of infantile megalomania and introjected educational rules was called *ego-ideal.*

The ego-ideal later became submerged in the newer concept of the superego. The relation between ego-ideal and superego was never clarified.

The Bergler-Jekels theory *assumes that the superego consists of two distinct parts: the ego-ideal and the "daimonion."* (See pp. 46–48.)

The latter term denotes the anti-libidinous parts of the conscience, loaded with derivatives of the death-instinct. The term is derived from Socrates' "daimonion": That philosopher believed that some kind of malignant spirit raved inside the personality. That mythological conception has—taking the death-instinct into consideration—a very real meaning.

The interconnection between ego-ideal and daimonion is this: The ego-ideal was originally created to maintain the threatened narcissism of the infant. It enshrines all the childish ideas of grandeur, all the promises the child gave himself of the great and wonderful deeds he would perform and achieve in this world.

Unfortunately for the ego, the daimonion takes the high-pitched expectations of the child, accumulated in the ego-ideal, very seriously. Mockingly, it presents the ego-ideal to the ego and asks: Did you reach everything you promised yourself? Since the ego-ideal practically never can be fully materialized in this real world, the ego-ideal thus becomes an instrument of torture.

Daimonion holds up to the ego the self-created ego-ideal like a silent mirror; and every discrepancy between ego and ego-ideal is felt as depression, dissatisfaction, guilt.

Derivations of the life-instinct, accrued in the ego-ideal, fight a losing battle with derivations of the death-instinct, symbolized in the daimonion. The irony in the situation is that the daimonion uses life-instinct—the ego-ideal—for its destructive purposes. The ego is caught in his own—and self-created—protective apparatus.

The superego, once established, is an *internal Frankenstein*, constantly ready to spring upon the poor ego. Still, there are certain restrictions—one could speak of "*rules of torture*"—governing that monster.

First of all, the superego is extremely formalistic in nature. It could—since it has the power—torture the personality simply because it is in the driver's seat. It does not, but adheres to the comedy of a *mock trial.* It always presents to the ego its ego-created dupe of an ego-ideal, asking the monotonous question: Do *you admit that there is a discrepancy between your ego and ego-ideal?* If that discrepancy cannot be denied, punishment in the form of guilt is imposed.

Why that comedy of intrapsychic justice is instituted, can only be dimly surmised. It is possible that the superego's cruelty is counteracted by tendencies of the life-instinct, forcing it to make the "compromise" in form. That assumption is based on theoretical considerations in cases of suicide where, according to Freud, "a pure mixture of death-instinct reigns in the superego." That de-fusion of instincts leaves the death instinct no longer attenuated by the life-instinct. Another reason for the superego's adhering to "rules of torture" is, perhaps, the fact that, because of the counteraction of the life-instinct, the superego must prevent a possible slave revolt of the tortured ego. Obviously the ego is more manageable when its "self-written check" is presented.

Second, the superego *never punishes* the ego *without proving that the varying forbidden wish is really harbored in the reservoir of unconscience wishes, the id.* Any denial is impossible because of the direct "pipeline" between superego and id. Precisely the fact that the superego knows so much of the person's innermost secrets, makes the unconscious conscience such a formidable enemy.

To compensate for that pseudo-restraint, the superego *does not distinguish between wish and deed.* The tragic result is that the internal "criminal law" is more severe than the external one, which does not prosecute sins "committed in thoughts." That "infernal—internal thought—police," as a witty patient called it, leads to most tragic consequences: *Nine-tenths of neurotic guilt pertain to unconscious fantasies only.*

Third, the superego *adheres ironically to "freedom of will,"* as far as the victimized ego is concerned. It pushes the victim indirectly—by relenting vigilance—into an impossible and self-damaging situation, turns the tables and asks indignantly: How could you do that? It acts, in these accusations, as if the action perpetrated were under perfect conscious volition.

Fourth, the superego camouflages its cruelty by *accepting "cultural standards"* fashioned after the specific environment. That makes it possible for naïve observers to make the faulty deduction that the individual is the product and mirror of his environment. Assuming for the sake of argument that the superego is basically interested in torturing the ego, what difference does it make whether the superego uses this or that prohibition based on specific taboos of the specific environment? The common denominator is still a series of "Don'ts."

On the other hand, the acceptance of the specific taboos—different in different cultural orbits—imposes an odd restriction on the superego. Anti-libidinous, as the inner conscience is, it is helpless against actions approved by the specific environment.

Fifth, the superego is impressed by success—though it is the typical *devaluator of success,* if it is incapable of preventing it in the individual. It is a well-known fact that many people are incapable of enjoying self-achieved victories. They start to doubt whether the expenditure of effort in the game has been "worth the candle." This is mostly the belated "contribution" of the superego.

Sometimes, that tendency goes so far that the superego makes fun of its own punitive executive organs. It acts like a gangster who extracts at gunpoint the signing of a detrimental document—only to show the victim later that the gun was really a camouflaged cigarette container.

Sixth—last, but not least—the superego is extremely *sensitive to real aggression,* when directed against His Majesty, the tormentor. Being constituted of malicious aggression itself, it understands one thing only: the fist with real power behind it. That is clearly visible in so-called normality as compared with neurosis. In normality, the ego has a good-sized quantity of real aggression at its disposal; hence the not-too-neurotic person has not too much to suffer under his inner tormentor. In neurosis, the balance of power is precisely reversed: The superego usurps the person's aggression and tortures the ego.

Even under the most favorable conditions, in normality, the ego uses a great deal of its psychic energy—mainly aggression—to ward off unjustified reproaches of the superego.

The superego is, thus, not simply a necessary restrictive institution, a necessity readily understood and approved. *It is the antihedonistic force in the personality, loaded to capacity with derivatives of the death-instinct.* The observation that it represents restrictions seemingly embodying only the specific taboos of a specific environment, is a mirage. That is the anti-libidinous blind for its punitive actions, attached secondarily as hitching posts to reality-restrictions. Its *prime movens* is the formula: *No pleasure.*

All of this applies to more or less normal people. The moment clear-cut *neurotic reactions* are involved, a different picture appears.

Neurosis is an anachronistic disease of the unconscious, preserving repressed infantile wishes, defense mechanisms, guilt. These old, normally relinquished, or, at least, modified tendencies are unconsciously perpetuated, though constantly counteracted by a severe superego. *The latter is, however, under neurotic conditions, meretricious and venable. Like a corrupt district attorney, it can be bribed, bought off, and appeased.* The intrapsychic currency is, of course, not money—the very young child does not yet know the value of money. The currency in the nursery is love and punishment. *Hence the inner conscience is partial to punishment.* The neurotic "deal" consists precisely in the tenacity of id-wishes, ego-defenses, superego-corruptibility. Simplified in caricature, the neurotic structure rests on a compromise like this: Under the conditions that the superego is bought off with consciously experienced depression, dissatisfaction, ego-restriction, the superego allows inuendos of unconscious pleasure—though not in direct form—screened by a defense mechanism against repressed wishes.[5] The superego gets his full share of punishment, the id receives attenuated wish-fulfillments, camouflaged in unconscious defenses. The neurotic pays an exaggerated fee for infantile, second-hand, substitute gratifications.

I believe that the influence of the superego exclusively pushes the analytic patient into treatment. I believe furthermore that the decision whether or not a patient is cured in analysis, depends on the analyst's ability to mobilize and utilize the patient's inner guilt.

The whole problem of "*working through*" is intimately connected with inner guilt.[6]

The phenomenon of "working through" was introduced by this term for the first time in our literature by Freud in 1914, in his

[5] Older analytic theories assumed a two-layer structure: Neurotic symptoms and signs were considered direct symbolic "substitute gratifications." I personally believe that a three-layer structure is involved: repressed wish-symbolic defense—defense against the symbolic defense. Only that secondary defense appears in consciousness as "strange" symptoms and sign. For a discussion of the problem see: "The Battle of the Conscience."

[6] First presented in a lecture before the New York Psychoanalytic Society, May 23, 1944. Published under the title "'Working Through' in Psychoanalysis." The Psa. Review *32*:449–480, 1945.

paper, "Recollection, Repetition, Working Through." [7] It belongs to the least-explored chapters in psychoanalysis despite the fact that in practice we are applying it during nearly every analytic hour. In the same way that we switch on the electric current without giving much thought to the problem of the theory of electricity, we are using in analytic therapy the working-through process without wasting much time on the theoretic basis of that phenomenon. Experience simply teaches us that we have to apply the interpretations of resistances to acceptance and renunciation of unconscious wishes, feeling of guilt, unconscious repetitiveness, and defense mechanisms *often* and *chronically* in the transference neurosis on varying or repetitious material until those interpretations finally work—and that is enough. Why this is so remains a riddle. In general the every-day analytic contribution to the theory of that phenomenon is, in beginners, a rather sterile feeling of impatience, which diminishes gradually as the analyst grows older, until finally he can bear the process of working through of resistances without inner rebellion as a part of his daily routine. When that time comes he really becomes something like an "experienced" analyst, and that gradually and painfully-acquired quality of not being impatient any longer during the working-through process is even more revealing of his being an "experienced" analyst than many other more conspicuous symptoms and signs of analytic maturity.

Interestingly enough, the feeling of impatience has been from the beginning associated with the phenomenon of working through, as Freud specifically mentions in his introductory paper. Freud relates that he was often asked for advice by analysts who complained that they had shown to their patients their specific resistances with no effect, the whole analysis standing still. That pessimistic expectation was, as Freud stresses, always unjustified. The cure was making good progress, but the physician was forgetting that simply naming the resistance could not result in its immediate disappearance. One has to give the patient time, says Freud, to work through that resistance by sticking to the basic rule. At the height of that resistance one finds, in common work with the patient, the unconscious drives nourishing that resistance. The patient now realizes the power of these drives in himself. The physician must simply wait and not hinder a phenomenon rolling up

[7] Ges. Schr. VI, pp. 118–119, or Collected Papers II, pp. 375–376. Hogarth Press.

automatically—if properly handled. That working through of resistances may be, as Freud admits, a tiresome task, but it is exactly that part of analytic work which has the greatest effect on the patient and clearly distinguishes analytic treatment from every form of suggestive therapy.

Freud mentions as the theoretic basis of the phenomenon the unconscious repetition which forces the patient to reproduce over and over again his infantile constellations. He further states means of overcoming the patient's unconscious repetition and changing it into a motive for recollection—the handling of transference. Finally, Freud compares the results of the working-through process to the cathartic abreaction without which the hypnotic treatment remained without influence.

We are thus forced to take into account, in addition to these affective experiences in *dosi refracta,* a purely quantitative factor in the understanding of working through. That conception has a similarity to certain physiologic experiments; for instance, the electric current must reach a certain strength before a muscular response ensues. Or, to put the idea still differently, the steady drop makes the hole in the rock ('*Gutta cavat lapidem non vi sed semper cadendo*"), of course, always bearing in mind that it happens only too often that, during the working-through process, additional, more deeply rooted material comes to the surface which gives the specific resistance a different meaning.

Later, in 1920, Freud made further contributions to the problem of working through in "Beyond the Pleasure-Principle." By introducing the idea of the "unconscious repetition compulsion," which works beyond and independent of the pleasure-principle, he made clear why the neurotic psyche clings with such tenacity to repetitiveness. From that conception follows also a hint of why the discontinuance of repetition of the active reproduction of passive experiences in the transference neurosis takes so long.

The working through problem has had a strange fate in our literature. There are simply *no contributions* to the study of it. It seems incredible that a problem with which every analyst without exception must deal for nearly as many hours a day as he works should not provoke a few ideas among hundreds of analysts all over the world. All of the authors of the some 200 papers on technique enumerated by Fenichel in his "Problems of Psychoanalytic Technique" mention, of course, the phenomenon, but none has anything to add to Freud's basic statements. Our literature must actually be devoid of contributions on the working-through problem, since not even our quotation specialist, Fenichel, could produce tangible evidence of some quotations, and could make use of only a single, lonely and not even published quotation of Rado, without reference to its source. Since Fenichel has been quoting the same statement consistently for 10 years, four times in three papers and books, without giving the source, the conclusion is permissible that he is quoting a casual remark, especially since this author quotes sources scrupulously in other instances. I could not find it in Rado's publications, and don't know what, if any, importance Rado himself attached to the remark. The quotation I have in mind is the following: [8]

> "The comparison of working through with the work of mourning (Rado) seems to me very apt. A person who has lost a friend must in all situations which remind him of this lost friend make clear to himself anew that he has this friend no longer and that a renunciation is necessary. The conception of this friend has representation in many complexes of memories and wishes, and the detachment from the friend must take place separately in each complex."

In other words, Rado's comparison applies Freud's ideas described in "Mourning and Melancholia" to the working-through process. This application of an old idea of Freud to the working-through process has its merits at first glance. We could imagine that parting from old wishes and their representatives must be consistently repeated, since "the detachment must take place separately in each complex." We could compare that process to light falling on a many-faceted object, only one facet being lighted at a time. That conception would account for the amount of time needed for illumination of *all* facets. Unfortunately, that idea presents us with two difficulties: First, it does not explain why the same situation must be worked through always again and again; in other words, it avoids the very problem to be answered. Second, it does not take into consideration the fact that the working-through process applies not to id-wishes alone. True, Freud stated originally that working-through is primarily necessary because of the id-resistance and the repetition compulsion. On the other hand, in "Problem of Anxiety," Freud names *five* forms of resistance (repres-

[8] "Problems of Psychoanalytic Technique," p. 80.

sion-resistance, transference-resistance, resistance to the renunciation of gain through illness, id-resistance, superego-resistance), and we know that working-through is necessary for at least four of them, despite the fact that one applies to the id, one to the superego, and two to the ego. Fenichel himself takes great pains to prove that working-through operates particularly upon the ego but only indirectly upon the id. In other words, the confusions are many when the quotations are few.

What we really need for the further understanding of the theory and improved practice of the working-through process are three things: First, a comprehensive theory of how the working-through process influences the superego. Since the decisive point of the therapy hinges, in my opinion, on the superego, the working-through has decisive effects there. Why and how? Second, a theory of details. The working-through process produces results via a along series of *affective* experiences acquired in detail-situations in the transference. Why is this so and of necessity? Third, a summation as complete as possible of types of mistakes exemplified in practical examples to provide a compass for steering away from pseudo-results of working-through.

In the following discussion of the problem I exclude at first, purposely, a whole series of possibilities of error. I assume that the interpretations given the patient are correct, that is, dynamically effective; furthermore, that the analyst understands the specific reason for the specific resistance. In short, I speak about an ideal case.

The working-through process has analytically the purpose of forcing the patient to make the transition from *intellectual to affective* understanding and acceptance. Since only the affective acceptance produces therapeutic results, the whole problem boils down to the question: How is that transition accomplished?

Let's start with a question seemingly beside the point, but which really contains the crux of the matter. Why do our patients come into psychoanalysis at all? The answer seems to be simple enough. They come because they suffer, are helpless, and want help. The objection immediately arises that many persons with the same or an even greater amount of suffering and feeling of helplessness who are no less aware of the existence of psychoanalysis and with equal means to undergo treatment, never come to us. Consequently, we see that something is required in addition to neurotic suffering, helplessness, knowledge of the existence of psychoanalysis, and the money necessary, to make a workable analytic patient. This something in addition which is an indispensable prerequisite is, I believe, an *at least potentially fluctuating unconscious feeling of guilt. Every* neurotic and perverse person has, of course, an abundance of unconscious feeling of guilt. This feeling is deposited in symptoms, personality difficulties, sense of depression, artificial ego limitations, and the outerworld rejection of certain types of neurotics and perverts.

The whole problem of prognosis depends on the ability of analysis to mobilize these feelings of guilt, to change their place of deposition, and to transform them in a productive way. The fact that in general we accept a patient at first only for a trial-period of from four to six weeks has the purpose, not only of finding out whether a neurosis or psychosis is present, as Freud suggested, but even more decisively of getting an approximate impression as to whether or not we shall be able to mobilize the feeling of guilt in the analytic procedure.

We are therefore immediately confronted with the problem of the existence of "the wish to get well" ("Genesungswunsch"). Let us at first recapitulate what is found in our literature on this problem.

The wish to get well, or the recovery-wish, presents itself at first glance as something self-evident, which seemingly requires no explanation. Freud mentions in his "*Introductory Lectures*" (Ges. Schr. VII, p. 454) the patient's wish to get well in discussing the question of the drives with which analysis works. Ferenczi and Rank postulate in "Entwicklungsziele der Psychoanalyse" that the wish to get well should be analyzed like a symptom. Nunberg in "Über den Genesungswunsch" (Int. Zeitschr. f. Psychoan., 1925) stresses the fact that the patient's wish to get well has two cores which are contradictory. One originates in the ego and expects from the treatment fight against inner drives. The other stems from the id and hopes satisfaction of exactly the same drives. Physician and patient are talking at cross purposes, since each understands by the term "psychic health" something completely different. The patient expects unconsciously from analysis something which analysis cannot give—the fulfillment of unconscious wishes. Nunberg emphasizes that the motives of neurotics producing the recovery-wish are as manifold as the motives of their respective diseases. The unconscious part of the wish to get well makes use of the transference to achieve satisfaction of the infantile drives in the present. The transference is mobilized through the recovery-wish and is substituted for it, more or less, during treatment. But recovery-wish and transference are not identical, though they may meet or the recovery-wish may even be substituted by transference. At the beginning and end of analysis they can be separated. In Nunberg's opinion, it is the mortified narcissism which activates the recovery-wish. The mortified ego-ideal provides the initiative for the creation of the recovery wish; the energy, however, stems from the reservoir of unconscious drives. Nunberg believes that the neurotic disease itself contains a nucleus leading toward recovery, just as in some organic diseases toxins produce antitoxins.

With the exception of the last statement, which could be misunderstood as describing neurosis as a sort of self-limiting disease which has at least the tendency to burn itself out automatically or to produce automatically counterforces, an assumption which I believe to be exactly opposed to observable facts, I agree with Nunberg's paper and believe it to be his best contribution to our literature, in spite of its being one of his earliest, appearing 23 years ago. In continuation of that paper in my contribution [9] to the Symposium on the Theory of Therapy, held at the XIVth International Psychoanalytic Convention in Marienbad, 1936, I pointed out that, in my opinion, the decisive rôle played by the unconscious feeling of guilt with regard to the wish to get well and analytic therapy in general has been underestimated. In that part of my paper I concentrated my attention on the last stages of analysis and the rôle of the recovery wish in these stages, stating:

> "as the analysis goes on, the unconscious sense of guilt is tremendously increased, for, in advanced stages of the treatment, the guilty feelings, which were lodged in the symptoms, depressions, self-provoked punishments, ego-limitations, etc., are activated, thus transforming the *bound*, unconscious sense of guilt into a *free-floating* one. When the analysis is far advanced, this sense of guilt, released from its former positions, temporarily increases the patient's sense of depression, his subjective uneasiness, and his aggressive impulses toward the analyst, although the symptoms have subsided. In its free-floating form it now fastens with all of its force on the reproach leveled by the patient's conscience, 'Why are you not well yet?' It

[9] Internat. J. Psychoanalysis, XVIII, 1937, parts 2 and 3, pp. 146–160.

is difficult to determine what part is played here by psychic-economic factors—the provision of a better outlet for the sense of guilt or indeed of any outlet at all. Of course, that part of the unconscious sense of guilt which represents the patient's reaction to his sexual and aggressive pre-oedipal and oedipal wishes is resolved by the analysis; besides, analysis destroys these wishes.

"This reproach of conscience, 'Why are you not well yet,' finds expression in typical dreams, in which the ego seeks to reject the superego's accusations. I proposed that we should call dreams of this type 'dreams embodying a sense of guilt in connection with recovery' (Genesungsschuldgefühlsträume').

"When analysis has been sufficiently thorough, two processes take place, parallel with this increase in the sense of guilt. In the first place, the patient experiences affectively and quite consciously the truth of the analyst's statement that his symptoms conceal an unconscious pleasure-factor. He even goes to the length of wanting his old pleasure back and disparaging the normality which is his goal. But in the final stages of analysis this confession of a long-denied pleasure has a purely theoretical value, for the old channels by which libido and aggression once found an outlet are closed, a fact which adds fuel to the flames of the patient's indignation. ('I feel like a stripped Christmas tree,' said one patient in this phase.) Second, in his infantile delusions of grandeur, the patient is deeply mortified by the ridiculousness of his childish wishes. One patient who had regressed to the oral level expressed this mortification concisely when he said: 'The neurosis dies of its own absurdity,' and 'I have to get well out of sheer despair; there is no other way out—you have spoiled all of my old pleasures.' This emotional utterance indicates three factors:
(1) an increase of the unconscious sense of guilt; (2) mortification of the infantile delusions of grandeur; and (3) the blocking of the old outlets for libido and aggression to which the patient formerly had access in his neurosis but of which, at the end of his analysis, he can no longer avail himself.

"Perhaps these factors . . . explain the lack of enthusiasm with which patients greet their recovery. One patient said to me in the final stages of his analysis: 'Health comes along like a poor country cousin. Nobody is expecting him and nobody is enthusiastic about him, but all of a sudden he arrives'. This is true, although sometimes our candidates for recovery have outbursts of enthusiasm, which very soon die away.

"The three factors which I have described, possibly explain, too, why many patients who are cured leave their analysis with a secret resentment in their hearts. It may be objected that this indicates that the transference has not been resolved or that the analysis of infantile wishes has not been searching or full enough. But this is not always so; even in the most favorable case there is a trace of resentment. Not even the analyst may with impunity lay hands on the infantile elements in the human psyche."

Contributions to the problem of the recovery-wish in our literature other than those cited above do not exist as far as I know.

I regard the unconscious feeling of guilt as the pivotal point of psychoanalytic therapy, and called it the *vis a tergo* of this therapy. I repeat that prognosis depends, *not* on the feeling of guilt as such, since therapeutically unchangeable neurotics have enough of it too, but on its at least potentially dynamic deposition. *Consequently, the whole process of working through is centered chiefly in the correct handling and mobilization of feeling of guilt.*

To make matters clearer, let us, by means of the analytic microscope, see how the three decisive unconscious provinces react to our therapeutic attempts with the vehicle of working through: [10]

1. Contributions of the id to the working-through process.

We can dispose of the id in this connection quickly. It behaves like Shylock demanding his pound of flesh. The id is *practically*, more or less, inelastic. Its contribution to the working-through process is threefold: First, it projects its wishes into the transference neurosis, following also the unconscious repetition compulsion, and secondarily, does everything possible to materialize its aims in the transference. To the extent that we can demonstrate these wishes and dispose of them in the transference, the id is involuntarily helpful. The id-resistance, however, makes us great difficulty because of its tenacity. As the third function of the id during the working-through process I shall mention later a queer rebellion in progressed stages of analysis, which is defeated by the superego.

2. Contributions of the superego to the working-through process.

In "Problem of Anxiety" (Ges. Schr. XI, p. 103), Freud calls the

[10] I would like to express my gratitude to Dr. H. H. Hart, who permitted me to use his work on Freud's quotations. I wanted a compilation of Freud's statements on free associations in connection with working through. The next day I received a list of 35 quotations. If one imagines the amount of work saved for an author—Freud's "Gesammelte Werke" consists of nearly 6,000 pages—one can judge the necessity of a work like Dr. Hart's. I hope that it appears very soon in print.

superego resistance "*the most obscure but not always the weakest form of resistance.*" That resistance, says Freud, stems from unconscious feeling of guilt or the unconscious need for punishment. According to him, it is adverse to every success and recovery of the patient in psychoanalysis.

That obscure but most powerful resistance is, in my opinion, the pivotal point in therapy. Analysts have till now made only two contributions toward the understanding of that resistance described by Freud. They have described the ways in which the superego becomes milder (for instance, Strachey), or they have, in a form of negative contribution, denied that that resistance exists at all (for instance, Fenichel, who attributes it to the ego). That negative contribution we can omit from our considerations, since denial of the existence of a problem is not a solution of it.

My opinion is that we have overlooked until now another factor in that superego resistance. I believe that under the influence of the working-through process one of the strangest things happen to that resistance: *an exchange of methods of torture.* By the way of explaining this statement, let's apply a modification of an often-used simile: The normal superego and the neurotic superego may be compared to the Swiss and Zaristic police, respectively. The Swiss police before the First World War were the most friendly and humane in Europe, but absolutely incorruptible. The Zaristic police, on the other hand, were the cruelest and most blood-thirsty, but they were corrupt. Paradoxically, one could say, therefore, that one could find access more easily to the cruel Zaristic police than to the humane Swiss police—via money. Of course, every comparison has its limitations. You cannot buy the superego with money, but you can "bribe" it, to use Alexander's term, with pain and depressions. What we want to achieve in psychoanalysis is exactly that *incorruptibility of the superego.* If we can destroy that mechanism of *habitual appeasement* of the superego, the neurosis gradually collapses. To use a popular catchword, the problem is to force the ego to accept the formula: "Appeasement like crime doesn't pay."

Let us assume that the id presents in the neurosis a wish; for instance, a voyeuristic one. The superego objects because of the liaison of this wish with pre-oedipal or oedipal tendencies. The unconscious ego then makes a deal, like the crooked lawyer pressed between his criminal client and a sadistic but corrupt district attorney. The stalemate between "I wish" and "I forbid" is overcome by the creation of a compromise—the neurotic symptom. To the id the unconscious ego says: "You cannot achieve your wish unless you disguise it and change it into the defense, e.g., exhibitionism instead of voyeurism and unless you pay for it." To the superego it says: "Allow this substitute wish in disguise and in unconscious phantasy only; you will receive your fee in unhappiness, pain, and the sense of depression." The neurotic symptom, for instance, agoraphobia, satisfies, therefore, the exhibitionistic wish as defense against the deeper repressed voyeuristic one. Since we show in analysis persistently wherein lies the "crooked deal," we force gradually the whole compromise to collapse in the long run. The question remains, however, as to how we achieve this and why the superego helps us. The usual answer is that even two criminals who are constantly exposed must change their methods. Yes, they must change their methods, but not their personalities. The idea that an habitually "wicked crook" becomes a benevolent friend of the people, approving their little pleasures, is a Hollywood fiction. It certainly does not apply to the superego. The situation where the superego is concerned is less humanitarian and more a matter of *psychologic barter.* What happens is simply that two processes of recompense are set in motion. First, the superego makes use of the analytic interpretation for purposes of torture. Second, at the end of analysis the superego, now made incorruptible by artificial means, is in certain respects cruel and antilibidinous as before, but exercises its regulatory powers in the direction of preventing even more aggressively the neurotic id pleasures. These two processes of recompense require some elaboration.

The chief characteristic of the superego is its lust for cruelty. Let us not forget Freud's statement: "*The superego seems to have made an one-sided selection and to have chosen only the harshness and severity of the parents, their preventive and punitive functions, while their loving care is not taken up and continued by it.*" ("New Introductory Lectures on Psychoanalysis.") That one-sided and cruel superego seems at first to use every dynamically effective interpretation in analysis for its torture purposes. Some years ago I published a paper in Psychoanalytic Review entitled, "On a Predictable Mechanism

—enabling the Patient Even at the Beginning of Analysis to Check the Veracity of Interpretations."[11] That test makes use of specific "dreams of denial," "*refutation dream*," in which the frightened ego defends itself against the analytic interpretations. In other words, every correct and dynamically effective analytic interpretation is taken up also by the superego with the purpose of tormenting the frightened ego. Unfortunately, there is one necessary prerequisite for the success of this test: The interpretations must be correct. The control described is not a *pons asinorum* and not a phenomenon which falls to one's lot automatically and without difficulty, as does the transference. It is perhaps superfluous to mention the fact that the control works both ways: The analyst, too, can check up on himself, since *incorrect interpretations never do provoke such dreams.* For details I must refer to the paper mentioned above. I would like to mention an example:

A man displaying oral regression is prevented from pursuing his profession because, for some "inexplicable reason," he fears his office. There is soon evidence to show that he is repeating a pre-oedipal conflict of defensive revenge with his wife (mother). The hard-working woman had supported him for years before marriage and had made it possible for him to complete his studies and to start on an academic career. Hardly had he begun to earn his living, however, when the anxiety in regard to his office appeared, and hence a disturbance of his working and earning capacity. I pointed out to him how he was reacting to the "good" mother imago of his wife, with an infantile conflict. Actually she stood for the phantasied "bad," frustrating, pre-oedipal mother. He wanted to avenge himself on her by denying her everything (money, comfort, social position). At this time began an often-repeated series of dreams. The patient remembered the content only vaguely. He knew it revolved around men's clothing, usually an overcoat. The patient did not know what happened to these articles of clothing. He saw them "perhaps"; "perhaps" they were packed up. He could only say with certainty that he never obtained the clothing; there was always a space between him and this clothing which had an indifferent effect upon him; he never owned them. He had no associations to the dream and asked ironically why I did not interpret the clothing "symbolically." One day he mentioned that one is always disappointed in one's family, particularly with the wealthier members. In connection with a quarrel he had with his wife, it occurred to him how badly her rich

[11] Vol. 30, pp. 19–32, 1943.

relatives had acted after the war. They had emigrated to a wealthy country around the turn of the century and had become quite prosperous. After the war our patient had visited these relatives, and had wished to have some new clothes made out of good pre-war materials in their factory. This was comprehensible, since in his country they were using poor substitutes. The stingy relatives not only allowed him to pay for materials and work, but also were responsible for his winter overcoat not being finished when he was ready to depart. Evidently in order to save the duty, he arranged to have a nephew bring the coat with him, since he intended to visit the patient in his country within the next few months. This promise was never kept. The nephew came, but stated that just this overcoat had been stolen on the trip.

This patient, at the beginning of his analysis, was weighted with the ever-increasing pressure of his own guilt-feelings, which through the analysis became mobilized and concentrated on one point. "Your innocent wife," I told him, "is receiving the brunt of a conflict with which she had nothing to do. You are projecting the revenge upon her which was intended for your mother." His conscience made use of this accusation, and the unconscious ego defended itself by declaring that the family was made up of crooks who denied him things and cheated him; hence he might be aggressive and denying. Accordingly the overcoat motif was used symbolically *to relieve feelings of guilt.*[12]

Further material is also collected in my paper, "A Third Function of the 'Day Residue' in Dreams," which appeared some time ago in Psychoanalytic Quarterly.[13]

We see, therefore, that even such a strong enemy as the torturing neurotic superego can be put to work *for* analysis. This queer fact is explainable by the structure of the superego. This part of our unconscious personality simply makes the most of every opportunity to torture the ego. This weakness of our enemy is only an initial advantage. Later, it increases the feeling of guilt and sense of depression to such a degree that the patient often has the tendency to leave analysis. At any rate using this mechanism may be compared to making a Hitler fight against himself, giving him inadvertently and with anti-

[12] The patient's aggression was but pseudo-aggression covering a deeper repressed masochistic wish.

[13] Vol. XII, No. 3, July, 1943.

Hitlerian purposes as "bait" a new argument which he misuses for his purposes of torment without realizing that he harms himself in the long run by his "greed."

This initial use of the analytic enemy *for* analytic purposes has the result that the superego in its known formalism does not simply torture the patient in general but takes up the analytic interpretations—for the purpose of torment, to be sure—and starts a campaign of "Confess, confess! " In other words, using the neurotic superego we elicit and achieve recollections of repressed material.

The whole process described is an unconscious one, it works automatically and does not require any knowledge on the part of the analyst or the patient. It cannot harm the analyst, of course, if he knows a little better what is going on.

The second recompense for the superego is at the *end* of analysis, when, after diminution or attenuation of preoedipal and oedipal wishes and after utter destruction of the constant bribing and appeasing of the superego with pain, unhappiness, and depression, the superego assumes its "normal" punitive function. In our literature a great deal of emphasis is placed on the fact that the superego becomes "milder" and "more lenient" under the influence of analysis. This phrase is meaningless unless properly interpreted. At best it must be taken, not with a grain, but with a pound of salt, as the following argument shows: *Before* analysis the stern *neurotic* superego allows the individual to fulfill his pre-oedipal and oedipal wishes in the disguise of defenses in symptoms, at the cost of suffering. *After* analysis the *normal* superego, though grown more tolerant, does not allow the cured individual to make use of his former neurotic wishes. It does, indeed, become more lenient and tolerant, but only on condition that the old wishes be renounced and normality be adhered to. The aggression of the superego is now directed against the id and to a much lesser degree, against the ego.

In other words, the incorruptible superego with which we provide the cured patient, when confronted with a repressed id wish, simply says "No," and that is final. The only outlet for the wish then is sublimation or harmless un-neurotic repression, or dreams, which are quickly forgotten and harm no one.

The poet H. Heine once made a bitter remark about a dying tyrant:

"Lächelnd scheidet der Tyrann,
Denn er weiss, nach seinem Tode
Wechselt Willkür nur die Hände
Und die Knechtschaft hat kein Ende."

There is no translation of this stanza. Loosely translated, it means: "The tyrant dies with a smile; he knows only too well that after his death tyranny changes hands only and slavery has no end." Perhaps something similar takes place with the very adaptable superego, a quality of adaptability of our conscience till now overlooked. The dying *neurotic* superego receives some consolation from the fact that its successor, the *normal* superego will be not less severe. From the nursery to the grave the tyranny of the superego is maintained and its continuity unbroken. Only its methods change.

We see, therefore, that the superego receives recompense and consolation in two ways, at the beginning and at the end of analysis. And what happens in between? It is difficult to isolate different phases in the metamorphosis of the superego, since they are, during the working-through process, interwoven in the Gordian knot of transference, resistance, and repetitiveness. For a long time the superego is our enemy, except for the unforeseen and involuntary help it gives us in the beginning. Very soon the old business of appeasing and bribing with pain and unhappiness is resumed, and the sense of depression even deepens. I would like to stress this well-known fact, which confronts us with such difficulty, since the patient and the environment hold analysis responsible for this increase of depression. This depression, strangely enough, has never been broken down into its components. Neurotic depression appears in the unconscious ego—indeed, it is a mechanism produced exclusively there—but the inner reasons for it and its genetic origin are different. We can distinguish seven forms of this depression, as enumerated in Ch. 1 (pp. 31–32).

The differentiation and working-through of these seven elements of neurotic depression in analysis is of paramount importance.

The working-through process has, therefore, very contradictory results. On the one hand, it strengthens the superego's instruments of torture; on the other hand, it lessens the superego's force. A straight line is not visible; the battle line fluctuates constantly. What is visible is that the superego, unable to continue the old neurotic practice of being bribed and appeased, accepts more and more the normal attitude, which, as I pointed out previously, contains certain torture-recompenses.

Summarizing our investigations about the role of the superego in the working-through process, we can state that the transformation of the superego is the decisive point in therapy, next only to the strengthening of the ego. That strengthening of the ego is analytically the most thoroughly explored part of the therapy, as is clearly visible in the results of the Symposium of the International Psychoanalytic Convention in 1936. Since it is so well known—the formula being "Where id was, ego should be" (Freud), I will discuss it no further, not even my own contribution to the problem.[14] To come back to the role of the superego, the factor which decides whether a patient can be cured or will remain, despite analysis, a lifelong neurotic is the potentially *dynamic* or *static* deposition of his feelings of guilt.

3. *Contribution of the unconscious ego to the working-through* process.

Freud mentions in "*Problems of Anxiety*" that three of the five types of resistance encountered in analysis belong to the ego. These three are the transference resistance, the repression-resistance, and resistance to the renunciation of gain through illness. It is therefore to be expected that the ego offers highly concentrated difficulties to our attempt of working-through. The simplest explanation for its offering these difficulties is that the unconscious ego, having created the compromise between id and superego, clings to that modus vivendi. After many bouts and conflicts, the unconscious ego has brought together his two tormentors, and now analysis comes along to destroy that neurotic balance.

The problem of working-through of ego resistance contains another well-known element which has also not been sufficiently stressed, the element of *anger*. We know that every person confronted with a new idea, especially one which affects him affectively, reacts at first with ironic or furious non-acceptance. There are various reasons for that reaction. First of all, his narcissism is offended, narcissism based on the idea that his learning days are over. In other words, to learn something new means unconsciously for the neurotic to be pushed into the passive

[14] For details see Internat. J. of Psychoanalysis, XVIII, Parts 2 and 3, 1937.

situation of being the pupil, and that is exactly what he resents, either narcissistically or as a defence against passivity. To learn something new about one's self is even more distasteful, since everyone considers himself a specialist in psychology in general and super-specialist of his own nature. To this frame of mind the analytic interpretations and reconstructions are a severe blow. They show the individual his complete ignorance of his own motives. The distaste for this enligntenment is so typical that, even in the process of admitting the truth of an interpretation, the patient will declare that the analyst has told him nothing new, since he has always felt the fact in question to be true intuitively. This reduces the analyst to the rôle of able formulator, like a linguist who has mastered the language which others can only stutter. That assertion, "I always felt it myself", is in general interpreted as contributory and evidence of the correctness of an interpretation, whereas in fact it is chiefly a form of narcissistic face-saving. Furthermore, it so often happens that the analyst gives the same interpretation for months without seemingly producing any affective reaction until, by chance, someone in the outer world puts his finger on the same place, when the idea "clicks." One example among many: A patient, a dentist with ejaculatio praecox, was told repeatedly that his whole marital relationship was based on the unconscious wish to disappoint his wife in repetition of the mother-child situation (pseudo-aggressive elaboration of masochism). For a long time he played the game of understanding and not understanding, of accepting and doubting, of ridiculing and deploring his "bad character". One evening he finished his dental appointments half an hour later than he had expected, and was anxious not to detain any longer his wife, who was awaiting to attend a party with him. But he then started some work in preparation for the next day, despite the fact that he could have done it in the afternoon or postponed it until the next morning. At that moment his wife entered his office and asked him indignantly what he was doing. Said she: "Every time I wait for you, you procrastinate and let me wait endlessly." At *that* moment my patient understood what my interpretation meant. We see once more that the patient believes that the analyst is biased; only the psychoanalytically-innocent by-stander is "objective". This non-acceptance of the analytic interpretation shows, not only the patient's distrustfulness, but his unwillingness to give the analyst the pleasure of being right (defense against passivity in the patient).

"An analyst," said an angry patient to me, "poisons the mind of his patients with little doses of what he calls 'interpretations'." The only correct part of that remark is the term "little doses", and that only because we are incapable often of applying big doses. In other words, affective understanding is not a solitary happening but consists of thousands of little incidents. The incident in itself may be forgotten, but a little scar remains.

There are in general two methods by which a neurotic person can learn something affectively:

1. The "*overwhelming experience*", which sweeps away like an explosion all doubts and objections and brings the affected person completely under the dominance of the dramatically superimposed new ego-ideal. Examples are religious or political fanatics, who, confronted with the necessity of digesting or explaining affective facts with which they are suddenly confronted and which they don't understand, resort often to complete submission to a miracle or hero, to whom they succumb because their psychic constitution predisposes them to that type of submission. Persons of that type gladly sacrifice ratio in order to retain at least vestiges of childish omnipotence via identification.

2. The less dramatic, long, tiresome, anger-laden, unheroic "*detail experience*", made up of chronically-repeated small instances. In this case the experience itself is quickly forgotten, since every such event produces a narcissistic lesion without giving even the consolation of a newly-acquired fanatic ego-ideal but, on the contrary, it forces the patient to accept at least partially ratio as the governing force and to renounce his magic omnipotence. There is a contradiction in itself, since affective experience of the detail type has the tendency to evade rational thinking. To draw conclusions from an experience which on the one hand offends the narcissism and on the other hand does not give the consolation of a super-imposed heroic ego-ideal to which one can masochistically submit and with which one can unconsciously identify, leaves the individual terrified with the power of facts, from which he quickly escapes. In other words, despite every affective experience, the ego tries to preserve the infantile megalomania. Since the described

detail-experience in the long run does exactly the opposite, it is painful, unheroic, and unconsoling. One of my patients quoted in this connection the Chinese proverb, "I have to swallow bitterness."

Unfortunately, the patient's analytic experiences, attained via the working-through process, are of the second, the unheroic type. Basically they involve the fight between pleasure and reality principles (Freud). As long as possible the child in the neurotic clings to the phantasy of childish megalomania. Therefore, we have no specific reason to be surprised that these detail-experiences must be repeated endlessly and are interrupted by long stretches of coldness, boredom, and anger.

Analysis is basically the last attempt to force the reality principle on an adult child. It achieves its goal through a summation of these affective unheroic detail-experiences. Each of these experiences offends the childish megalomania, the basis of the pleasure-principle. For example: A patient tries to provoke the analyst's anger in the transference. The analyst disappoints him by showing him, a) what he repeats, b) how he is fooling himself about his real motives, c) that the analyst will not play his game by becoming angry, and d) that the patient hopes to achieve masochistic pleasure. The disappointment is not only of libidinous aggressive elements but also of megalomaniac ones. The result is that the patient represses the whole distasteful experience. "You cannot blame one for trying" is the formula for his next attempt. It is a long, long rebellion.

Another problem, however, is also involved, the problem of the *detail* itself. I personally believe that the unconscious personality in general and the neurotic one in particular are incapable of learning except through detail-experiences. There are only quantitative differences between neurotics and normal persons in that respect. Why is it so? First of all, it can be remarked that the adult's position toward details is full of contradictions. On the one hand, he is highly impressed by the ability to draw broad and correct conclusions from details, as found, for instance, in the great diagnostician or the great detective. On the other hand, the intelligent adult has in general a kind of contempt for exaggeration of details, demanding a proper sense of proportion and a broad point of view. An example of this is found in the ridicule heaped upon a certain woman patient, who, when asked her psychologic impression of the play, "Hamlet", which she had just seen for the first time, remarked that the actor who played Hamlet must have been left-handed, since he always held the skull in his left hand in the churchyard scene.

Psychoanalysis has complicated the problem of details by proving what important conclusions may be deducted from minutiae, as proven in Freud's "Psychopathology of Everyday Life". We can speak of the "rehabilitation of detail" through analysis. Incidentally, Stendhal hit intuitively upon the importance of details even before analysis, declaring, "Il n'y a d'originalité et de verité que dans les détails."

Taking into account the "rehabilitation of the detail" through analysis, we can state that details are conclusive insofar as they give hints of the situation as a whole. They may be indicative, but on the other hand, may be misused for incorrect and neurotic conclusions. The story told by a well-known neurologist comes to my mind to illustrate the difference: A stingy patient had to have a lumbar puncture, which was performed with great skill. "What do I owe you, Doctor"? he asked. "Fifty dollars", was the answer. "What! Fifty dollars for five minutes' work"! exclaimed the patient indignantly. "You are mistaken," answered the doctor, "For five minutes work one dollar; for knowing where to stick the needle—forty-nine dollars."

To clarify the terminologic question concerning details: We know that there are *no* details as such for the neurotic person as far as his conflict is concerned. For him the socalled detail represents the concentration and incarnation of all of his problems. The patient, of course, prefers to call something a detail and wants to contrast it to the "greater problem". He also may use terms like "bagatelle", "trifle", or "nonessential". I am using the term "detail" to denote the difference between the perception of a situation in its objective importance and the patient's personal aspect. The patient's personal aspect is his only experience laden with emotions. For obvious reasons, the patient prefers to dwell upon his psychic *microcosmos* as a kind of hide-out. What he is actually hiding is the conclusive interconnection between his microcosmos and his most disliked *macrocosmos.* I repeat: I use the term "detail" only in a *linguistic* sense, in order to distinguish between the entire situation (Gesamtsituation), which is inaccessible to the patient from the affective level, and the emotionally-charged detail-situation.

The adult's approach toward details is the purified result of many repressions, and we encounter it mainly as resistance in analysis, without explaining why *affective experience must go through the channels of details.* This phenomenon is explainable only if we go back to the child's psychologic reaction toward disappointment. We know that the child is apt to draw far-reaching affective, *general* conclusions from little incidents. For instance, a child of 3 or 4 years, confronted with a specific disappointment or reproach, reacts with a *general* feeling of hatred. The child does not react as an adult would, with the attitude, "I like you in general but dislike your behavior in this particular instance." The child's reaction is immediately a generalized, though transitory one, and involves, as P. Federn would say, the whole ego. Here we meet with a seemingly hopeless impasse. If the child's tendency toward *affective generalization* is correctly observed, our difficulty is increased in explaining why, on the other hand, every affective experience in analysis must go through the *channels of details,* in a repetition of the childhood experiences. We might assume that in that specific point psychic development stops in childhood, an assumption which cannot be so, since we see that not too neurotic persons, sometimes euphemistically called "normal" persons, are in one at least quantitatively higher degree capable of acknowledging not only detail experiences. Since that solution does not satisfy, we have to find some *specific* reason for the neurotic's clinging to detail experiences.

I am not ashamed to admit that it has taken me years to understand that contradiction in the "*theory of details*". I have finally arrived at the following solution. It is true that the child draws *generalized* affective conclusions from *specific* disappointments. What is overlooked, however, is that his feeling of guilt is immediately mobilized against that generalized conclusion, since the persons toward whom these negative feelings are directed are mother and father and their representatives. Consequently, the child is torn between the generalized "I hate you" and the superego reproach, "Mother is good to you in general; you should love her even if she disappointed you in this instance." The child's aggression, mobilized through the mother's offense against his omnipotence, wants to assert itself *despite* that feeling of guilt. Consequently the ego *must magnify and deepen the specific disappointing detail* to prove its case. Since the specific detail is thus used as defense against a superego reproach, it is increased out of proportion. The child clings to his *specific* disappointment, showing it obstinately and using the formula: "You can say what you want; that small disappointment was *real*." *In this way the detail becomes the basis and pattern of every affective experience.*[15]

I regret to bother the reader with such a complicated detail as the "theory of details", but I sincerely believe that without understanding the problem of details, the working-through process is theoretically unintelligible. I suspect that the "theory of details" presented here has even clinical importance. In a few stagnant cases of endless repetition in which I applied it, the results were surprising: *The feeling of guilt was increased.* I don't dare to be more specific on that point because of lack of sufficient experience with regard to it; but I have the impression that the practical application will give us a powerful new weapon for the discontinuance of neurotic repetitions in seemingly "hopeless" cases. Of course, it does *not* substitute for the regular "working-through"; it is simply a device to be applied with working-through and after all attempts of working-through have failed.

To return to the practice of working-through, it is a frequent mistake of beginners to be proud in the first months of analysis that the patient *seemingly* accepts affectively the analytic interpretations in a specific case. The patient speaks in the language of the analyst. This is a positive transference-mirage which changes overnight if the negative transference appears. Some analysts are *so* eager to find affective response that they sometimes forget what they otherwise know only too well—that every patient goes through a whole series of transference phenomena, playing the whole scale of his repetition-repertoire. For instance, a patient accepts interpretations in order to be loved; he rejects them if he hates in the transference-disappointment. On the other hand, he rejects obvious interpretations when he is afraid of the analyst, the device being positive transference under negative disguise. One form of pseudo-acceptance is especially difficult to discover: The patient

[15] One could object to so "circuitous" a deduction by simply stating that the child's conflicts are "small fry", anyway. This argument is wrong. It is true, of course, that the child's conflicts *appear* to the adult to be ridiculous detail-conflicts, but not so to the child himself. Analysis has proven the old idea of "small child—small conflicts" to be erroneous, emphasizing the fury and vehemence of conflicts in childhood. Every fury of which the adult is capable is but an attenuation of childhood fury.

accepts, seemingly affectively, interpretations on a narcissitic-love basis. His formula is as follows. "I know you don't love me because you don't love anybody but yourself. I am like you—love me"! [16]

Some colleagues have the strange idea that the repetition of feeling in itself in the transference is the curing factor. Of course, such a nonsensical proposition was never published, but in continued analyses one sees that that idea is sometimes represented. These colleagues have, as one could call it, the *cafeteria idea* of analysis. There is no self-service in psychoanalysis; we know that the repetition in the transference is only a special case of the transference-addiction (to use Ferenczi's phrase) of neurotics in general. The difference is that we interpret and utilize these affective repetitions, using interpretations and the working-through mechanism. If the repetition of feeling *per se* would be helpful, there would be no need of paying an analyst; the patient projects his conflicts anyway, in the outer world and, more, he spends his life with that affective repetitiveness. These colleagues remind me of the old story of the surgeon who believed the operation to be over when he had washed his hands in preparation for it. Since I have encountered that queer assumption in the continuation of three analyses, I find it worth mentioning. As a representative example of that fallacy, I might mention the case of a patient with psychogenic oral aspermia, treated first by a colleague in another country. The patient was told that he was to tell everything which he had on his mind. He did this for some time, while the analyst remained as silent as the Sphinx. The patient was orally regressed, and repeated in the transference his pre-oedipal oral-refusal. Since the analytic technique required the patient to *give* words and the patient's speciality was unconscious *refusal*, visible in his withholding of sperm in his aspermia, the result was that his conflict increased. He grew more and more despondent, forced himself to talk, since he believed that the talking in analysis would affect the cure, and became finally highly agitated. Every analytic appointment was "hell", as he put it. One day he sent his wife to the analyst for information, saying, "He does not tell me anything; perhaps you can get something out of him." The analyst explained to her that the patient was making excellent progress, since, to quote him "he is so angry with me." That fury was linked with working-through,

[16] See my study "Plagiarism," Psychoan. Bewegung, 1932.

which was explained to the woman as a simple mounting of fury. In other words, the cafeteria idea once more.

Another misuse of the correct working-through process consists of wasting time. A few patients have reported that in previous analyses the analyst would remain silent, as usual, and would interrupt the patient only at the end of the appointment, simply to announce that the patient had wasted time, since all of his so-called associations in the last 50 minutes—there must be magic in that number—were worthless. Or, if the patient was silent all of the while, the analyst would inform him at the end that his refusal to speak was a sign of resistance. One wonders if these correct observations could not have been made earlier. The whole problem of silence on the part of the analyst, and especially on the part of the patient as resistance, cannot be discussed here; I give an account of that problem in my paper, "On the Resistance Situation: The Patient is Silent".[17]

To return to the subject of the correct use of the working-through process, the term, "affective acceptance" of an interpretation should be used, in my opinion, only after the patient has exhausted all of his repetition-repertoire and even that repeatedly. In other words, affective understanding and the approaching end of a successful analysis are more or less synonymous.

The element of anger, mentioned before, comes to the fore even in the last stages of analysis. Some patients behave in this transitory phase as if they had been deprived of something. "I feel cheated out of something," complained a patient of mine in this situation.

We see that for a long time in analysis the neurotic ego behaves like a *trapped animal*, which, forced from one corner, seeks another seemingly ad infinitum. One day the neurosis collapses.

Until now I have been speaking of the ideal analytic situation. The analyst knows what he is talking about, understands the case and the level of libidinous-aggressive development to which the patient has regressed, or on which he is fixated, and applies correct, that is, dynamically effective interpretations and reconstructions. We know that this situation is often found. Often, however, in a specific case, the analyst does not conform to these three indispensable conditions. An unfortunate but typical example is the case of the orally-regressed

[17] Psychoanalytic Review, 1937.

patient who is treated by the analyst as an hysteric neurotic. When the patient "doesn't give in," the analyst, not realizing that he is on the wrong track, blames lack of sufficient working-through for the failure. We must, therefore, distinguish precisely between *legitimate* and *illegitimate* use of the working-through process. That process is often used as an excuse and a scapegoat for the analyst's own insufficiencies.

The working-through process is disappointing to the patient, not only in the length of time it requires, but also in the amount of cooperation it asks of him. Every patient harbors the naïve idea that analysis should be some kind of automaton: You throw in a few dollars every appointment, push a button, and health or at least "progress" neatly wrapped falls out. He regards the need of his cooperation indignantly, since he believes the analyst should do all of the work for which he is paid. On the other hand, in certain phases of analysis he regards every contribution of the analyst indignantly, too, considering him a parrot who always repeats the same thing. Since the unconscious wishes in a specific case can be reduced to a few elements and only the defences and resistances are manifold, the analyst must discover these few wishes in their manifold disguises during the working-through process. The patient, far from understanding that it is senseless to blame the translator for the repetitious and unimaginative contents of the book he translates, turns the tables and accuses the analyst of his lack of imagination.

What about cases in which, despite sufficient and extensive working-through, a matter of long duration, at best, the patient does not change? First, we have to admit that we cannot cure all of our patients. Furor therapeuticus is not less dangerous than therapeutic nihilism. When, after two, three, or four years of correct working-through of the correct—mind you, correct!—interpretations and interpretations of resistance, the patient has not changed, we must admit the hopelessness of the situation. Often, however, the analyst makes of such a case a narcissistic sanctuary. He will not admit his defeat. He will not even send the patient to another analyst, a procedure to which many colleagues and myself adhere. In my opinion, that should be followed as a matter of course in the event of such a standstill, since the possibility cannot be excluded that the analyst's personality or his failure to detect the problem in the specific case may be responsible for the failure.

Instead, he continues the analysis, with some illusions, every passing year making the situation more hopeless. We know through Freud that the element of time is not represented in the unconscious. However, that disregard of time is overdone, it seems to me, when applied to analysis, which, unfortunately, must be measured also in terms of that commodity. The prolongation of these hopeless analyses is dangerous, not only because it pushes some analysts into an unjustified therapeutic pessimism, some being really haunted by unsuccessful cases or the memory of them, but also because, and this is more important, it results, without the analyst's volition, in making of the patient a propagandist against analysis. To admit defeat after "only" four years of treatment seems to be a rare analytic virtue.

What is going on theoretically in these hopeless cases? The patients do understand thoroughly the interpretations; they indulge no less thoroughly in all of their repetition-repertoire in the transference; and still they make no progress. Something is missing, and that missing factor is *not* that of sufficient working-through. In certain phases every analytic patient misuses analytic interpretations for his masochistic and resistance purposes. But these hopeless cases make of a transitory phase a permanent one. They simply express pre-analytic conflicts in analytic language and believe that they are doing enough. They are not; they are simply playing with unassimilated words. They continue the old conflicts in a new language, which, since it does not penetrate, is meaningless. In other words, when the strong push stemming from the superego is not dynamically visible, nothing can be achieved. The deposition of the feeling of guilt is static instead of dynamic. The old appeasing of the superego with depression, pain, and unhappiness continues—ad infinitum. When the vicious circle between neurotic wish and neurotic punishment is frozen, so to speak, and the feeling of guilt cannot be mobilized, even the best analysis is powerless. Two additional factors for therapeutic failure might also be mentioned. One is the unconscious feeling of magic omnipotence which every neurotic enjoys. I am of the opinion that many an analysis fails because we are not capable of destroying that childlike sense of omnipotence.[18] The other is the unconscious repetition com-

[8] See my contribution to the Symposium on Theory of Therapy, XIVth Int. Psychoan. Convention, Int. Journ. Psycho-an., 1937, and my paper, "Thirty Years

pulsion, which in unsuccessful cases remains fully under the influence of the id, whereas in successful cases it is "libidinized",[19] as Nunberg says. Those who are interested in these complicated factors are referred to Freud's "*Beyond the Pleasure Principle.*"

Working-through is often connected by the patient with *masochistic misuse* of that process. Frequently the patient is incapable of bearing that prolonged process without using it for purposes of self-torture. The typical outburst, "I am a hopeless case," must be analyzed in the same way as a symptom and not, as is often done, countered with suggestive reassurances.

Boredom is even more often associated with working-through. I cannot go into that problem here, since it implies a study of boredom.[20] True, in every analysis comes the moment when both physician and patient are "fed up" with the constant repetition of the material. That is rather a good sign. One has to console oneself that two persons coming together for therapeutic reasons have not the object of amusing each other.

After Ferenczi's Formulation of the Stages of the Reality Sense," Psychoanalytic Review, Vol. 32, No. 2, 1945.

[19] See Nunberg's contribution to the Symposium, Int. Z. F. Psychoan., 1937, p. 64.

[20] "On the Disease Entity Boredom (Alysosis) and Its Psychopathology." Psychiatric Quarterly, 1944, No. 3.

5

Orality and the Myth of the Superior Male

ONE OF THE results in my own mind of the "Breast Complex in the Male", published in 1933,[1] has been a re-evaluation of man's psychologic development. If the premise corresponds to observable facts, namely that the male child overcomes the trauma of weaning via Freud's "unconscious repetition compulsion," leading to *active* repetition of *passively* endured experience (in order to overcome a lesion in narcissism), then the typical male's "superior" and supercilious attitude towards women corresponds to what is really a frantic defense mechanism. The identification of breast and penis has been well established in analysis; the "unconscious repetition compulsion" not less widely publicized; still nobody has connected both facts. This had been done in the Breast Complex. The resultant claim was that the male child denies via identification of breast = penis the narcissistic wound of the offense inflicted upon infantile megalomania: instead of being the *passive* recipient of milk, it becomes the *active* dispenser of urine (later sperm). The child borrows strength via identification with the pre-oedipal mother.

Years later, these ideas were amplified when I wrote a book entitled *The Hoax of the He-Man.* The fate of this book shows the extent of the emotional dynamite involved in the problem: not only did it not find a publisher, but the reactions of the rejecting editors could be subdivided into distinct classes:

a) deeply offended neurotic he-men. These people were furious and angrily objected that no proof has been submitted that women are "superior" to men. My objection that this was not intended at all, only man's shaky foundation clarified, was emotionally rejected.

b) deeply offended neurotic he-women. These career women would

[1] "Der Mammakomplex des Mannes" (in coll. with L. Eidelberg), Int. Ztschr. f. Psa., 1933, No. 4.

never admit to what they were really doing: subjugating their husbands. Since man's inner weakness is woman's best kept secret, these hypocritical ladies shouted: "What, one child more in the family—the husband? No, thanks!"

c) enthusiastic aggressive shrews who misunderstood the deduction as giving them ammunition in their neurotic fight against the species man. Being somewhere conscious of the emotional background, they, too, did not dare to accept the book.

Well, the poor He-Man finally did see printer's ink—though in simplified form. In my book *Divorce Won't Help* (Harper, 1948) one of the chapters is called *The Myth of the Superior Male,* and contains the essentials.

Once more, the whole tragicomedy of the neurotic gamut, cloaked in emotionalism, ran its course. The book received in general excellent reviews; but what interests us in this connection is the reception which greeted the He-Man. For the most part, he was overlooked; few of the reviewers seem to have noticed him. Those who did, were either surprised, without commenting, or they were fighting mad. Especially a few female reviewers objected. To quote:

"For people who want to measure their normalcy Dr. Bergler writes: 'A simple yardstick for recognizing lack of neurosis is the ability to work, to love (tenderly and with normal potency retained), to have normal social contacts and interests, to enjoy one's hobbies.'

"This seems a good yardstick, except for Dr. Bergler's definition of 'tender love.' To show a patient that there is 'more to love than sexual pleasure,' he tells him, 'the lover's ego-ideal which he has projected on his beloved, is, after all, nine-tenths self-love. His over-evaluation of his beloved is simply narcissism, self-love in projection.'

"That is to say, you never selflessly love a person, never wish him to develop the best that is in him for the sake of his own fine qualities. . . . ."

In other words, narcissism was misconstrued as meaning "selfishness," and emotional difficulties which are embedded in man's make-up, as lack of "true partnership." [2]

Another female reviewer used my book for straightening out her

[2] For theory of tender love see my paper (in collaboration with Dr. L. Jekels) "Transference and Love." Imago, 1934.

unsettled accounts with analysis, and provided her readers with specific advice on how to resist in analysis. Besides, she had this to say about the He-Man:

"Feminine readers must now ask themselves: Do we *want* men to know what fools we make of them? What will happen to our real power if the psychoanalysts begin exposing it as the ideal state of things, to be known as 'tender love' and achieved at great expense of *Angst* and money on the psychoanalytic couch? Dr Bergler, who anticipates a future of great marital clinics when 'the psychiatrist's service will be taken for granted in the same way that the dentist's is today,' may even be defeating his purpose by writing too many books (this is his sixth). For $3 a wife can stay home and feel even more tenderly toward her great infantile boob of a husband than she does already."

To put a little more unconscious irony into her conscious high-pitched irony, the lady invokes Freud as witness for her resistance against Freud's psychoanalysis. The trick is old, but seems to convince some people in an acute anti-analytic conflict: by admiring the *dead* Freud, and spitting at his *living* pupils, the proof is given that no resistance toward analysis (meaning personal conflicts) is involved: unfortunately, the only trustworthy analyst is—dead. Stephan Zweig did something similar in his essay on Freud; [3] this did not rescue Zweig, though, from neurotic suicide. Obviously, it is easier to misuse printed paper than to convince the more recalcitrant unconscious.

But what counts are facts, and not emotional rejection pointed by irony, misunderstanding or anger. Even reviewers will find out what Voltaire knew long ago, "A witty saying proves nothing."

And these painful and stubborn facts do indicate that man is the weaker, woman the stronger sex. This is not only psychologically true, biologic facts point in the same direction. To adduce a statement from Boyd's famous *Pathology:*

> There is a higher mortality for the male throughout all periods of life. This cannot be explained away, as is commonly done by references to overwork, industrial hazards, abuse of alcohol and tobacco, venery, etc. for the difference in the sex mortality is most striking in intra-uterine life and during the first years of childhood. There appears to be an inherent weakness in the male, a sex-linked inferior-

[3] Here the excuse was that Freud was too busy to analyze all neurotics.

ity, so that by comparison with the female he is a weakling at all periods of life from conception to death. This holds true throughout the animal kingdom, the males being shorter-lived. As Allen remarks, the price of maleness is weakness, and the woman is far from being "the weaker vessel."

The pre-oedipal phase (though many people seem not to remember that Freud described that phase in 1931), proves that the first relationship of the human being is that between himself and a woman. That fact alone puts the male at a disadvantage: years later, he will have to play "big shot" with the image of a person who changed his diapers, witnessed his potty actions, his first attempt at crawling on all fours! The objection that the woman (or succession of women—we live in the age of one divorce to three marriages!), the now grown-up baby will have to impress, is not identical with mother and nurse, is only superficially correct. For the inner personality, the identity not of objects but images of the genus woman, remains an entity. And if the candidate for He-Man has good-sized neurotic depositions, the wife will be but a continuation of the triangle: mother—nurse—female teacher. In passing, I draw attention to the fact that Dorothy Parker's dictum: "Men seldom make passes at girls who wear glasses," may be using the image of the traditional schoolteacher as a prototype for the girls who wear glasses.

There are basically two possibilities: the boy can accomplish an identification with the *image* of the "*kind, giving* mother." Then he will give freely—tenderness, love, money. Or, he performs neurotically the identification with the *image* of the "*bad refusing* mother", to whom he becomes masochistically attached, then he will be forced to erect inner pseudo-aggressive defenses and *refuse* freely—tenderness, love, money. He will become a masochistic injustice collector and live on the basis of layer II of the "mechanism of orality."

Of course, psychic development does not stop on the oral level. The neurotic He-Man will try to reach the oedipal level only to be pushed back in his regression to the oral Styx.[4]

This reversal of rôles (*parasitic baby—giving mother*) explains a series of facts always taken for granted. For instance:

[4] See Chapter I.

How is the transition between parasitic baby and "*family provider*" accomplished?

Or: Why do men consider women "inferior"—isn't the *penis pride but a defense* against the more deeply repressed breast envy?

Or: Why is the male objection against *woman's equality* so vociferous?

Or: Why does the typical man call his wife "*baby*"?

Or: Why has the typical man such an inner need for *deprecation* of housework and *cooking?* Isn't his rejection a reminder of early nutritional dependence?

Or: Why does the He-Man consider his wife a *parasite* for whom he works himself to death?

And so forth, and so forth.

The most important fact, emerging for man's life as residue of the pre-oedipal phase of the "breast complex," is the desperate rescue attempt into the anal and phallic phase. Having carried his oral passivity into anal passivity with a few autarchic attempts,[5] the boy plunges head on into the oedipal phase. Here, a triple *disclaimer of passivity* is possible:

(1) Father does something "terrible" to mother—mother on the receiving passive end.

(2) The mother of the oedipal time isn't dangerous at all—she is castrated; hence no reason to be frightened of the "septet of the baby fears" pertaining to the "pre-oedipal mother."

(3) The oedipal mother is a duplica of the baby's passivity: mother is passively penetrated by the penis (as once upon a baby time the baby's mouth has been "penetrated" by the nipple), the active doing in this penetration is done by father.

By identifying and borrowing strength from father, the boy reduces the oedipal mother to an image of his own passive self. The triumphant reversal is perfect!

But the grandiose borrowing of strength from father collapses, too: the oedipus complex is, as Freud proved, shattered by the castration complex. Hence, passivity is reinforced.

The amazing fact remains that the child has borrowed inflated strength twice: first from mother, later from father. This wholesale

[5] See Chapters I and II.

borrowing did not solve his problems, but as sham it remains paradigmatic for a lifetime. The child first uses identification with mother as *crutch;* later, it uses exactly that crutch as *stick*—to beat up on the "weak woman": he feels superior in his penis-pride! That the latter is but a defense, is easily eradicated from memory.

The whole irony of the superior male is visible in the last years of life. In the late forties and early fifties, typical organic diseases start to manifest themselves. Whether the husband is advised to avoid overexcitement (bloodpressure), or stop strenuous sport, or observe a diet, or abstain from alcohol or smoking (heart) or sweets (diabetes), his wife takes over the execution of the doctor's orders. Observe the man in that situation and you see a child-like and not mature attitude: the infantile cheating starts all over again. There is seldom mature resignation and adaptation to reality factors discernible. The man who shouldn't drink does so behind his wife's back. The man who must stop smoking seems to believe that his enemy is not the coronary disease but his wife who refuses the cigars. In short: He-Man pushes his wife once more into the situation of the refusing mother! He-Man, your name is irony!

The poor He-Man actually lives above his emotional means; his superiority rests on a conspiracy of inner negation. I consider that fact of paramount importance for the understanding of man, the "glory and the shame of the universe," to quote Pascal.

I shall not be surprised if even serious scientists should call the description of the hoax of the He-Man "feministic" and un-Freudian. Yet science, including psychoanalysis, is not static but dynamic. Since the majority of people (including the so-called scientists) think statically, one has, if one mingles with them, to be prepared for every objection from the arsenal of static thinking.

6

Twenty-Seven Clinical Pictures of Oral Regression

THE VARIETY of clinical pictures encountered in oral regression is extensive and at first glance confusing.

The sheer number of orally regressed people is amazing. *I have the impression that the bulk of neurotics has a rendezvous with orality.* That undigested orality prevents people from making the grade in more superficial neuroses, not to mention relative normalcy.

Imagine a closely guarded border. Many want to escape, few accomplish the aim. All those who are sent back remain inside the hated border. No wonder that the mass of those who remain is an incongruous company. They have only one thing in common: they cannot pass the border, though they want to escape. Even many of those who do escape are later returned—by force. In this mass of unsuccessful emigrants are all shades and types of people. That accounts for the different pictures they present.

To complicate matters, the reality of a neurosis never corresponds to simplifications of textbooks. Every neurotic presents a composite picture. The skill of the therapist has to find the main problem which makes the patient "tick and click." The danger of being dragged into dead ends and camouflaged side-roads is great. To find and to find quickly, for that matter, the "main switch"—is the decisive point.

1. The Oral Character-Neurosis

The orally regressed personality is characterized by dominance of the "mechanism of orality" with its triad. These neurotics are chronic "*injustice-collectors*," running around with a great assortment of "chips on the shoulder." Unconsciously, they are constantly provoking a "kick in the jaw." Having thus utilized the ever ready aggression of the other fellow (whether the latter's aggression is real or compensatory does not matter), they feel "terribly abused," and fight, seemingly in justified self-defense (their own initial provocation being thoroughly repressed) and "righteous indignation," the self-constructed enemy. As a final act, they pity themselves consciously, once more oblivious of the fact that they smuggle in a good sized portion of psychic masochism in that self-commiseration. If one listens to them, such terrible injustices can happen only to them—the poor and innocent victims of other peoples' meanness.

Oral personalities are in general pessimists. Insofar as they appear to be optimistic, they apply their hopeful expectations in the wrong place—only to be even more deeply disappointed by the outcome.

From time to time, they utilize "magic gestures," in mute dramatization of how badly they were treated, whereas they themselves are so "nice."

Oral personalities are strangely unappreciative: if you do them a good turn, they take it for granted. They wake up—so to speak—only when they complain.

They are inwardly *submissive* when confronted with a "*stronger*" person (meaning one capable of kicking them); strangely *cruel* with a person *weaker* than themselves. That dichotomy is once more at first glance confusing: it represents but a defensive cover. Constantly accused by their inner conscience of passivity, they reverse the rôles, making a show of alibis—hence in the "cruel edition" the proof is submitted "I hate passivity . . ." Another confusing phenomenological aspect is the "provocative technique" of psychic masochists which should not be put in the same basket with "real" aggression.

Phenomenologically, they represent contradictory types: from the cold, taciturn, reticent type, to the easily excitable, logorrhoeic, "boiling over" complainer. Inwardly, all of them complain: the facade is different.

The *sex life* of these sick people is very frequently disturbed: they are either refusers in sex, or suffer from premature ejaculation or aspermia. The female of that species is typically frigid: mother (projected upon the exchangeable man) "refuses" her pleasure. It is practically impossible to live in peace with them: with great ingenuity they will ferret out the weak spot and provoke long enough until they cash in on their badly needed "injustice." The *marriage* partners of these people are either a reduplication of themselves: another "injustice collector" is chosen unconsciously. Or, in rarer cases, the partner is chosen after the principle of an alibi; then the mate is provoked so long until he (or she) provides the necessary amount of injustices.

The *inner motto* of these neurotics is: *"Please give my daily dose of injustice."*

Frequently combinations with one or more of the symptoms and types described in the following pages are encountered.

It is of prime importance for the understanding of orally regressed personalities to keep in mind that *these sick people live psychologically on the basis of their pet-defense: pseudo-aggression.* Hence these neurotics frequently impress the naive observer as being "aggressive." That aggression is, however, only defensive pseudo-aggression. The "aggressive" refusal covers the *defense against the masochistic wish to be refused.* Of course, one cannot expect the wife of such a neurotic to understand that his refusal in sex is—a defense. For her, the aggression in being refused sex, money and tenderness is real enough. The same holds true for the husband when confronted with a sexually refusing wife.

Typically, these neurotics harbor what I call an *"elastic fraud corner"* in their psychic make-up. Basically, it is the old megalomaniacal idea of "being an exception," as Freud named it in another connection. Having suffered so much, such an "exception" can allow himself to cut the corners with respect to the usual moral requirements. The "fraud corner" is elastic and leads sometimes to rather fantastic stretching, which, in turn, produces masochistic results.

The general *mood* of oral neurotics is gloomy pessimism—by projecting the "cruel, bad mother" of their distorted fantasy outward, they expect the worst. The camouflage, though, is sometimes extensive. If one scratches the surface, *psychic diapers* are invariably encountered.

Oral neurotics are frequently misjudged as—parasites. That confusion arises from taking at face value the *defensive* "wish to get," covering the deeper repressed craving for "being refused." The clinical proof is simple: were the wish to get solid, these neurotics could be satisfied by achieving their aim. They are *not:* they *always* feel refused.[1]

[1] For elaboration, see "Samuel Johnson's 'Life of the Poet Richard Savage'—A Paradigm for a Type," first published in American Imago IV, 4, 1947.

2. Premature Ejaculation

K. Abraham's classic study explained ejaculatio praecox so convincingly that with few exceptions further studies have not even been attempted. The strange thing in Abraham's results has been that further investigations simply had to confirm his findings though they showed that a deeper motivation is hidden behind the facade, correctly observed by Abraham.

I believe [2] that the deepest layer in premature ejaculation is the masochistic wish to be refused. To counteract that conflict, the defensive layer of pseudo-aggression is reinforced. In unconscious identification of penis-breast, sperm-urine-milk, vagina-mouth, they "*spill the milk before it can reach the mouth.*" Moreover, these psychic masochists with a vengeance counteract the secondary reproaches of inner conscience, pertaining to pseudo-aggression, too, by the secondary inner alibi: "I don't want to refuse, I give *immediately*." But this precipitated ironic "giving" is a mockery of giving, since as a result the woman cannot derive pleasure in the sex act without the amount of necessary frictional movement, which, of course, is lacking in these neurotics.

If one is not familiar with the pseudo-aggression of these neurotics, and interprets in analysis mainly the "hostility" towards the woman, the analysis *must* fail.

One has to admit that the pseudo-aggression of these neurotics is very impressive—at first glance and to the uninitiated. Here are a few examples.

A man 54 years of age entered analysis, apparently because of an "actual conflict." Although he held a very good business position, he had started a liaison with the sister of a charwoman in his office, which licensed him to inspect and kiss her buttocks and masturbate. He was not restrained from so doing by knowledge of the social difference between them or of the hysteric disposition and loquacity of the woman. Unconsciously, by means of this association, he not only satisfied ex-

[2] See my studies: "Ejaculatio Praecox". Psychiat. an Neurol. Bladen (Amsterdam) 1937.—Ch. IV of my monograph "Psychic Impotence In Men" (Huber, Berne, 1937).—"A Short Genetic Survey of Psychic Impotence" I and II. The Psychiatric Quarterly *19*:3 and *19*:4, 1945.—"Newer Genetic Investigations on Impotence and Frigidity," Bulletin of the Menninger Clinic *11*:2, 1947.

hibitionistic (scopophiliac) tendencies [3] (an affair in the office!), but also apparently hoped for a scandal. When the dénouement was too slow in developing, he unconsciously tried to hasten it. On the last working-day before Christmas, he distributed in the office little presents in public, intentionally passing over the charwoman and her sister. The latter made a public fuss, and went so far as to telephone the patient's wife and tell her all of the details. His wife, 40 years of age, immediately came to his office, called him to account, and threatened to divorce him at once. A family council was hastily summoned, in which were two brothers of the wife, whom the writer had treated years ago. Through their advice, the divorce was postponed and the delinquent was sent to be analyzed "as a punishment." In analysis, the writer found that the patient had suffered from ejaculatio praecox from the days of his puberty, and had had no intercourse with his wife for the past 10 years, substituting for it masturbation. The analysis revealed the patient's oral fixation and defensive fantasy of revenge. He was indignant over having to "give" by supporting his wife and 80-year-old mother, who lived with them. This indignation caused him unconsciously to wish for a situation which would prevent his supporting them. If, because of his liaison, he had been prematurely pensioned, seven years before he could legally claim a pension, his rather high income would have been greatly reduced, thereby forcing the two women whom he unconsciously "hated" (defense against masochistic attachment) to restrict their expenses considerably. In harming them, he did not mind harming himself; indeed, he wanted unconsciously to injure himself as a punishment for his pseudo-aggression. As a matter of fact, in the months preceding his entry into analysis, he had used a means in addition to that of his compromising relation with the charwoman to provoke a severe conflict in his office. He had made a mistake in the very complicated work in which he was an outstanding specialist, for which his firm had had to pay damages. Had he pursued such a course at that time, when the prevailing trend was to cut down expenses, he would very likely have been pensioned before his time.

[3] Exhibitionistic (scopophiliac) tendencies play an important part in all patients troubled with ejaculatio praecox, and are always at the disposal of the patients' *pseudo-aggression*. For details see the writer's previously mentioned essays.

This analysis took place in pre-Hitler Austria where employees of large concerns were entitled to full pension after 35 years of service.

The neurotic attitude of another patient suffering from ejaculatio praecox may serve to illustrate how dominating is the pseudo-aggression of denying as defense against underlying psychic masochism. This man had intercourse only with prostitutes of the lowest type. Asked for the cause of his strange predilection, he replied that he was incapable of spending large sums of money on women. If he happened to hear that he had paid even 20 cents more than was necessary, he became depressed. His greatest pleasure was to cheat a prostitute of money, but since such cheating led invariably to disputes, he had recourse to the following expedient: He would visit the prostitute at 10 a.m., a time at which she was idle. Since prostitutes were most superstitious in this patient's country, and would not allow their first customer to go away for fear they would earn nothing all day, he succeeded with ease in securing intercourse for a "ridiculously cheap" price. The fury of the prostitute at being underpaid was for him "the best part of the whole thing." The fact that he used his ejaculatio praecox only as a means of pseudo-aggression was made especially obvious by one affair. A prostitute to whom he often went praised him one morning for the rapidity with which he had completed the act. "You are finished at once. I call that good. The others take half an hour before they are through," said she. In having intercourse with this prostitute the next time, he experienced his first technically normal, undisturbed intercourse.

The defensive pseudo-aggressive attitude of these neurotics permeates their whole personality: they are refusers, misers, querulous people in every respect. They shift their inner masochism to that pseudo-aggression.

Premature ejaculation has recently received a boost from an unexpected source: Dr. Kinsey does not consider it a disease. Naively, he accepts the rationalization of those neurotics who claim that the symptom is rather a sign of their real sexual excitement, even their alleged superiority. Kinsey's argument (given in a scientific discussion) was rather curious: "Look at the bull!" Thus a "biologically" shaky argument was adduced, which fell flat when I countered "Look at the dog where duration of intercourse is much more protracted."

The analytic prognosis of premature ejaculation is excellent, even in the most severe cases—provided the oral substructure is analyzed.

3. Psychogenic Oral Aspermia

My discovery of the disease entity "psychogenic oral aspermia," started quite appropriately with a clinical observation, a hunch as to its importance, secondary disbelief in the correctness of my deduction, finally, preliminary ironization by experts, to whom I submitted my suspicions.

The beginnings were quite humble: I treated 20 years ago a patient who entered treatment because of blushing, shyness, inability to come in contact with women; he never even attempted intercourse. After working through his feminine identification (negative Oedipus), his scopophiliac tendencies, etc., the patient became potent but did not ejaculate despite prolonged frictions. An organic difficulty could be excluded, because he ejaculated during masturbation and in his wet-dreams. That neurotic symptom has never been described in our literature. I consulted two of my colleagues. The first told me ironically, one should not believe everything a patient reports. Since the symptom of psychogenic aspermia does not exist, the patient was pulling my leg. The second expert informed me that my diagnosis of the case must be wrong: obviously the patient suffered from a severe obsessional neurosis where the symptom of protracted ejaculation is sometimes encountered; the patient's statement that he never ejaculated must be an exaggeration. My insistence that the patient definitely did not suffer from obsessional neurosis, was dismissed as my lack of experience.

That experience taught me that clinical experience in older colleagues frequently means only "to know the known," but not the unknown. It also implies lack of respect for the not yet catalogized coupled with the disparaging remark: Does not exist.

The further "saga" of "psychogenic oral aspermia" can be read in the literature dealing with that strange disease.[4]

[4] Details in "The Psychic Impotence in Men" (ch IV. C). "Some Ejaculatory Disturbances not Hitherto Described," Int. Jour. of Psychoanalysis (London) 1935.

The patient at first achieved intercourse without ejaculating. Being a good observer, he reported the following concomitant circumstance: during protracted intercourse, he developed oversalivation. That symptom convinced me that an "autarchic" oral substitute of ejaculation was installed: he produced and gave himself the fluid and of himself. (The spiteful connotation of spitting was defensive.)

The whole "refusal" of sperm seemed extremely "aggressive." In the identification of penis with maternal breast, and sperm with maternal milk, these people "refuse" to give because they had allegedly been "refused." *It cannot be emphasized enough that this vindictive refusal is a secondary manifestation, cloaking a deep masochistic attachment.*

The patient was finally cured from his aspermia. I heard repeatedly from him; the last time a few months ago. During all these years (nearly 2 decades) the aspermia did *not* return; he is the father of a child.

The next case, I observed, added a detail to the oral substructure: an over-dimensional pseudo-aggression, identifying ejaculation with bursting of a bomb:

An analyst of high standing, who had read my paper on ejaculatory disturbances, sent me a patient, a man of thirty-four, whom he had been treating for the past three years and whose analysis he was now obliged to break off for external reasons. When he began his analysis with my colleague, the patient had been married four years and, with the exception of a few unsuccessful attempts at coitus, he had not had any sort of sexual contact with his wife. The failure was due to his incapacity for erection and to his wife's indifference and repugnance to sexual activities. After four years he decided to be analyzed, because both husband and wife, although they had no desire for intercourse, were very anxious to have a child. My colleague told me that analysis revealed first of all the oedipus fixation and consequent castration anxiety. After only six months of treatment he became capable of erection and "from a sense of duty" he utilized his potency

"Further Observations on the Clinical Picture of 'Psychogenic Oral Aspermia'" Ibid. 1937. "A Short Genetic Survey of Psychic Impotence." The Psychiatric Quarterly 1945. "Newer Genetic Investigations on Impotence and Frigidity," Bulletin of the Menninger Clinic, 1947. (March).

for the defloration of his wife and a few attempts at coitus, but ejaculation was invariably totally absent. Moreover, the impulse to perform coitus, in itself but feeble, died out completely, so that, from the seventh month of analysis to the end of the third year, he was incapable of sexual intercourse. My colleague said that, in spite of two-and-a-half years spent in working through the analytic material, the analysis "stuck," for reasons which are not apparent. After reading my paper on ejaculatory disturbances,[5] however, he surmised that the ejaculatory disturbance had an oral genesis and in the final sessions before the analysis was broken off he indicated this to the patient.

The continuation of the analysis with me provided abundant confirmation of his conjecture: oral defensive hatred of the pre-oedipal mother occupied the foreground. This explained why, after only six months of analysis with my colleague, they had been able to record a partial success: the phallic element in the disturbance of potency had been overcome by correct interpretation and the working-through of the oedipus complex. Of course, it was impossible for interpretation of the phallic and anal elements in that complex to loosen the underlying oral fixations of the pre-oedipal period. The demonstration of the "breast-complex" made a very strong intellectual impression on the patient, but he very soon rid himself of it and skilfully countered my interpretation of orality with my colleague's interpretation, which laid stress on the oedipus complex. This fierce resistance to the interpretation of orality struck even himself as suspicious. In his arguments he constantly recurred to the oedipus complex and made merry over it, saying ironically that, in spite of an analytic interpretation extending over three years, he really had nothing against it. A dream which he had during this phase illustrates his attitude:

He was in a street car with his wife. Suddenly he heard a newspaperboy crying a special edition. He got out, bought a paper and threw it away in a fury when he found it contained nothing of any interest whatever. Wishing to go on with his journey, he got into a taxi, and the driver, instead of taking him to my house, persisted in going in the opposite direction. . . . The patient added that the place

[5] "Some Special Varieties of Ejaculatory Disturbances not Hitherto Described." Int. Journal of Psychoanalysis (London), XVI, 1935.

where he got out was the very point at which his uncle had met with a fatal accident.

The boy selling the special edition was a mocking reference to the second analyst: the patient knew about my paper, which had caused his first analyst to send him to me. The statements which I made there were treated ironically and nullified by means of an allusion to the oedipus complex: he got out at the place where his father's brother died. His ironical suggestion to me was: "You had better pay attention to my wishes for my father's death, which have made me ill, and not bother about your stupid 'new discoveries,' which have as little in them as a fraudulent special edition, the only object of which is to lure people to spend their money." Nevertheless it was clear that his conscience was reproaching him with wanting to shirk the analysis owing to resistance, an accusation which he refuted by pointing out that he *wanted* to have coitus with his wife (riding together in the electric street car), acquitting himself ironically with the reflection: "It is not my fault if the driver (physician) always takes me in the wrong direction." So it is the analyst and not the patient who is to blame for insisting on unimportant interpretations and making the second analysis (as the patient expected) a failure. He thus succeeded in refuting the accusation of his conscience: "You want to give up the analysis because of the oral interpretations," and in fulfilling the wish of his id, namely, to escape from analysis, i.e., to retain his infantile oral wishes for defensive vengeance. In fact, the dream represented a wish-fulfillment *and* refutation of reproaches of conscience.

Jekels and I have proven, in our paper read at the XIII International Psychoanalytic Convention in Luzern,[6] that the "day's residue" has a double meaning: it covers unconscious wishes (Freud) *and* represents a superego reproach. Every dream "runs," according to that conception, on "double rails"; it fulfills unconscious wishes *and* rebuffs the reproaches of the inner conscience. These two apparently banal elements in the dream I have quoted: the "taxi" and the "particular place" at which the patient got out, led to the conclusion that these elements conceal a latent reproach of conscience, for it could not fail to strike us as remarkable that the patient confessed so openly his wish to kill his father, even when we take into account the tendency to divert

[6] Published in Imago, 1934 and Psychoanalytic Quarterly, 1940.

attention from other material. *Qui s'accuse—s'excuse:* this is a truth which is evident in all "genuine" books of Confessions [7] and it is applicable here. Actually, the element "taxi" contained the gravest possible accusation of conscience against the patient's ego, for, in analysis with me, after quite a short time, it became clear (much to his surprise) that the transference in his first analysis was by no means simply a father-transference, as appeared at first sight. He projected on to his first analyst, during three years of treatment, above all, his unconscious fantasy of the bad, phallic mother. In a manner typical of orally regressed neurotics he put the mother in the wrong in the most sweeping fashion, deriving from every injustice which he experienced, i.e., fantasied, the right to commit fresh aggressions and thus establishing a vicious circle. Although my colleague at first objected, the patient had insisted on coming to his analysis at a quarter to eight in the morning, saying that it was his only free time. He annoyed the physician by making him get up unnecessarily early for this morning appointment, and he himself was always late, a fact which the analyst regularly interpreted as resistance. Now it turned out that the patient took a taxi every time, "because it was already so late," although the distance between his house and that of the analyst was so short that in other circumstances he would never have gone to the expense of driving. In a total of nearly seven hundred and fifty sessions he never mentioned this fact, and calmly let the analyst put it to him that it was resistance which manifested itself in his arriving late. The meaning of this behavior was twofold: (1) he revenged himself on the analyst, whom he deprived of sleep, and gratified a pseudo-aggressive impulse

[7] In his *Confessions* (1850) Heinrich Heine makes fun of all confessions in book form, and says about Rousseau: "For instance, I am convinced that Jean Jacques did not steal the ribbon which caused a chambermaid to be unjustly accused and dismissed, costing her her reputation and her situation. . . . Probably there was another offence of which he was guilty, but it was not theft. . . . Nor did he send children of his own to the Foundling Hospital but only the children of Mademoiselle Thérèse Levasseur. Thirty years ago, one of the greatest German psychologists pointed out to me a passage in the *Confessions*, from which it seems certain that Rousseau could not have been the father of those children. The conceited old growler preferred to let himself be thought a barbarous father rather than bear the suspicion that he was altogether incapable of fatherhood." *(Heine's Werke,* Aus. Bong, XV, p. 22).

by "keeping him waiting" (a reversal of the childhood-situation with the mother), and (2) he subtly put the physician in the wrong, thus: "I sacrifice money (the taxi) for you as a proof of love, and, on the top of that, you reproach me instead of praising and loving me." Therefore (this was the corollary of his unconscious reflection) "I have a right to be aggressive." The "trick" lay in causing the analyst, who did not know that the patient was spending money on taxis, always to interpret a proof of love as resistance—a *quid pro quo* contrived by the patient himself by his suppression of material! [8]

The element "taxi" was further determined as follows: The first dream which he reported in his analysis with my colleague and which could not at that point be interpreted contained a declaration of his intention to lead the analyst by the nose. This was symbolized by driving in all possible directions in a taxi. Besides this, motors in general played a prominent part in the patient's thoughts and feelings: he was enthusiastic about driving and said it was one of the few things which he had "mastered perfectly." If any of his relatives lent him their car, they were amazed at his assurance. Driving was one of the few "aggressive" (active) actions which he consciously permitted himself, precisely because it was not recognizable as aggression.

As the analysis went on, it provided abundant confirmation of the conjecture that, in the transference, the patient was reproducing his masochistic relation to the bad, sadistic mother of the pre-oedipal period. For instance, he suddenly remembered that his first analyst used to strike him as being like a spider, sitting behind him and "lying in wait" for everything he might say, although consciously he respected and rather liked this physician.[9] When I asked him if he ever told my colleague about the idea, he said: "No," explaining that it was only in the second analysis that he became really conscious of it since I spoke to him much more than his former analyst and so this impression did not occur so frequently.

[8] Asked why he never told the real truth about his coming late, he appeared taken aback and said it was strange that it had never occurred to him to excuse himself thus. He added that he had not kept anything back on purpose.

[9] The dream I have quoted contains a reversal of this situation: the patient sat behind and directed the driver. There are, besides, unconscious feminine elements here. Lastly, both the driver and his fare represented parts of the dreamer's personality.

The idea of the "devouring spider" (some female spiders devour the males after coitus) was typical of the patient's whole unconscious relation to women. When we reconstructed the period of his early childhood we found that he had always thought of his mother as an aggressive, nagging woman, constantly demanding love and interest, while his father was a quiet, rather weak man, under the thumb of his wife. In later years he engaged in bitter conflicts with his mother because of her inordinate demands on her children's love and respect. For example, she expected her grown-up children, who were no longer living at home, to pay her a long daily visit, and when they explained that there were real difficulties, such as the claims of their work, she indignantly declared that they were simply making excuses. As a young child the patient was ostensibly devoted to her, but in reality he attributed to her every possible bad motive. For instance, when a cousin who lived with them as an adopted child had a fall on a climb in the mountains and, sometime later, the patient's mother in quite another connection blamed him and his sister for not caring to climb, he thought to himself: "Of course, she wants me to have a fall too, simply so that she can brag about how sporting her children are." At the same time he evidently had pangs of conscience about his own unconscious aggressive impulses against his mother, as the following recollection showed. At the time of the food shortage during the First World War, the family was having meat at a certain meal. The mother served the meat and the patient had the impression that his portion was "unfairly" small and he looked covetously at her plate. She, however, misunderstood his glance and said: "Don't trouble about me, I have got enough." This scene is typical and so is the fact that the material for the conflict was oral.

It is not easy in a brief account to convey the impression made by the patient's outward demeanor. I think I can best compare him with a block of ice. There emanated from him a strange indifference and coldness; he was silent, rather morose, very correct and entirely inaccessible, and his "calm" drove those around him frantic. "When other people would explode, you are as calm as ever," his wife used to say to him. She misunderstood this tranquility, not perceiving the aggression behind it, and she summed up her opinion of him as follows: "It's no use talking to you."

The patient displayed the following characteristics which are typical of *all* cases of oral regression:

(1) Adherence to the "*autarchist fiction,*" the disappointment allegedly inflicted by the phallic mother is reacted to with an obstinate struggle for alimentary and general independence.

(2) An incapacity for the normal attempts at restoring the damaged illusion of omnipotence by means of object-relations and love: the sole relation to women consists in an unconscious, aggressive determination to put them in the wrong (that is to say, in *revenge on the mother*) and in an *unconscious, masochistic enjoyment of being unloved.* Secondarily, this relation is extended to everyone with whom the individual comes into contact, irrespective of sex.

(3) The unconscious aim it not to fulfill the wishes but to *perpetuate the disappointments* of childhood (psychic masochism).

(4) The result is "*oral*" pessimism; every situation is unconsciously so arranged as apparently to justify the pessimist's expectations. Through the aggression of others he derives relief from his sense of guilt, and a justification for fresh aggression on his own part—a *vicious circle of psychic masochism.*

(5) The *deepest wish* of persons suffering from oral regression is to be refused. Compare this situation with the normal one. Normally, the early disappointments of weaning are overcome via identification with the phallic mother and *active* repetition of *passive* experiences—what Eidelberg and I called the "breast complex." In our joint work "Der Mammakomplex des Mannes" [10] Eidelberg and I explained that, normally, children master the trauma of weaning by reproducing *actively* what they have experienced *passively,* in accordance with the unconscious repetition-compulsion postulated by Freud. From being the passive recipient of his mother's milk the child becomes the active bestower of urine (later, semen). The purpose of this reversal is that he may free himself psychically from the trauma of weaning and preserve the infantile fiction of omnipotence which was jeopardized. The narcissistic mortification suffered in this very early period continues to act as a stimulus in his unconscious throughout life: even in the coitus of normal men we can detect traces of this attitude. Through identification with the phallic mother the man, in the sexual act, puts the woman in place of the child, i.e., of himself in an early stage of

[10] Int. Z. f. Psychoan., 1933.

development. Ejaculations is equated with the jet of milk and acquires the unconscious significance of a "magic gesture." Thus in coitus we have once more the active repetition of a passive experience, namely, that of the infant at his mother's breast. If the individual fails thus "normally" to surmount the "breast-complex," the penis retains the significance of the breast and neurotic symptoms make their appearance.

Following this line of thought about the "breast-complex," I gave it as my opinion that one of the possible results of a failure to surmount the pre-oedipal, oral mother-fixation is total absence of ejaculation: The penis refuses to perform its normal function: from defensive motives of revenge on the woman (covering masochistic attachment), identified by the patients with the phallic mother, ejaculation (milk—urine) is entirely absent. For in ejaculation they should do psychically precisely that which they assert that the "castrating," phallic mother refused to do for them as lavishly as they wished, namely, to cause a fluid to flow from the breast (penis) into the mouth (vagina).

It is of great importance to understand that the *aggression* displayed in genital refusing of sperm is but a *pseudo-aggressive defense against an inner reproach:* What you really want is to be *refused* so that you can enjoy that refusal masochistically.

In studing the mental processes of our patient let us begin with the technique by which he put in the wrong the woman whom he identified with the phallic mother. The patient had married a virgin with a repugnance to everything sexual. In theory she assented to coitus simply because it was a duty to be "normal." The most harmless acts designed to evoke initial pleasure were repudiated by her as "beastly." Above all, in intercourse she wanted to play the passive part of a woman who is forced by the man. The patient, on the other hand, expected his wife to take the initiative in coitus and to help him, i.e., to stimulate him manually and introduce his penis into her vagina. Thus it came about that for years he abstained from all sexual activities and said not a word on the subject to his wife (oral stubbornness). He interpreted the fact that she "gave" him nothing and refused to seduce him as indicating not merely sexual inexperience but an evil disposition, which led her to refuse from sadistic motives that which he wanted and justified him in letting loose upon her the pseudo-aggressive impulses whose real object was his mother.

Superficially, it looked at first sight as though all this simply amounted to phallic castration-anxiety due to the oedipal mother-fixation. Yet one could not but be struck by his determination to force his wife into the role of the wicked woman who refuses what she should give and especially by the fact that he did nothing to mend matters. Moreover, the patient's passivity was of a different kind from that met with in neurotics of the passive-feminine type, as was apparent in his onanistic practices at puberty. He would fasten various objects, e.g., a toothbrush, a nailbrush, a bath-thermometer, etc., to the *sulcus coronarius* with a piece of string and masturbate by swinging these objects. But he never let himself go to the point of ejaculation. The mechanism was even clearer in another of his habits: he would masturbate by causing a jet of water to play on his penis. (The oral substructure of this fantasy became obvious when he said that he had sprayed water into the urethra by means of a syringe.) The unconscious fiction was: "I am not doing anything; I am passive, someone else is responsible." This fiction enabled him to drive a car and go skiing. The idea was that he did not control the mechanism: the "responsibility" lay with the mechanism itself.

In the transference he projected on to the analyst the same fantasy of the bad mother who sadistically drains the infant dry. We have an instance of this in his concealment of the fact that he regularly took a taxi to the analyst's house. He continued on the same lines in the second analysis, but with this difference, that his oral behavior was interpreted to him. He construed silence on the part of the analyst as a "refusal to give." A specially clear instance of this was contained in the following situation. One day, immediately before he should have come for analysis, he rang me up to say that he would not be able to come. During the whole of that day he wove around this incident the following fantasy: I would give the time reserved for him to someone else and he would make a "row" because it was not fair. His logical faculty told him that I could do as I liked with my free time but, affectively, his standpoint was that I must wait for him at all costs. Here he was forcing me to play the part of his wife, whom he punished by keeping her endlessly waiting. On another occasion his fantasy in a similar situation was that I would reproach him for not coming at all or for being late. This last fantasy he produced only when he actually had been hindered and it really would have been unjust to reproach him. (Cf. his mother's real behavior when her children excused themselves from coming to see her.)

It was very characteristic that in his dreams the patient managed to emphasize the malice of the woman who refused to give (the phallic mother sadistically perceived), but always representing her in the situation of having more than enough.[11] The accusation of withholding what she should have given was the more well founded and telling since there was no question of her not having had enough; it was simply that she was wicked and malicious. The situation of super-abundance, which in dreams generally took the form of the overflowing of vessels, had two variants. In the first, the patient refused to accept the fluid (reaction by means of the autarchist fiction), while in the second, some external impediment prevented him from receiving it. The latter situation served as an argument to allay his unconscious sense of guilt: "If the woman is so malicious, I have a right to be aggressive."

This brings us to the second problem of our patient's ejaculatory disturbance, the fact next in importance to the breast-complex. I refer to the idea of *ejaculation as a punishment.* Unconsciously he had a positively shattering idea of ejaculation. He thought of it as something *like the explosion of a hand grenade* which blows a man to bits. His unconscious sense of guilt led him to expect that this would be the result of ejaculation in his own case. Expressed in the terms of the patient's unconscious, ejaculation meant blowing the woman to pieces, and bursting oneself as a punishment for one's aggression. Thus his refusal of ejaculation was not only due to the inhibition imposed by his sense of guilt upon his aggressive impulses against the woman, but was also a kind of self-protection.[12] It was characteristic that in the

[11] The patient reacted to his revengeful impulses by a reinforcement of the autarchist fiction, as is seen in the following dream: "A scab had formed under his left rib, and when he scratched it off a third nipple made its appearance." The interpretation of this dream showed that it contained a reference to the story in Genesis, in which Eve is created from one of Adam's ribs. This expressed his view that the woman was a nonentity, for it proved that he was not indebted to his mother even for his birth; in fact, on this theory, the position was reversed. Moreover he went one better than his mother in the matter of breasts (nipples), for he had three of them! In my paper on Grabbe I mentioned the so-called "manna-dreams," which are always based on the wish to be independent of the mother (and later of the father) for food.

[12] This latter also took the form of identification with the woman.

second analysis, when the twofold aim of his aggression (covering masochism) was made clear and he had begun to attempt coitus, a particular type of dream tended to occur, in which the effects of his aggressive impulses were diminished. He now dreamt that hand grenades ("egg-bombs") were thrown without exploding, or that he was the only civilian in the war area and so was not called up, or that he was in a battle and the bullets either missed him or ricochetted harmlessly, etc. These consolatory oral dreams of ejaculation were based on the formula: "aggression is allowable since it does not necessarily kill." He thus satisfied the pseudo-aggressive wish and at the same time refuted the superego's accusation of "murder". He constantly shifted the blame attached to psychic masochism, to his pseudo-aggression.

When the patient first attempted coitus, he could not do it with his wife, for she herself was sexually abnormal and unfortunately the whole of his unconscious defensive hatred was concentrated upon her. After the second analysis had been going on for some months, he decided to make the attempt with a succession of prostitutes. The history of the various stages which he passed through was very remarkable. He was invariably capable of erection but, at first, coitus was continued from ten to thirty minutes without achieving ejaculation. He would then generally interrupt vaginal friction and cause himself to be manually stimulated until ejaculation occurred. For some months he was able to achieve ejaculation through manual stimulation by the prostitute, but not in vaginal coitus. In the next phase the patient continued coitus until he felt the first sensation of semen. This did not, however, as is normal, intensify into the second sensation which is no longer under conscious control, but spent itself without the occurrence of ejaculation into the vagina. There were other occasions when the patient, who often had no inclination for coitus when actually in bed with the prostitute, caused her to stimulate him manually till the first sensation of semen occurred, when he "utilized" for coitus the excitation achieved extravaginally. At first, however, the excitation died away, while erection persisted. The *first* time that he achieved a vaginal ejaculation it was in the following difficult way: vaginal friction was continued for ten minutes, coitus was then interrupted and sexual excitation was intensified by manual stimulation for one or two minutes, when the first sensation of semen occurred. Coitus was resumed for one minute with intensifying excitation, culminating in the second sensation of semen, ejaculation and orgasm.

The difficulty which I have described was peculiarly hard to overcome: in coitus the excitation invariably died out, in spite of the occurrence of the first sensation of semen and of the persistence of erection. There was no intensification of sensation and ejaculation could be achieved only by means of manual stimulation. Another point was that movements on the woman's part disturbed the patient; he required his partner to be completely motionless. His rationalization of this requisition was as follows: the prostitute was simply going through a farce of sexual feeling. Though there was a certain amount of truth in this, his real reason was quite different. He wanted to "give" the woman no enjoyment in coitus, and any sign of pleasure on her part roused him to "silent" fury.[13] At the same time her immobility signified the death which he desired for his partner and corresponded to necrophiliac tendencies in himself.

The stimulus of sexual relations with prostitutes gradually died away and the patient turned again to his wife. But it recurred with fresh force when he began to play off the two women, or two types, against

[13] The following details show how deeply rooted in revenge on the woman was the patient's attitude. In sexual intercourse he had erections suggestive of priapism, which disappeared only gradually after ejaculation. Evidently the reason for this, apart from the fact that he actually remained unsatisfied, was that his unconscious murderous impulses had insufficient outlet in such aggression as he could perpetrate on the woman in coitus. The same was true of the long-drawn-out process of intercourse, lasting as much as half an hour: in fantasy he was attacking the woman, indeed, "bursting her." The following are some of the thoughts which occurred to the patient during coitus. "If I get no pleasure out of it, at least I will see that she is burst to bits." Again, he asked once during fellatio, "What happens if it suddenly goes off?" referring to the possibility of ejaculation occurring unexpectedly. The double meaning of the words used: "to *burst* with anger" and "a gun "*goes off*" is evident. His craving to obtain something orally (as defense against the wish to be refused) continually broke through. Touching the breast of a prostitute, he said "very nice, but there is nothing inside!" Another time he offered a girl five shillings less than he had paid her the first time they had been together. This made her indignant. "Yes," said the patient ironically, "I shall give you five shillings less every time, and in the end *you* will give *me* something on top of that!"

one another—wife and prostitute.[14] On the one hand, he degraded his wife to a harlot, and, on the other, he vented his hatred of women in "playing off one against the other." In coitus with his wife another disturbance now arose. The patient began to suffer the symptom of "unperceived ejaculation," which in these cases evidently represents a typical passing phase in the analysis of aspermists. This phase consisted of the fact that the patient ejaculated but did not feel it. It was only when his wife definitely asserted that he had actually "spat" (which was the term for ejaculation used by this sexually abnormal woman) that he could be convinced, by viewing the contents of the vagina, that ejaculation had really occurred. After this, moreover, the priapistic erections disappeared.

I need scarcely say that the separate phases in the clearing-up of the patient's ejaculatory disturbance did not follow a straightforward course. Relapses, periods of depression, in short, the ups and downs of every analysis were not lacking. The patient's reaction to his incipient normality has been by no means one of unmixed enthusiasm; at times it has taken the form of marked aggression.

The patient was finally cured, divorced his wife, remarried and had children.

The problem of impotence is clinically so important that a short survey [15] of all types of regression is indicated.

Reviewing the psychoanalytic literature dealing with the problems of impotence we find in some points general agreement, in some a series of unclarities and contradictions, in still others, completely blank spaces indicating *terra incognita.*

No analyst doubts that fixation on the level of the positive Oedipus is responsible for a simple case of hysteric impotence. If a man unconsciously identifies the sexual object with his mother, the inner conscience objects, with the result that impotence automatically results.

Disagreement starts, however, if we deal with a case regressed to the negative or inverted Oedipus. In this case the boy identifies unconsciously with the mother and wants to be overwhelmed sexually by the

[14] In this there was at bottom a reference to the two breasts.

[15] Excerpts from a paper read before the Topeka Psychoanalytic Society April 27, 1946. Published in condensed form in Bulletin of the Menninger Clinic 11, 2, 1947 under the title: "Newer Genetic Investigations on Impotence and Frigidity."

father. In later life this man builds up as inner defense a compensatory "he-man" attitude, runs from one woman to another, speaks contemptuously of them. His potency often fails him despite his braggadocio. In our literature this type is designated as "passive-feminine" or "unconscious homosexual." The latter term is responsible for a great deal of confusion. Some authors believe that this type of hysterical individual—had he a perversion and not a neurosis—would become a full-fledged homosexual. Clinical experience proves that this reasoning is fallacious, since perversion homosexuality has a completely different genetic basis; namely, oral regression.[16]

Partial agreement is to be found in anally regressed cases. The basic investigations of Freud, Jones and Abraham on obsessional neurosis have been verified time and again. As far as the problem of potency is concerned, it is interesting to note that obsessional and compulsive neurotics often have—"mechanically"—a good potency. The erection does not fail them, the neurotic disturbance uses—as far as potency is concerned—as hitching posts, doubts and fears pertaining to venereal disease, impregnation, mysterious damage to the penis, etc. Often the coitus is protracted, the orgastic potency is regularly disturbed; only in severe cases of obsessional (compulsive) neurotics does the erective potency fail them, too. The fact of orgastic disturbance in these cases is easily explained: these neurotics believe that sex is something "dirty", that is, anal and "sadistic."

At this point the confusion starts. How are we to explain that anally regressed neurotics are on the one hand very sadistic in their conscious sexual attitudes, fantasies and daydreams, and at the same time full of self-damaging tendencies? The usual explanation is that the original aggression is counteracted by an overdimensional feeling of guilt. I personally believe that a three-layer structure is involved. The *end result* of the infantile conflict was anal passive submission. This first layer is vetoed by the severe inner conscience which forces the unconscious ego to mobilize pseudo-aggression as a defense. This second layer, too, is contradicted by the superego with the result that passivity is established as the third layer because of inner guilt.

For example: an obsessional patient had, among many other symptoms, the obsession to think about the telephone number of his divorced

[16] Sec. No. 12.

wife and often felt panic lest he forget the number. He had been divorced for twenty years (more precisely, his marriage had been annulled because of his complete impotence), had not seen his wife in two decades, did not know where she lived, or even if she were still alive. The obsessional idea was connected with a telephone number of twenty-years standing; he knew that in the meantime the telephone numbers had been changed, but never dared look up the number in the telephone directory. The obvious interpretation was that he unconsciously wished evil to his wife and his superego reproached him because of these death wishes. The inner defense offered his superego was: "Call her up and you will see that she is still alive." In other words, the interpretation assumed, as usual in our literature of obsessional cases, a repressed aggressive tendency and an overdimensional feeling of guilt because of that aggression. How was one, however, to explain that a man so deeply masochistic should fight inwardly only against reproaches of aggression, executed via omnipotence of thoughts, and not defend himself also against reproaches directed against his psychic masochism? It seemed more likely that his aggression was but pseudo-aggression and that the really decisive reproach of his inner conscience pertained to exactly the opposite wish, namely, psychic masochism. One could, therefore, assume that a three-layer structure was involved:

1. A wish to be mistreated, counteracted by a superego reproach;
2. First defense mechanism of pseudo-aggression ("I am not masochistic in relation to my wife; on the contrary, I want to kill her.");
3. Rejection of that defense, too, by the superego, continuation of reproaches, resulting in establishment of a second defense by the unconscious ego: "I don't want to kill my wife; call her up and you will see that she is unharmed."

The advantage which the unconscious ego derives from the three-layer structure is that, by constantly fighting on a specious front, it can cover and preserve the dynamic wish. Of course, the "return of the repressed material" (Freud) takes place; in reproaching himself, the obsessional neurotic enjoys exactly the basically forbidden wish: psychic masochism.

If we interpret only their aggressiveness to obsessional (compulsive) neurotics suffering from potency disturbances, they at first object, but soon accept the interpretation and actually look flattered and smile when we draw their attention to a new aggression. When, however, we show them the passivity behind the mask of aggressiveness, that is, their pseudo-aggression—or, as the purist would call it, "aggression used as defense against passivity"—the picture is quite different. They become angry and depressed, or repress the interpretation with great regularity. They constantly stress their aggressiveness and regularly overlook the passivity behind it. The whole analytic battle then centers around constant exposing of this pseudo-aggression. In other words, what the analyst has to guard against is a *danger encountered on all levels of regression: not to confuse the defense mechanism with the underlying wish.* Many an analysis can fail on exactly that point.

In orally regressed cases there exists the greatest unclarity; to use the word "confusion" for the present state of affairs is an euphemism. The majority of authors believe that the *wish to get* ("oral greed") is the content of that regression. The minority—and I have to admit that I am responsible for that formulation—believes exactly the opposite; namely, that the basic wish in these cases is the masochistic elaboration of the wish to get: *the tendency to be refused.*

"What sort of people are these?" one could object. "If a child is refused candy, for instance, he will, when he grows up, eat as much candy as he can stomach, to make up for his early disappointments." True, he will, if he is normal. If, however, he develops an "oral" neurosis, he will repeat the situation of being refused. Obviously, for these neurotics the wish to show up the pre-oedipal mother as a disappointing, "bad" and refusing monster is more important than their original wish to be given.

On the oral level, the fantastic fact is clinically observable, that penis and breast, vagina and mouth, sperm, urine and milk are unconsciously identified. Following is a clinical example: a patient suffering from pseudo-imbecility remembered that as a child of seven he had often witnessed gypsy women nursing their children. Watching them—especially the breast—greatly excited him sexually, and suggested the game of inserting a long straw into his penis, putting the other end to his lips, and drinking his own urine. In this game, he played at once the roles of mother and sucking child, clearly establishing an "autarchy."

The result of the prevailing misconceptions concerning orality, is that the two main symptoms and signs of "penis neurosis" on that level—premature ejaculation and psychogenic aspermia—are interpreted as aggressive refusal, whereas they constitute but pseudo-aggressive defenses against a deeper repressed wish to be refused.

It is, of course, true that oral neurotics have to wish to deny. Everybody lives psychologically on the basis of his pet defense mechanism. And this unconscious defense mechanism happens to be, in oral cases, pseudo-aggressive denial of the masochistic wish to be denied. Therefore, pseudo-aggressive elements dominate both in ejaculation praecox and in aspermia. In both cases fluid is denied: in premature ejaculation the "milk" is "spilled" before it can reach the mouth (vagina)—*ejaculatio ante portas*—or a few seconds after insertion, when the woman can derive no pleasure because of the short duration of coitus. In aspermia, refusal of fluid manifests itself more directly since these neurotics always take it for granted that it is sperm which interests the woman most. The ironic twist consists in the fact that the majority of women are frigid anyway and rather enjoy protracted though spermless intercourse. Characteristic of the exaggerated stress oral neurotics lay on sperm and for their underestimation of frictions, are their reactions when it is pointed out to them in analysis that their alleged revenge on the woman is rather a blessing to her. The reaction is surprise, then anger and fury.

The pseudo-aggressive defense against masochistic attachment produces characterologically the typical symptom of playing off one woman against the other. Here is a grotesque example. A patient of this type always had two mistresses though his potency was poor. One day he tried to have intercourse with mistress No. 1, had an erection, used a condom, but found that his erection collapsed after a few movements without ejaculation. He took off the condom and deposited it in the drawer of his night table without thinking. The next day, he repeated the performance with mistress No. 2. He reached for a condom and "by chance" got the used one. "In this moment I experienced the greatest pleasure of my life. If both girls only knew. . . ."

Premature ejaculation is the most typical of all types of potency disturbances. It is known from Karl Abraham's classic study that an urethal-anal wish to soil the woman is unconsciously discernible. It is also known how often enuresis can be found in anamnesis. All this is clinically correct. The question remains, however, whether the aggression displayed in the symptom is real or pseudo-aggression. I believe the latter.

The patient's conflict arises from the fact that, being an exquisite psychic masochist (layer 1 of the "mechanism of orality"), he is constantly reproached by his inner "district attorney" (superego), which forces the unconscious ego to furnish an "alibi." This alibi is pseudo-aggression, namely refusal. This alibi, too, is rejected by the superego, which in turn reproaches the ego for malicious refusal of sexual pleasure to the woman. A new defense is then set up "I don't want to refuse; I give immediately." But this precipitated giving is really a *mockery* of giving, since pleasure is refused to the woman. The man with premature ejaculation behaves like someone who shows a hungry person a plate of delicious food, but throws it out of the window before the hungry one can reach for it.

The feeling of guilt pertains to two reproaches of the inner conscience: to the basic masochistic wish to be refused and to the pseudo-aggressive covering of refusal. The analyst who interprets only the aggressive component in these cases plays—without knowing it—the game of involuntarily strengthening the patient's defense mechanism. In severe cases, he will meet with failure and then blame everybody but himself.

What about cases in which the interpretation of the aggressive component *only*, leads, nevertheless, to successes? There are all types of premature ejaculation. Some are not oral in genesis, but hysteriform. In these cases even the incorrect interpretation will help. In other cases the patient's unconscious is so afraid of losing the whole neurosis, that it gives up the symptom only to save the more important characterologic part of the neurosis. In complicated cases no success is possible if one does not reach the end result of the infantile conflict—namely psychic masochism concentrated in the wish to be refused.

The second disturbance of potency encountered on the oral level is "psychogenic oral aspermia." The genetic basis of that queer aspermia is a variation of the mechanism of orality. The denial and refusal of sperm has the same reasons as in cases of premature ejaculation, namely, pseudo-aggressive refusal covering the wish to be masochistically refused. The specific feature in these cases is that these patients unconsciously identify ejaculation with bursting of an explosive charge. In their refusal to ejaculate, they protect the woman and themselves, from being burst. To use a simile from the news of the day, the problem with these patients is to convince them that ejaculation and the atomic bomb are different things.

4. Oral Type of Frigidity

Frigidity is a complex phenomenon and differences of opinions about it start already at the definition. I wrote (in collaboration with Dr. Hitschmann) the first Freudian monograph [17] on frigidity and defined it as follows:

> "Under frigidity we understand the incapacity of a woman to have a *vaginal* orgasm. It is of no matter whether the woman is aroused during coitus or remains cold, whether the excitement is weak or strong, whether it breaks off at the beginning or the end, slowly or suddenly, whether it is dissipated in preliminary acts, or has been lacking from the start, The *sole* criterion of frigidity is absence of vaginal orgasm."

The Bergler-Hitschmann definition of frigidity is by no means generally accepted. Many colleagues believe that clitoric arousal is the most a woman can get from the sex act. Why they consider coitus and not masturbation the sexual basis of marriage, is not clear.

Here, too, popular opinion, which considers a woman frigid only if sex-rejecting in general attitude, can muster strange arguments from scientific defenders. To name but three:

> "Two psychoanalysts have *invented* (!) what they call the vaginal orgasm and call frigid the hottest woman who cannot have one (whatever it is)."

This sentence can be read in Professor G. L. Kelly's booklet "Sex Manual," on page 42.

And the remedy, recommended by Kelly? He accuses men of sexual ignorance if they try to achieve an orgasm in the woman in the vagina, and recommends rubbing of the clitoris during intercourse, or positions

[17] "Frigidity in Women." American translation. Nervous and Mental Disease Monographs N. Y. 1936. (Austrian edition Ars Medici 1934; French edition Denoel & Steele Paris 1936; Japanese edition Tokyo Institute for Psan. 1937; Swedish translation in preparation.)

which bring man's organ in contact with the clitoris, quoting a professor of physiology who advised "Ride 'em high."

Nobody denies that with specific techniques artificial penis-clitoris contact can be established. To postulate that, or even clitoris masturbation during intercourse, as normal prerequisites, as Kelly does, seems to me an extreme concession to frigidity making out of woman's neurotic inhibition a virtue, blaming the victimized man to boot. The argument that only clitoris excitation can produce orgasm is mechanistic; orgasm is a psycho-sexual reflex. Tragically, even artificially produced clitoric orgasm does not have in the psychic economy the same effects as does vaginal orgasm.

The inner disbelief in psychogeneity of frigidity goes sometimes so far that even authors who in "certain cases" recommend analysis, recommend for other cases—ointments. An example is the otherwise interesting paper of A. P. Hudgins, "The Frigid Wife." [18] He speaks favorably of "glycerine-camphor ointment with a trace of creoline" which "produces a sensation of heat and is sometimes helpful." The ointment is applied over the area of the clitoris and vagina.

The latest defender of clitoridian orgasm, nay, denier of vaginal orgasmic capacity in the woman, is to be found in Kinsey's report. Here we read:

> "—there is a *widespread* but certainly *unfounded* opinion among psychiatrists, which is repeated among other clinicians involved in marriage counseling, that *there is such a thing as a vaginal orgasm* which is something different from an orgasm achieved through clitorial stimulation." [19]

Kinsey announces that Volume II of his series will be devoted to that problem. It is amusing to observe that the statistician Kinsey even exaggerates the number of psychiatrists ("widespread opinion . . . repeated by other clinicians") who accept the Bergler-Hitschmann definition of frigidity. We hope Kinsey has statistical proofs for that statement; neither I, nor Dr. Hitschmann, are conscious of the fact that our theory has been so widely accepted.[20]

[18] The Medical Times, December 1945–January 1946.

[19] Kinsey report, p. 576.

[20] We summarized our opinion on frigidity in our joint paper "Frigidity in Women—Restatement and Renewed Experiences," The Psa. Review 1949, I, commemorating the 15th anniversary of our monograph.

What is wrong with the clitoric theory? If one presses its proponents for an answer as to what they understand by emotional satisfaction, for instance, if they include in this term orgasm experienced, not during *coitus*, but *after* coitus, in the clitoris, through masturbation with the help of the man, one would receive the laconic reply that it is unimportant where and when the sexual tension is released, provided it is released at all. Pressing the proponents of the clitoric theory still further one learns that they have either no precise conception of the entire vaginal orgasmic capacity of the woman, or deny its existence altogether, having the unexpressed view that the woman is really sensitive only in the clitoris, needing no orgasm-like release and being satisfied with a general excitation.

It is difficult to understand why the proponents of the clitoric theory speak of coitus rather than of masturbation as the basis of normal sexual behavior. Actually, according to the clitoric theory, sexuality for the woman is masturbation *a deux*, while the general custom is to regard masturbation as infantile and coitus as the adult form of sexual satisfaction. Furthermore, we know that a large group of neurotics remain masturbationists throughout lifetimes, whether they consciously find more pleasure in this or whether they lead a "double sex life," an unsatisfactory "alibi coitus" and a more satisfying, though guilt-laden masturbation. A further objection to the clitoric theory is that, according to it, one would have to designate pathologic cases such as the following as "normal": a masochistic patient who lets herself be beaten by a sadistic man and attains orgasm through cunnilingus only; or a patient who performs fellatio on the man lying on his back while he slaps her with all of his force on her buttocks, then masturbates her for half an hour to achieve clitoridian orgasm. The formula "Orgasm is orgasm," independently where, and how achieved, is wrong, and does not correspond to clinical facts.

The question arises whether the difference between vaginal and clitoridian orgasm is not overstressed. Perhaps it is really important only that the woman succeeds in obtaining some kind of satisfaction. Optimists may even express the hope that when a woman is aroused at the clitoris by preliminary acts, this arousal will be intensified during coitus. Here one runs into a factor that is neither theorized, classified, nor of terminological nature. I am referring simply to an anatomical factor. When studies on topographical anatomy are recalled, one will be reminded that for purely anatomical reasons the clitoris does not come into contact with the penis during coitus. Here again is an indication of the truth of the words coined by Freud, "Anatomy is fate." Thus, there can be no mechanical intensification of arousal of the clitoris through friction during coitus, and the transfer of the arousal from the clitoris to the vagina is purely psychological, that is, an unconscious factor. Women know that, as their substitute techniques prove. They try to maintain the illusion of enjoying sexual intercourse vaginally by holding the thighs closely together, thus establishing artificial contact between penis and clitoris, or they pretend to be highly excited, producing acrobatic movements only to achieve the same aim of penis-clitoris contact. Other women resign, and put on an act only for the benefit of the partner; still others ask directly before or after the man's ejaculation for clitoridian massage. Another group constantly blames the man.

I analyzed, for instance, a "big business man," married for 23 years who consulted me because of premature ejaculation. Asked how long his intercourse lasted, he answered: "Approximately 30 to 40 minutes." I congratulated him on his good potency, stating the empirical fact that normal intercourse lasts from two to ten minutes. The patient had understood as premature ejaculation his inability to protract intercourse until his wife's orgasm came. Since she reached one, seldom enough, only after an hour, she accused him of having premature ejaculation. The patient wanted to leave immediately after receiving the information. "Then I don't have premature ejaculation," he exclaimed triumphantly, jumping from the chair. "Sit down," was my answer, "you suffer from something worse." I was referring to the man's pathologic masochistic attachment to his frigid wife, who made him swallow all this nonsense for a quarter of a century, exploited him financially on a grand scale and induced in him a strong feeling of guilt because of his alleged sexual inadequacy.

Clinical experience proves that the great majority of neurotic women never experience vaginal orgasm. Every symptomatic neurosis, whatever the level of regression, is accompanied by a sexual disturbance. There is only one exception from that empirical rule: some cases of agoraphobia can experience vaginal orgasm. The reasons are unknown.

Even more puzzling are cases of characterologic neurosis; in these, normal orgasm is often, by no means always, possible. No satisfactory answer can be offered for that state of affairs.

How can one diagnose frigidity? There are only two facts both tested time and again, which can be used as guides. The first is that the *involuntary contractions* of the pelvic and perineal muscles at the end of the sex act is the *one and only sure criterion* that a man can use to determine whether the woman is frigid. A man can be deceived by a clever woman in many things—in love, sensitivity, sexual interest, alleged pleasure in intercourse. In only one thing she is helpless—the production of involuntary contractions. Over the muscles involved in these, she has no conscious control. Inasmuch as the man feels these contractions at the penis at the end of the act, any attempt at simulation is impossible, provided the man is informed about this fact. It is superfluous to say that men are in general ignorant.

The second fact leading to discovery of frigidity is much less reliable. The absence of glandular lubricating secretion produced at the entrance of the vagina before and during coitus is a sure sign of frigidity; the converse, however, is not true. The presence of the secretion does not exclude the presence of one of the many forms of frigidity.

It is impossible to enumerate here all possible and known forms of frigidity. In our monograph on frigidity, written sixteen years ago, Doctor Hitschmann and I enumerated eighteen forms. I could add a few other forms. I prefer to give a short survey of the points of agreement and disagreement according to the genetic level.

There is agreement concerning hysteric cases, covering the positive and the negative Oedipus. If a woman identifies the sexual partner with the father, or unconsciously wants to act the part of the man, the result in both cases is frigidity. The same misunderstanding exists, however, as far as female homosexuality is concerned, in accusing the negative Oedipus as a causative factor. The situation is analogous to male homosexuality—an oral genesis, complicated with some additional factors.[21]

Few differences of opinion are encountered on the level of anal regression. Here, however, the difference between interpretations as-

[21] Sec. No. 13.

suming a two-layer structure versus a three-layer structure, is as unsolved as previously stressed in cases of obsessional impotence.

Complete disagreement is visible in orally regressed cases. The problem has, if possible, even greater practical importance than in the symptomatology of impotence. An unexpectedly large percentage of frigid women are orally regressed. True, outward appearances often suggest a hysteric case; unfortunately this is but a palimpsest fooling the inexperienced observer, including some analysts. In our literature, cases are mentioned in which the frigid woman is unconsciously afraid of intercourse because she attaches deep masochistic connotations to orgasm. These cases are undiagnosed oral cases.

Orally regressed women unconsciously identify penis and breast, vagina and mouth, sperm and milk. The inner reproach of conscience is: "You want to bite the breast"; the inner defense: "I cannot bite since I don't feel anything in my mouth (vagina)." In other words, the inner battle is apparently fought on the second pseudo-aggressive level of the "mechanism of orality." This layer, however, covers the dynamically decisive wish to be refused. And these women, indeed, satisfy in their total frigidity the wish to be refused sexual pleasure. These women still unconsciously identify the husband with the "refusing mother." Hence, every sexual disappointment bolsters the basic fallacy: mother refuses!

The whole problem of frigidity is complicated by the fact that some "*character neuroses*" do not show the symptom of vaginal frigidity. If a woman chooses, three times in succession, neurotic men who ill-treat her—the orgasm she experiences is far from being a certificate of psychic health. Or, if a woman adheres to the "condition of the forbidden" (frigid in marriage, orgasmic capacity preserved in a clandestine relation) neither is that orgasm a proof of psychic health. Naive overvaluation of orgasm as *only* yardstick of health leads clinically to erroneous conclusions.

5. Specific Type of Promiscuity

The "seducer" and the promiscuous woman with "sex on my own terms," enjoy in the eyes of naive contemporaries the aura of a special patent for happiness and smartness.

The sober facts are that we are dealing clinically with a specific type of impotent men and cold-frigid women who use a specific preventive unconscious "trick."

The wolf is an impotent man who can maintain his shaky potency only in the initial stages of a relation with a woman and then loses "interest" quickly and regularly. Were he to stay with the woman, his potency disturbance would become painfully apparent. To avoid the fiasco, he jilts the woman, to repeat the identical performance with the next "victim."

This preventive technique is, of course, unconscious. At bottom, the "wolf" is a neurotic inflated sissy.

The promiscuous woman has her illusions too, though of different kind. Her frigidity is quite conscious to her, the reason is unconscious. She stubbornly believes that somewhere in this universe an imaginary satisfier does exist—the problem is to find him. Hence the persistent search.

Both, wolf and wolferette alike, are "injustice collectors": every object of their choice disappoints them. Both live on the basis of the pseudo-aggressive defense (layer II of the "mechanism of orality"): wolf lets the object of his dissatisfaction fall, not less disgusted than does the promiscuous woman. Both emerge defensively "victorious" from their everlasting fiascos: *they* have said good riddance to the discarded "lover."

Grotesquely, wolf and wolferette are the unhappy prey of each other. The reason is that the "wolf" has the reputation of great sexual experience which, in turn, attracts the promiscuous woman who hopes in vain that the "professional" will make her feel, where the "dilettante" failed.

The wolf, on the other hand, finds in the promiscuous woman an "easy to get" object and push-over for his Leporello-list: the more normal woman gives him a wide berth.

Both, promiscuous men and women, are cheated cheaters: their pseudo-aggressive defense works at the price of dissatisfaction.[22]

[22] There are also other, more superficial reasons for promiscuity; the camouflage is frequently hysterical in appearance. The "real" wolf and wolferette are orally regressed, whatever the trimmings.

6. Pathologic Blushing (Erythrophobia)[23]

Pathological blushing has been the subject of many psychoanalytic papers[24] in which it has always been considered a hysterical conversion symptom of a 'Befangenheitsneurose' ('embarrassment neurosis'). A displacement from below upward phallicizes the face, whereby unconscious exhibitionistic and punishment wishes are satisfied. It is also known that those given to this kind of blushing are therapeutically difficult of access, narcissistic, and self-contained, and not infrequently express ideas that border on paranoia.

In spite of the bad therapeutic results obtained, the erythrophobic patient is not resistant to therapy. The fault lies rather in our technique. In the first place, if we demonstrate his phallic and exhibitionistic trends to an erythrophobic patient[25] we obtain more abundant evidence of their presence. Though we may be happy to find such confirming material, we are really taken in by a complicated unconscious defense mechanism of the patient. For, strange as this may be, the exhibitionism analytically observable in the symptom of morbid blushing is not primary at all, but secondary. What is primary is an excessively strong voyeur component, which is secondarily warded off by means of the exhibitionism.

The question of the origin and development of the voyeur component takes us back into the pre-oedipal period. Since Simmel's Wiesbaden paper, we know that looking is a variant of oral devouring; that the 'eye and ear are introjection organs for the adequate digestion and

[23] Paper read before the XVth International Psychoanalytic Congress, Paris, France, August 1938. Published in The Psa. Quart., XIII:1, 1944, under the title "A New Approach to the Therapy of Erythrophobia."

[24] Cf. References on scopophilia, Freud, Franz Alexander, Therese Benedek, E. Hitschmann, H. Christoffel, Michael Josef Eisler, S. Feldman, Otto Fenichel, Josef K. Friedjung.

[25] In the literature on the subject, very little distinction is made between fear of blushing and morbid blushing; both are inaccurately subsumed under the concept erythrophobia. In this section I deal essentially with the symptom of morbid blushing and do not enter upon the anxiety problem, since that would involve a tedious discussion on the theory of anxiety. See on this matter Ch. III, No. 7.

assimilation of optical and acoustic perceptions'.[26] To what degree devouring with a glance is primary or is a substitute for devouring with the mouth cannot yet be decided. In any case, once it is brought to our attention, we find in erythrophobic patients a strong oral and aggressive component, originally related to the mother's breast,[27] as excerpts from the case history given below clearly show.

In its subsequent career, this oral component encounters the bounds set by maternal prohibition. All of the child's multiform tendencies of devouring, tearing, biting, handling and gazing at the breast are understandably checked by the mother. This leads to the damming up of the oral component, to aggrievement at the blow to the baby's assumption of omnipotence and to reactive revenge. In boys, one solution [28] of this conflict is a defiant exhibitionism, somewhat according to the formula: 'I don't want to look at the mother's breast; I want to show myself.' The organ defensively displayed is the entire body (Lewin), but particularly the penis, the cheeks, and the buttocks.

In the oedipal phase, the original breast significance of the cheeks (maternal breast-penis) is fused with the phallic penis significance of the head: 'It is not true that I am castrated and have no penis; on the contrary, my penis is as big as my head'. In this mechanism of denial, the boy takes care of the feeling of defiance and revenge against supposed castrators (mother, later father). Symbolically displaying the penis, he also defends himself against unconscious feminine wishes of the negative oedipus complex (penis as 'amulet').[29] Yet this mechanism of denial through phallicized exhibition and pseudo-aggression finally succumbs to repression and is replaced by the symptom of erythrophobia, in which the aggressive and exhibitionistic wishes are no longer conscious. Incidentally, the exhibitionistic tendency that

[26] This point of view is taken up later by some authors, as Christoffel, Fenichel, Servadio.

[27] It is interesting that in a very significant case history published by Therese Benedek the oral, pre-oedipal substructure of erythrophobia is plainly visible in the material, although in her theoretical conclusions the author clings to the oedipal conditioning of the symptom and the entire illness.

[28] See in relation to other conflict solutions Bergler and Eidelberg, "The Mammakomplex des Mannes." Int. Z. f. Psa., XIX, 1933, pp. 547–83.

[29] Ernest Jones, "Nightmare, Witches and Devils." New York, W. W. Norton & Co., 1931.

was warded off is smuggled into the symptom: by blushing the erythrophobe makes himself really conspicuous, i.e., exhibits himself. It is also noteworthy that traces of the original voyeuristic wishes themselves are included in the final symptom. In the first place, according to Freud, every exhibitionist unconsciously identifies himself with the voyeur, and by this detour enjoys voyeur pleasure. In the second place, the erythrophobe projects his own wishes to peep upon his surroundings. As virtually all analytic observers stress, these patients have pseudo-paranoid ideas of being watched and observed. Thus peeping pleasure finds surreptitious satisfaction along all projective by-paths of identification with an onlooker, buttressed by the moral alibi, 'Others, not I, are looking.' The erythrophobe makes use of others as a mirror in order to look at himself with a clear conscience.

Here are three clinical examples of the extraordinary interplay of original voyeurism and secondary exhibitionistic defense.[30]

A patient, described in more detail below, occupied a box one evening at a circus performance. While watching two women trapeze artists demonstrate their skill she suddenly became 'dizzy', covered her face with her hands and cried out very loudly, 'I can't look at it; please tell me when it's over.' Voyeurism was warded off by means of exhibitionism: by attracting the attention of those about her, the patient exhibited herself. But this defensive exhibitionism was itself warded off as the patient blushed, grew ashamed and self-conscious because the scene she provoked was consciously very painful to her.

An erythrophobic patient stated that in childhood it was very distressing for him to sleep in the same room with his mother. He said that even at the age of three-and-a-half he felt ashamed. At any rate, he clearly remembered the following scene: the outer wall of his bed, made of netting, and therefore permitting a free view through the interstices, was turned towards his mother's bed. He would always cover this outer wall with his top sheet and covers for the night. Officially, this was a proof that he was not watching his mother undress; nor by inference, in the oedipal period, was he watching parental coitus. At the same time, exhibitionism—lying half naked without cover—was

[30] The fact that both parts of scopophilia are used as defense, has been stressed first by the author, in coll. with L. Eidelberg, in "The Mechanism of Depressionalization", Int. Z. Psychoan., 1935.

here used as a defense against the original voyeurism. In the third layer, the exhibitionistic defense too was warded off: he felt ashamed whenever his mother would cover him in the morning.

While being analyzed, another erythrophobic patient had the following experience. At a mountain cottage, he met a lady whom he thought he knew. He stared at her, against his usual custom, but could not remember where he had seen her face before. Suddenly it occurred to him that she might be a patient he had frequently seen at my office on leaving. The thought was distressing to him. He looked away but in the next few minutes behaved very exhibitionistically: he spoke loudly, began to sing, opened his shirt, put on another sweater, etc. The lady, not understanding what was going on, reported to me: 'The man behaved as if he desired to attract attention, although at the same time he was rather embarrassed and quite red.' Again we see the same set of facts: the primary desire to stare is secondarily warded off by means of exhibitionism ('as if he desired to attract attention to himself'), and at a tertiary stage the exhibitionism itself is warded off ('rather embarrassed and quite red').

To preface a consideration of the theoretical and therapeutic consequences of the three-layer structure of the symptom of erythrophobia, the following excerpt of a case history is presented.

A thirty-year-old lady came to psychoanalysis for erythrophobia. The symptomatology was typical. Whenever she would come upon some acquaintance unexpectedly or would have to wait on a strange customer at her husband's business, she would become embarrassed and her face would grow blood red. (More precisely: her cheeks grew red, her forehead remained unchanged.) A very similar thing would happen if some man looked at her in public, in a cafe, a theater, etc., or if she was seated in her automobile when it was not in motion. She would become fearful that she could not get the motor going and that she would make a fool of herself as a driver. If she needed to go to the toilet in a restaurant and did not know its location, she would avoid looking for it, preferring to wait until she got home. She rationalized as follows: 'I don't want to be stared at. It would make me feel insecure, I might stumble ('fall'—prostitute fantasies), turn over a table and attract attention.' Officially, therefore, everything was avoided which might attract attention, but exhibitionism was thereby unconsciously smuggled in at every point. Although she dressed very decently, her whole appearance had something indefinably pretentious and attracted attention.

The infantile situation was described as follows: her energetic mother was the 'dearest and best woman' in the world, but her father was passive and without interest in anyone or anything. During her mother's long illness—she died of cancer of the breast—the patient cared for her with the utmost sacrifice. With her mother she was more a good friend than a daughter; her mother had indeed married young and had long retained her youth, so that she and her daughter were often taken for sisters. Since her mother's death, the patient had been in constant fear lest she too die of cancer of the breast. She would anxiously watch her breasts, was disturbed over every harmless pimple, and constantly bothered the doctors.

'My great misfortune is that I am not a man,' the patient openly declared. Till her sixth year she was an only child; when a brother was born. 'From that day on I was through, nobody bothered about me, everything centered around the boy, it was always thrown up to me that I was only a girl.' The patient was deeply aggrieved by her demotion. She felt an 'honest hatred' for the system of male-dominated culture and for her brother. From a cheerful, friendly child she turned into a 'shy, unfriendly, retiring stay-at-home' who very soon found only one joy—reading. 'I swallowed books, nothing else interested me at this time.' Obviously, her brother's existence, or rather his penis, contributed greatly to the oral regression.

The patient at first denied any childhood or pubertal masturbation. Her later sexual relations were always of the same type: the man must be beneath her mentally, a weakling, and sexually inadequate; he must arouse her pity. The patient was very presumptuous sexually and considered herself superior to men, whom she designated as 'stupid, clumsy and backward.' In sexual matters she had to train them. Yet, despite all her finesse, she achieved at the very most no more than clitoris orgasm. On the other hand, she would arrange it so that she could complain of unjust treatment, and ingratitude. Twice she fell in love with men despite (unconsciously because of) the fact that they had lost their means; then their families rejected her. Through clever unconscious provocations she succeeded in being wronged by a person or a group of persons, and then she exploited this masochistically in a big way.

Women she intellectually rejected. They were, she held, stupid, petty, mean, malicious, and interested only in clothes and intrigue. She considered herself to be different. On the other hand, she found the upper part of the female body very beautiful, especially the breast. 'The first thing I look at in a woman is the breast.' Then hesitantly, 'After which I compare it with my own.' And the triumphant conclusion: 'So far I have not yet found a woman with a bosom more beautiful than mine.' This vanity about her breasts—and it was a veritable infatuation—was disturbed by the constant fear that she would fall victim to cancer and 'go miserably down to destruction like my mother.'

The symptom of blushing appeared when she was still in elementary school. To break her of this 'bad habit' and for the sake of 'practice' and 'strengthening her will,' her mother would send her on errands to various shops. The opposite result was achieved.

The patient entered her analysis with a preconceived resistance: she could not believe that she might unconsciously hate her mother—an idea she had picked up from reading. Soon some dreams with unequivocal death wishes against me and her mother startled her. Gradually she had to admit that she was filled with savage aggression and she saw then the essential connection between this aggression and the unconscious guilt feelings, which led to a need for punishment. She saw too how she sexualized this feeling of guilt, how masochistic she was, and how she was always reconstructing the situation of being wronged. Nonplussed, she honestly admitted that she was sexually 'most strongly disposed' when she suffered some bodily pain, e.g., during her chronic neuralgia. This struck her as strange since her husband, on occasions when he suffered from bodily pain, had reacted quite otherwise.

But in part the patient's understanding of her psychic masochism, which she thoroughly assimilated, was accepted tendentiously because of resistance. The patient adopted an attitude of hostility and rejection towards all interpretations relating to her scopophilic impulse; she fought such interpretations with a cool 'very interesting' or a dubious 'but that is very complicated.' She would deliberately bring forward information given to her in the interpretation of masochism, would apply it in studying her husband and her surroundings, and would constantly find new confirmation in her own life. Unconsciously, she went through the old game: playing off one interpretation against the other, one being tendentiously emphasized, the other completely neglected.

Her childhood story showed that her mother had been the center of her chief conflicts. The mother, whom the patient always presented as a gracious 'friend,' was in fact full of aggression towards the child: she cursed her own 'stupidity' which had brought her a child so much too soon, who had hampered her enjoyment because of its demands, and she was maliciously critical of her daughter. She would constantly find fault with her daughter's appearance, with the color of her hair, with her complexion—the patient as a child had plump cheeks, like 'milk and blood' (the German equivalent of 'peaches and cream'),—with her manner of speaking, etc. Thus there grew up in the child the feeling of not being loved, or rather of being inadequately loved, along with an immense hatred of the mother, which, however, had quite other causes that were practically independent of the mother's behavior and reached back into the pre-oedipal period. The following is a reconstruction of the conflict (with a certain degree of probability) around the patient's scopophilic impulse:

1. The child wishes to gaze at the mother's breast (gazing a substitute for devouring, touching, fingering, sucking). This later brings a sharp rebuke from the mother, producing in turn a severe lesion of the child's narcissism (pre-oedipal).

2. Attempts are made at reparation; the original voyeur wish is denied and supplanted by exhibitionism: 'I don't want to look at all; on the contrary, I want to show myself.' Instead of her mother's breasts, are chosen—after complicated permutations in psychic substitution—her own chubby cheeks (pre-oedipal). In the oedipal period, the lack of penis is denied through exhibition of the face (penis).

3. Then ensues a warding off of oral and phallic exhibition, repression, formation of the symptom of erythrophobia.

Each of the three phases here sketched lasts for some time with gradual transitions. The following supplementary material is to be noted. The patient subdivided the entire male world into two groups: the 'lookers' and the 'nonlookers', depending on whether the men in question looked at her sexually, a matter of great importance to her. If they gazed at her sexually, she would grow quite ironical and contemptuous of them. She would coquettishly display her bodily form so as to compel being looked at. Despite her marked simplicity, she would dress strikingly. In fact, she was quite a coquettish woman, even though neurotically inhibited. She constantly visited every possible variety of physician, would undress for examination with an almost conscious pleasure (the doctor serving to relieve her guilt feelings), and repeatedly exposed herself elsewhere 'innocently' to attack, admitting that she was playing with fire. She could record a whole series of typical occurrences connected with the scopophilic impulse: men compromised themselves for her sake, frequently by looking through keyholes, etc. Consciously, all this was rather distasteful to her; she reacted to such occurrences with great moral resentment.

What was the sense of this chronic exhibitionism? Without doubt she satisfied her desire to show herself, even though this component, as has been pointed out, was secondary and a defense against her original desire to look. On the other hand, the men by looking at her relieved the guilt feelings she had for her own desire to look: 'Since everyone else is doing the same thing, I am exculpated.' It might indeed be said that every 'nonlooking' person represented a grave reproach of conscience. But these people were men and with these men the patient identified herself on pre-oedipal and phallic grounds. In this direction is to be found one of the approaches to the patient's strong unconscious homosexuality, at bottom determined pre-oedipally.

The patient, by exhibiting herself, played the part of her mother through identification, in this way emphasizing the 'malice' of the mother's denial: 'To strange men you show yourself without restraint, but not to your own child.' Here there is a connection with the typical behavior of oral people, to which I have called attention: they constantly bring the mother of early pre-oedipal days into the situation of denying, despite the greatest superabundance, in order to be able to be pseudo-aggressive without any feelings of guilt and to exploit the denial masochistically.

In later years, the mother and daughter would go walking together, would coquette with men, and then jeer at them. The game was started by the patient to demonstrate the mother's malice: 'You show yourself to every strange man, but not to me.'

As an apparent contradiction, the patient said that her voyeurism was uninhibited on one single point: she could look at every woman's bosom without embarrassment. As an explanation we might in general appeal to the quantitative factor in the symptom formation, and to the fact that even in the best of cases the symptom is an *attempt* to settle inner conflicts which does not always succeed entirely. But because of their unmeasurability, quantitative factors should always be the last refuge. We must question whether looking at the breast really did satisfy primary voyeurism, for the looking may have been a defense. This supposition, once it had arisen, could not be dismissed. In fact, it is probable that the patient's looking at women's breasts might reassure her that the breast was still there.[31] The patient was thus defending herself against the chronic latent reproach of conscience—'You want to bite off your mother's breast'—establishing the intactness of the breast she was looking at, and identifying her mother with other women. In addition, the patient satisfied aggression against her mother: she said that she always found her own bosom to be the most beautiful.

To consider now the patient's harassing fears that, like her mother, she would die of cancer of the breast: at such times, she was immediately compelled to think of amputation of the breast. Her fears were greater by comparison than the usual fears in such cases. But if the supposition is correct that the patient's libidinal and aggressive interests had been concentrated from earliest times on the mother's breast, an explanation lies close at hand. They are the consequences of her unconscious feeling of guilt: 'You wanted to tear off your mother's breast; as punishment the same thing shall happen to yours'.

How thoroughly the defense against the patient's fantasied disappointment with her mother was directed towards the narcissistic restitution of the impaired fantasy of omnipotence and defiant revenge, are indicated by the following details. The patient was a passionate drinker of milk, which she consumed by the quart. The implied defiance of her mother was: 'I don't need *your* milk.' Similarly, we may regard the above-mentioned warding off of disappointment, 'I want to look', as a disavowal, 'I want to display myself.' With this patient everything

31 Very much as many agoraphobes refute their compensatory death wishes against their 'companion' through the constant necessity of having that person with them, i.e., through that person's bodily intactness, as Helene Deutsch has shown.

was based on hate-laden defiance and exaggerated independence; the possibility of kindly, good-natured relations with others was altogether spoiled. For her the statement certainly holds that man lives less by his drives and impulses than by his defense mechanisms and his attempts at narcissistic restitution.

It is difficult to exaggerate the pseudo-aggressive component in the symptom of erythrophobia. Thus, for example, these patients often have the strange unconscious notion that the woman's breast contains blood. Whether this represents a primary theory or a secondary one making use of the patient's own aggressions against the mother's breast, is difficult to say, although the latter seems to be the more probable. In the full-blown symptom there are thus included unconscious aggression against the breast (growing blood-red) and unconscious punishment therefor. On the other hand, red cheeks often serve as bait; erythrophobic men, in female identification, utilize them in unconscious femininity. And finally it must not be forgotten that blushing is often held to be a sign of beauty. Recall Lessing's words in Nathan the Wise: 'Blushing makes even the ugliest so beautiful, shall it not make the beautiful still more beautiful?'

As evidence of the oral substructure of the patient's malady, we have a suddenly emerging remembrance of a tale told by her mother. When the patient was a child, her mother had told her that as an infant she had long been given to screaming violently. The family doctor was puzzled until a consulting specialist explained: "The child is famished," and ordered a milk fattening cure. For this reason the patient was kept on a fattening diet in later years, which, among other things, led to her plump, chubby cheeks. This factor, bound up with a real oral disappointment of the suckling infant due to the mother's mastitis, while certainly not the sole cause of her malady, might very well have had a good part in it. The essential point could well have been the unfavorable psychic utilization of the orality and its voyeuristic derivatives; yet the constitutional reënforcement of orality and the real disappointment during the period of suckling must not pass unregarded. An interesting detail relating to the choice of her own cheeks as substitute for the maternal breast must be mentioned. The patient, as we have noted, had full cheeks as a child which people always would tell her, looked like 'milk and blood' ('peaches and cream'). Every visitor would pet them, make friendly remarks on their size, color and firmness. As the patient was brought up with great regard for modesty, her cheeks were virtually the only part of her body permitted to be exhibited. Naturally it is not implied that this is the entire explanation for the selection of the cheeks. Very probably other elements played a part, e.g., displacement from below upwards, mentioned by all analytic writers on the subject, i.e., the later penis identification from the oedipal period. In the pre-oedipal period, however, the pre-oedipal significance of the penis as a breast should be considered. In this connection, I point to a game played by another patient in his seventh year. He again and again saw women suckling their children. This excited him sexually and led to the following: he took a long blade of straw, stuck it into his own penis, put the end to his lips and drank his own urine.[32] Here the psychic utilization of the conception of the penis as breast is unmistakable. The pre-oedipal stage is also indicated by the fact that two cheeks made use of psychically in blushing are in obvious correspondence to the two breasts. Further, it should be emphasized that the oral-receptive desire finds expression in the fact that while the cheeks do not secrete a fluid like the breasts, they have the mouth lying between them and the mouth can *devour*. Thus this desire insinuates itself into the defense against the earlier fantasy of being "devoured". Finally, it should be stressed that the choice of the cheeks emerges gradually, and the existence of exhibitionistic forestages of the whole body, the penis, the buttocks, etc. may be demonstrated.

The three-layer structure here indicated for the symptom of pathological blushing has already been postulated in the case of another malady, likewise connected with the scopophilic impulse. In depersonalization, Eidelberg and I have stated that an anal-exhibitionistic impulse is repressed and built secondarily into a reactive narcissistic voyeur wish: 'I don't want to show myself at all; I will look at myself.' The morbid self-observation of the depersonalized we attributed to unconscious voyeur desire. This defense is also repressed and leads in a third layer to a new effort of the unconscious ego: 'I don't look; I observe myself for the sake of conscience. I do not enjoy myself; I suffer.'

As to the therapeutic consequences arising from the three-layer

[32] For details see "Zur Problematik der Pseudodebilität" (loc. cit.) and Ch. VI No. 9.

structure in the special case of morbid blushing, it would appear that the hitherto customary interpretation of phallic exhibitionism is, to say the least, inadequate. Brought forward by itself, it does not break down the symptom. On the contrary, it bolsters the unconscious defense mechanism. In my opinion, it is always necessary to point to the defensive character of the exhibitionism in the symptom and to show that this exhibitionism is a protective wall, a sort of moral alibi, against the still more forbidden voyeur wishes. If this is done consistently over a long period of time, the prospects of therapy are essentially improved.

It is also a mistake to believe that the pseudo-paranoid ideas expressed by these patients constitute an excuse for lack of therapeutic success. These ideas must be properly understood. At bottom, it is a question of an alibi for looking at one's self through projection: 'I am not looking at myself; the others are doing it.'

7. Writer's Block.

Early psychoanalytic studies by Freud, Rank, Sachs, Reik, Brill, considerably advanced the knowledge of the artist's motivation. Instead of the rather naive preanalytic assumption that the artist expresses his *conscious* wishes in a camouflaged form, analysis proved that *unconscious* wishes and fantasies were presented. The contents of these fantasies were, according to all but one of the authors, quoted above, oedipal in scope. Only Brill stated that pre-oedipal material was used, and suspected that "chewing and sucking of nice words and phrases," hence the oral getting desire, was the contents of the poetic outlet.

My own studies [33] on the psychology of writers led to the result that I suggested—on the basis of clinical material comprising *thirty some cases*—a substantial revision of current views. I arrived at these conclusions.

[33] "Talleyrand-Napoleon-Stendhal-Grabbe," Int. Psychoan-Verl. 1935. "A Clinical Approach to the Psan. of Writers," Psan. Rev. *31*:1, 1944. "The Danger Neurotics Dread Most: Loss of the Basic Fallacy," ibid. *33*:2, 1946. "Psychoanalysis of Writers and of Literary Productivity," in Roheim's Psan. and the Social Sciences, Int. Univ. Press 1947. "Further Contributions to the Psan. of Writers. I and II." The Psan. Rev. *34*:4, 1947 and *35*:1, 1948. "This Typewriter to Hire—Psychology of the Hackwriter," The Psychiatric Quarterly, 1949. "Writers' Block and Unconscious Sources of Literary Productivity" Psan. and the Social Sciences, Int. Univ. Press, 1949.

1. I came to the conclusion that the writer does *not,* in his work, *express his unconscious wishes and fantasies,* as had been assumed previously; but rather that, under pressure of his unconscious guilt feelings, he gives expression to his unconscious *defense against these wishes and fantasies.*

2. My clinical experience taught me that the writer does *not* suffer from a "shameless urge to reveal himself," that is, from the *exhibitory* impulse which, since Rank, has been asserted by every psychoanalytic biographer. On the contrary, I could prove that every writer, on the deepest level of his being, is a *voyeur* who utilizes his exhibitionistic tendencies as a defense against these scopophiliac impulses.

3. The basic unconscious difficulty in writers is an *oral-masochistic conflict* with a *specific defense twist* in his unique "solution." However, according to my conception, the writer's type of neurotic orality is not greediness or a wish "to receive" in repetition of the child-mother situation, but rather a spiteful desire for *oral* independence. By this, the artist *identifies* himself with the "giving" mother out of defensive pseudo-aggression toward her, and thus eliminates her. He achieves oral pleasure for himself through "beautiful" words and ideas. In its deepest sense, it is a desire to refute the "bad" pre-oedipal mother and the masochistic "disappointments" experienced through her, by establishing an "autarchy," *acting a magic gesture.* The peculiar solution of the writer (and every real artist) is the fact that he—and he *only*—acts in his productivity *both roles (mother—child) on himself.* No other neurotic or normal "solution" is known in which a person makes out of the *duality* (mother—child) a *unity:* every neurotic and normal person needs for the acting out of infantile fantasies *two* people. The writer (and artist) condenses this duality into—one person. He thus makes of the typical neurotic duality—a "*one person show.*"

The writer's alibi before his conscience, is peculiar and specific for him. He denies the oral-masochistic attachment to mother by intrapsychically *denying her mere existence.* His unconscious argument runs something like this: "How can I be accused of masochistic attachment to mother, when mother doesn't even exist? How can I be accused of the wish to be refused, when my wish is to get?" In his giving to himself, the defensive alibi-wish is dramatized!

4. I found myself forced to conclude that many psychoanalytic biographies were constructed on a fallacy, namely, on analogy. Very few writers were actually analyzed, but a great amount of analytic experience was gathered from analyses of neurotics. Because in these *clinical* cases the oedipus complex was found to be the basis of hysteric and compulsive neuroses, and because in *writings* of unanalyzed writers the oedipus complex also could be discovered, the analogy was obvious: In both—in neurotics and writers—the oedipus complex seemed to be decisive. That was fallacy by analogy. Clinical analysis shows that, in writers, orality is the basic element. The analysts of the first decades were struggling for a recognition, as it were, of the oedipus complex; hence they were delighted to find evidence of it in the writings of famous men. What they erroneously concluded was that these writings revealed the unconscious wishes of the writer. They overlooked the possibility that the oedipus complex could be used as a defense against more deeply imbedded oral material.

5. In contrast to the "approach by analogy," I found that the *clinical approach*, that is, a psychoanalytically unprejudiced attitude in a clinical analysis of writers, led to therapeutic results. This statement is based on clinical analysis of thirty-six writers.

6. The writer's productivity denotes that his alibi of "overcoming" the oral-masochistic conflict has been accepted by the superego—temporarily at least. When, however, this productivity fails him and he becomes victim of writer's block and sterility, at that moment the superego rejects the alibi, claiming "You still want to be refused!" To counteract that reproach, the alibi is unconsciously reinforced by pronouncing the defense: "The indictment is unjustified! *I* want to refuse and not be refused." Thus, the unproductive writer is caught in his own defensive net: by dramatizing his refusal, he satisfies the need for the stronger alibi. But—and here the tragedy of unproductivity starts—the alibi makes him sterile: he no longer can give words and ideas.

The specific features, characterizing productive writing, have these interconnections:

1. Before the writer is technically capable of writing, he must develop a "plot." A plot presupposes "imagination"; and the basis of the latter is sublimated voyeurism. Normally, in the process of writing, *voyeurism is changed into exhibitionism,* simply because by writing down his

story, the author exhibits before publisher and reader. Hence, the transformation of voyeurism into exhibitionism, is essential.

In cases in which the superego does not accept the alibi and accuses the writer of infantile sexual connotation (of being an infantile Peeping-Tom), the alibi is "lack of imagination," hence sterility results.

2. The writer must convince his inner conscience that he is *not interested in his original wish, but only in the defense.* For instance: A patient of mine wanted to write a comedy in which a man accepted the sacrifice of his wife only to learn that his whole life thereafter was made miserable by her resenting her sacrifice. Let us assume that the man had written that aggressive comedy and that one hundred years later a psychoanalytic biographer would make a study of the famous author. He would come to the conclusion that the author was an exceedingly aggressive person to whom nothing, not even sacrifice, was sacred. Actually, however, the patient was a very passive, severe hypochondriac. What he expressed in his work was not his aggressive id-wish, but the defense against his passivity via pseudo-aggression. The moment the alibi is not accepted, sterility sets in.

3. Enlisting of the reader as "*accomplice in crime*" must be successful. Every work of art contains implicitly an invitation to the reader or spectator to partake in the writer's inner guilt. The writer unconsciously reasons: "If people approve of my work, they accept its unconscious contents, too; my guilt is therefore shared by them and lightened." This mechanism of expiation, first stressed by Rank and Sachs, must be modified insofar as the reader is invited to share the writer's inner defenses and not his inner wishes directly.

4. Very strange is the fact that an *objectively psychologic correct evaluation of the material* presented, *must correspond to the alibi*, which makes the writer write. If it doesn't, the writer must, out of inner necessity, write psychological trash.

For instance: A fine writer published a book describing an "injustice collector" in the making. Afterwards, he became sterile and produced but one short story, depicting a "perfect murder." The element of guilt was fully excluded—an inner impossibility and unpardonable literary and psychological error.

Analysis of the "silly mistake" revealed, that the writer became so frightened of his own psychic masochism (though described in his novel as if the hero were but the innocent victim), that he had to reinforce his defensive alibi. That defense consisted of pseudo-aggression and aggressive negation of guilt. Hence, the "mistake" in the subsequent story.

What differentiates the *typewriter-operator* from the *real writer,* is his unconscious psychological insight, coupled with his conscious ignorance of the real motives. Ironically, one could say that the last person to ask for explanation of his own dramatis personae, is the writer himself. He will give some silly rationalizations. Still, he will (if he is a real writer) describe correctly the psychological actions of his marionettes. This occurs only if the inner defense he has to furnish before his forum internum corresponds to inner facts. The coincidence of both factors makes for a "real" writer. Basically, he solves his inner conflict in this "self-cure" and even gets paid for it, very much in contradiction to the typical neurotic who has to pay the physician for his cure.

In any case, a blank head, a blank sheet of paper, connected by a typewriter, manipulated by shaky or determined fingers, does not automatically constitute the phenomenon "a writer."

Analysis of writer's block is, in my purely personal opinion, successful only on condition that the above stated oral mechanisms are applied.

If they *are* applied, one can promise to the patient with 100% surety that analysis will "open the literary safe." One can add: "What we will find in that safe, is another story." In other words, we don't guarantee "Genius," we just guarantee that the writer will be capable of writing. Oddly enough, in no other neurotic difficulty can we be so sure of success!

If the mechanisms enumerated above are *not* applied, and writing is explained on the phallic and anal levels, the analyst only maneuvers himself into more troubles than he bargained for, and the writer-patient will remain—unproductive. I know of cases in which the patient was told that he was no writer at all and "guided" into some tangential profession. In other cases, analysts told their "cured" patients with writing block that they will "perhaps, or perhaps not," write in later years—shifting the blame to impersonal Fate. In one other case of a female writer, the analyst—confronted by the patient with my publications—

stated that the latter do not apply to her, because my examples dealt with orally regressed neurotics, she, however, represented a hysterical one. That diagnosis was wrong; not less the definition of what constitutes a writer. A writer is a person who unconsciously tries to solve his (her) inner conflicts via writing. Hence, a person is, psychologically speaking, a writer whether or not he is successful or unsuccessful in that endeavor, did or did not ever write even one line, published or did not publish that line. It represents a psychologic attempt at solution of conflicts, and it is not the analyst's business, nor is it within his competence, to decide ("how like a God") whether or not the patient has the "stuff," making for a successful writer. It can happen that the writer whose writing block is analytically removed, decides *not* to devote his energies to writing—that's his business and depends upon his appreciation of reality factors. The analyst's job is simply to remove the writing block.

I observed in the continuation of an analysis an especially tragic case in which an exceptionally gifted writer "lost" his writing ability through analysis. The man's oral neurosis had been misunderstood by the first analyst as being a hysterical one. The transference was one of the "devouring mother" type though interpreted as oedipal father projection. The patient played a diabolic-masochistic joke on the naive analyst: he unconsciously preferred the pseudo-aggressive grievance against the analyst to—writing. The continuation of that analysis showed the neurotic reaction on the patient's part, and the analyst's misunderstanding of the transference situation.

It may be rightly objected that in the above exposition a decisive factor has been completely overlooked: congenital talent. Freud has never failed to stress that, psychologically, we can understand only the superstructure of the artist. Without allowing for talent, i.e., the constitutional factor, an explanation of the artist's personality is, according to Freud, incomplete.

I personally believe that the biological part of the mysterious ingredient "talent" can be defined in writers more precisely today. It consists of a quantitative increase of oral tendencies and their derivative: voyeurism. Both are biologically conditioned. In other words, I do not believe that a writer can be a writer without this specific, biologically-conditioned admixture. The psychic superstructure of writing can be more easily described, as has been tried in this section. Still, the results are "strange":

> " 'Tis strange—but true; for truth is always strange,
> Stranger than fiction."
>
> Byron, *Don Juan*

Quantitative increase of orality and its derivative, voyeurism, do not constitute per se the phenomenon, a writer. Obviously, something else is necessary: oral regression and a specific technique of coping with this regression. The writer has not passed through the danger zone of orality unhurt; on the contrary, he fights desperately to master his childhood situation. He uses a specific technique—specific for him only—to overcome the deep disappointment experienced through his mother. Intrapsychically, he denies her existence and thus the possibility of being disappointed by her. He makes her superfluous by acting unconsciously her part as well as his own in the autarchic giving of words and the autarchic receiving of words as accepted substitutes for earliest "gifts" (milk, love, attention). Obviously, strong narcissism is a prerequisite of his technique, as is the queer ability to transform voyeurism into exhibitionism, which depends somewhat on narcissism. The psychological part of "talent" is related to these peculiar mechanisms of reparation of masochistic fantasies or experiences. The latter half of the formulation: "The literary safe can be opened analytically; what will be found there, is another story," refers to the fact that the mechanism described as peculiar to writers may or may not be the leading mechanism; if it is not, the "writer" is not a real writer. Generally, it is, if a genuine sublimation can be developed.

A writer of distinction, whose "durable fame" has been conceded by the not too benevolent critic of *The New York Times*, gave, after being successfully analyzed by myself, an interview to a metropolitan newspaper in which he realistically described the trials and tribulations of his writing block:

> "Although . . . . . is the author of seven books, among them an international best seller, entitled . . . . ., he considers . . . . . (his new book) as his first book. That's because—in the first place —Mr. . . . . . has been silent as a tomb for seven years; and—in

the second place—through the rack of those long, lean years Mr. . . . . . feels he underwent a change, and consequently, has started anew. *What happened during much of these years was this: he would sit down at his typewriter and thereupon his mind, heart and hands would become paralyzed. Later he got himself psychoanalyzed* and the seven lean years have given over to what he hopes is the beginning of at least seven fat years (Biblically speaking). Mr. . . . . . is now, and naturally enough, *a convinced Freudian*. . ."

That writer admitted his analytic success openly and gave the permission to use his name which, however, I have declined to do. But the statement is illustrative of the success which *can* be achieved by *every* analyst, treating writers, provided he takes the trouble of acquainting himself with the oral substructure of writer's block.*

A famous writer who underwent analysis with me and whose writing block had been removed, stated correctly that the fate of the writer should not be dependent on any particular analyst's "acceptance or nonacceptance of newer findings." He was a friend of another gifted writer whose analyst told him that he was no writer at all and who consequently gave up writing to become a huckster. The previous publisher of the latter writer was horrified, and wrongly claimed that analysis "destroyed his writing ability." "Look what's going on," complained my patient, "analysts are their own worst advertisers among writers." I consoled the patient with a fact which I once heard in a lecture given by Professor Jellinek, the famous Viennese specialist for medical electropathology. Jellinek related a case of an electrical accident which "killed" a worker. A physician, who had been called in, declared the man dead, *without* ordering protracted artificial respiration. The co-workers of the "dead" man were more optimistic and tried the new method of revival for hours, working on his arms, to bring back respiration. The man *was* finally revived, a human life rescued. Later, the physician who wrote the death certificate was asked why he did not apply that new technique. He answered: "I did not believe in the new theory. . . ."

* There is only one remote chance of removing writer's block with superficial phallic interpretations: if the patient, having projected his own fantasies of magic omnipotence on the analyst, unjustifiably suspects the latter of finding the "deeper secret." This amounts to a "success because of unconscious fear" and is not of long duration. See pp. 337–38.

8. Pseudo-Humbugs and Hucksters

I suggested in 1946 the use of the term "pseudo-humbugs" ("pseudo-bluffers") [34] for neurotics who, though objectively successful, are constantly accused by their respective inner conscience of being a fake, a humbug, a bluffer.

The material presented consisted of 4 advertisers, one journalist, one dramatic critic.

Their analyses proved that all these six people were "writers manqué," who used a specific modification of the mechanism characteristic of creative writers. Whereas the writer changes a voyeuristic wish into the exhibitionistic defense (writing means exhibiting before publisher, reader, etc.), in pseudo-humbugs a different solution is unconsciously found: *the transition occurs, but only on condition that —humbug is displayed.* In other words, a caricature is set in motion. The result is that real artistic productivity is prevented, but its caricature, for instance advertising, is not. What is shown is constant mockery stemming from the sadistic inner conscience (superego). Thus we see why pseudo-humbugs are usually frustrated writers and artists.[35]

The combination of oral-masochistic tendencies and the *specific* solution of the scopophiliac ones gives us the clue to the type of pseudo-bluffers. Men of this type also contribute to the understanding of the tragedy of "not taking one's self seriously." The pseudo-humbugs are habitually under pressure of their inner feeling of guilt that they are humbugs. Seemingly, one of the prerequisites of living in peace with one's conscience is the superego's acceptance of one's work as real and serious. The moment the superego does not accept the work as such, it reproaches the ego, with disastrous results. One could say that the pseudo-humbug does attempt a self-cure, but achieves only a self-cure in—humiliation.

Interesting are the different devices with which the pseudo-humbug

[34] "Psychopathology of Pseudo-Humbugs and Pseudo-Bluffers," The Psychiatric Quarterly Supplement *20*:1, 1946, pp. 14–22.

[35] One could object that perhaps some of the pseudo-humbugs are simply lacking in creative talent. That is possible; their superegos behave, however, as if they were guilty of misuse of their given talents.

of the advertising variety tries to prove to himself that his constant inner reproaches are unjustified. From what I could observe, I would say that that type of neurotic uses the four following inner defenses:

1. *Paternalistic attitude.* The advertiser behaves as if the product he is handling is created, not by manufacture, but by advertising. *He* "makes" it.

2. *Contempt for the public.* The pseudo-humbug has a deep-rooted contempt for the common man whom he wishes to reach, is full of irony toward him. He reminds one of a bit of cynical advice which a famous critic gave to dramatic writers: The writer must pretend to be as stupid as his audience really is, so that the audience can believe itself to be as smart as the writer allegedly is.

3. *Cynicism.* Cynicism is a specific defense mechanism. Years ago the writer could prove [36] that the "mechanism of cynicism" has the following structure: Constant pressure from ambivalence and equally constant pressure from the punitive superego, which penalizes this very ambivalence, so that the "unconscious compulsion to confess" (Reik) becomes the motive power of behavior. The unconscious ego of the cynic relieves itself of this conflict resulting from the crossfire of an id-striving and a superego-prohibition by means of repartee couched in the same form as the original thrust of the assailant. It attempts to prove that *other people possess the same ambivalence.* These "other people" are conceived as part of the subject's own projected superego. The cynic's attack is apparently directed toward this external-world moiety of the superego; in reality the cynic is defending himself against his stringent internal superego, unconscious, and perceptible to him only in the form of a sense of guilt. The rabid behavior of the cynic does not spring from his aggression; it is the expression of a desperate defensive warfare against his "internal enemy," the intrapsychic superego, and it permits the battle to be transferred to "foreign territory." The cynic treats the external world with the same aggressiveness with which his own superego treats his ego. At the same time, the cynic attacks his superego in and via the external world, somewhat according

[36] "Psychology of Cynicism," Psychoan. Bewegung, 1933: "Obscene Words," Psychoan. Quart., 1936; Chap. I of "Talleyrand-Napoleon-Stendhal-Grabbe," Int. Psychoan. Verlag, 1935.

to the formula: "I strike others but am aiming at myself." Basically, every cynic asks the outer world (here, projected superego) to admit that it is no better than he.

4. *Pessimistic outlook and doubts concerning stability of "talent" and "productivity."* All pseudo-bluffers are inwardly full of pessimism, springing partly from their undigested orality, consciously rationalized with doubts as to the continuance of their specific productivity in the form of "ideas." Very typical are their prognoses in connection with "government interference." One of my patients constantly predicted, with malice toward everyone, including himself, that the "unhappy time will come when most of the profits will disappear, because products will be tested objectively by the government, and only those passing the test will be allowed to be popularized." The more solid concerns abstain, even today, from too unscrupulous advertising. Another patient spoke with bitter irony of a manufacturer who wanted his product to be advertised as a "life prolonger." He countered objections to this with actual sales figures, achieved through advertising, which ran high. Said the patient to the writer: "First you make a million dollar baby out of nothing, and afterward you have to use your own fake as objective proof. . . . Do you understand why I call my profession a lot of hullaballoo?"

The feeling of being unjustly treated (See "Mechanism of Orality") was constantly stressed by these patients, and used as an alibi for their "fake" professions. This was very obvious in the four advertisers. The journalist mentioned before had a similar approach. The dramatic critic justified his malicious aggression toward younger creative people in this fashion, using self-created artistic "standards" as an excuse for tearing down their work "on principle." Characterologically, some of these six patients were borderline cases of "psychopathic personalities," not too trustworthy in general. The majority had correctly functioning egos, but, as is usual with orally regressed persons, were at times capable of strange pseudo-aggressions of which they were justifiably ashamed in moments of self-reproach. Sexually, all six had potency difficulties or orgastic disturbances.

The pseudo-humbug suffers from a complicated neurosis, basically in the sphere of scopophilia [37] and is curable analytically. He does not lose his "creative" ability in analysis, as he fears; he can be restored to inner satisfaction and may sometimes even become a writer or artist.

9. Pseudo-Mental Deficiency (Pseudo-Debility).

In 1932, at the time I published my study on pseudo-debility,[38] little was known about that disease-entity. A series of authors had devoted their attention to intellectual inhibitions,[39] but only three authors had made a study of pseudo-debility specifically. In his work on character formation, Abraham drew attention to the taking in of knowledge as oral substitute (orality denoting in his opinion the "sucking-in" attitude), Landauer and B. Bornstein enumerated a series of mechanisms; the later author concluded "that some *not clearly understood* disturbances of the oral phase" are to be blamed.

The case I observed started his analysis with a female colleague because of peculiar reasons: he consulted first a male analyst with the complaint that he did not dare ask a prostitute to urinate into his mouth; to acquire the necessary courage, he wanted analytic treatment. The analyst sent the patient to the female analyst where he remained for a series of months; he became more agitated, especially after a short interruption caused by the woman's giving birth to a child. He became unduly familiar with her (used the pronoun "Du") and developed a truly pathological jealousy of her baby (he called the latter "Herr Saügling," Mr. Baby), and, what is more important, started to attack his mother bodily when angry. The colleague suggested a change of analysts, which the patient immediately agreed to.

In the first interview with me, the patient acted quite rationally, claimed to understand that the transference with the colleague became too "hot" and that his fear was "too big" for him. In his behavior

[37] Scopophilia has been, until now, a stepchild in psychoanalysis. The writer suggested that three neurotic entities in which scopophilia plays the decisive role, depersonalization, erythrophobia, and boredom, should be subsumed under "scopophiliac diseases." See "On the Disease Entity Boredom (Alysosis) and its Psychopathology." Psychiat. Quart., *18*:2, 1944.

[38] "Zur Problematik der Pseudo-debilität," Int. Zeitschrift für Psychoanalyse XVIII, 1932, pp. 528–538. Abstract in Int. Journal of Psa. XIV, 1933, pp. 408–410.

[39] Freud, Aichhorn, Federn, Rado, Laforgue, Klein, Tamm, Zulliger.

on the couch, he presented a rather peculiar picture: He trembled, sweated, and commenced his "associations" with the shouted battlecry: "Don't understand! Don't understand!" This one and only contribution of the patient was wholly anticipatory: there was nothing to understand, since I did not even open my mouth. Every attempt at explaining something was hopeless. To complicate matters, the patient's mother appeared on the scene, informing me that she had decided to transfer the "boy" (he was at that time 23½) into a psychiatric institution—at the advice of her family physician. I warned her against that procedure, whereupon the woman—she owned a big bakery—countered with the remark that she had no reason to have confidence in analysis. First, out of a "harmless idiot," the colleague made a "raving and dangerous" idiot. Second, a therapy which works with "words," cannot be any good, because it contradicts "sound business": "If a customer buys a loaf of bread in the store, I give him a few friendly words, too. Do you think he wants to pay for friendly words alone?"

All this happened after three appointments—the situation looked hopeless. In this quandary, I had an "intuitive" idea, the meaning of which I could not explain. I felt that one should talk for days and weeks with the patient, completely disregarding his shouting of "Don't understand." This I did; it was like telling a child fairy-tales. The patient himself, did not take part in that procedure. I gave him hundreds of simplified examples from analyses of fearful patients; I could just as well have chosen the theme of the weather. In later years I have been always amused at the ethics prompting me to choose medical examples. . . . In any case, *talking* seemed to me the remedy. Why, I could not explain. The patient listened silently; every time I interrupted my tale even for a second (e.g., to light a cigarette) he started his shouting contribution "Don't understand."

This went on for weeks, till one day I used an example from an analysis in which a patient misunderstood the term "resistance." I was interested in this patient's case to find out to what degree of human "stupidity" analysis was still effective. I chose from the waiting list of the clinic, among 2000 people, one with a low I.Q.[40] In this analysis, I told the patient once "You are under the influence of your resistance." The patient answered, "You are quite right, one should

[40] Described in "The Battle of the Conscience," pp. 154–158.

have a good resistance." He misunderstood the word, relating it to "resistance against infection."

That example was countered by my new patient with the remark "What a dope; he must have known what resistance means." This was the first statement the man had made—the ice was broken!

In evaluating theoretically what I did intuitively, I came to the conclusion that the patient projected upon the first analyst the image of the "bad mother" who *refuses* and to whom he was masochistically attached. That masochistic tendency was counteracted by inner guilt, hence the pseudo-aggressive tendency of the alleged *wish to get* had to be established. Hence, his demanding and jealous attitude.

At the time he came to me, he expected punishment for these wishes and defenses. In shutting his ears and shouting "Don't understand," he reduced from the start every connection ad absurdum, more, he acted out a demonstration of "You cannot achieve anything with me." What the patient was really afraid of, was not any punishment, but a break-through of his pseudo-aggressive defense. Preventively, he reinforced the aggressive defense. My giving attitude confronted him with a new problem: "Mother does not refuse; on the contrary, she gives." He now seized the opportunity of a new *defense:* "That's exactly what I really want—to be given." On the basis of the defense a temporary modus vivendi had been established!

The life history of the patient, especially his neurotic evaluation of reality, gave later (after that preparatory phase, clinical analysis could be conducted) abundant proof for these conjectures.

The patient was the son of an aggressive domineering mother and a bored, dissatisfied father. He was the second child; his one-year-older sister suffered in her childhood from infantile paralysis. The boy disappointed both parents with his "stupidity"; both punished him severely. Both parents found in the child a scapegoat for their unhappy marriage: the father hated his profession, and spoke about his years spent in military service during the war as the high point in his life. The mother was deeply disappointed with the boy for whom she dreamt of an "intellectual career." These dreams had been rudely interrupted as early as the first grade: the boy was expelled from school because of masturbating during school hours. The parents were so "disgusted" with the child that they sent him away from home, to a school in a hamlet where the school teacher was at the same time the owner of the boarding house. Here he remained from his 7th to 11th year; he repeated the old provocative pattern: he could not grasp anything, nor could he retain in his memory anything. Stigmatized as a "moron," he knew the feelings of the rejected child, unhappy about the lack of "home life." In compensatory spite he stated that he preferred to be away from home.

During these years away from home, an incident occurred which threw light on his sexual fantasies. He observed at the age of 7 a gypsy woman suckling her baby. This excited him sexually, and he produced the following game: he put a long straw in his penis, took the end in the mouth, urinated and drank his own urine. In this game, penis and breast, milk and urine, are clearly identified. He acted *autarchically:* giving mother and accepting baby!

The patient's whole life seemed to be concentrated on oral *getting:* he was a voracious eater, drinker and smoker, always sucking on something. His conscious motto was "the important thing is the juice." He had no conscious interest in the breast "nothing comes out of it," he complained. His occupation in the movies was sucking the fingers of the girl. Some asked him ironically "Do you think something will come from it?" His wish to be urinated upon by the woman as sex equivalent, belonged in the same category.

His relationship to his mother proved that these wishes were not to be taken at face value. He constantly provoked refusal and was full of pseudo-aggression towards her—allegedly because of her refusal ("Mechanism of Orality"). He was constantly demanding—at times where his mother's "No" was to be expected. Every refusal was masochistically exploited. On the other hand, he claimed that he would rather "bite his tongue," than ask his mother for a favor. His practice was quite different: he asked in order to be refused. During these conflicts, he was "terrified to death," and once compared his situation with a "rabbit hypnotized by a snake."

The predominance of oral demanding was thus a defense against the reproaches of his conscience, accusing him of the masochistic wish to be refused. As *defense* the wish to get had been reinforced. Equally reinforced was the pseudo-aggressive defense: after his father's death, the patient became officially manager of the bakery and gave exaggerated production figures to the income tax office, just to "make my mother pay."

His pseudo-debility had different reasons.[41] The decisive one was the identification of taking in of food and taking in of knowledge, a fact first viewed in our literature by Abraham. (Poets knew that equation long ago; see, for example, Goethe's Faust: "to suck on wisdom's breasts.") In his refusal to "take in" knowledge and information, he acted out pseudo-aggressively his defense: "I don't want to be refused, *I* refuse." Behind that thinly veiled aggression toward the parents, was hidden a deep masochistic regression: he played for high stakes, since having been considered an "idiot and moron," was not exactly pleasant.

At the same time, he demonstrated in his stupidity "See, how my mother starved me?" Grotesquely, he had even consciously fears lest his mother throw him out of the business, thus "throwing him to the dogs and leaving him to starvation."

The degree to which he masochistically reduced the mother to the role of "refuser," was visible also in a trick he played with himself when visiting prostitutes. He stipulated the price of shilling 10, Austrian denomination, paid with a bill of 20—"to get something from the girl." The "gift" of the change was—his money. His urolagnic tendencies were similarly explainable, at least on higher levels, where urine already had the derogatory connotation. He thus proved to himself how bad woman is!

It was amazing to what degree the patient changed in analysis. The "moron" later became the director of a Viennese bakery in another country, where he introduced Viennese rolls.

In a series of other cases I found similar oral-masochistic tendencies as basis of pseudo-debility. The disease *is* curable.

10. Retirement-Neurosis.

"Retirement neurosis" is a term coined by myself in collaboration with Dr. Olga Knopf in our study "A Test for the Differential Diagnosis between Retirement Neurosis and Accident Neurosis." [42] We defined

[41] In the original study a series of seven reasons is enumerated.

[42] The Journal of Nervous and Mental Diseases, Vol. 100, 4, 1944, pp. 366–380.

that type of neurosis as characterized by the following symptoms and signs:

(1) A *young* and organically *healthy* person concentrates consciously all of his energy toward achieving an "independent income" at the young age—the twenties or early thirties, subordinating all other interests to that goal.

(2) The desire for retirement is not influenced by special predilections in the use of free time. *The goal is purely negative;* to be undisturbed in "doing nothing."

(3) In strange contradiction to the high-pitched and exalted expectation that the true enjoyment of living should start with an "independent income" is the fact that a person of the type we have in mind has a pronounced financial modesty. He is satisfied with a *very small income,* but one which is not dependent upon work.

(4) After achieving his "retirement paradise," such an individual *does not know what to do with his time,* does not enjoy his leisure; on the contrary, sinks more and more into neurotic *depression* or hypochondriac symptoms.

(5) If the independent income or pension is withdrawn (through bankruptcy or inflation), this person is *incapable of making a new start* and remains a flop and a failure.

(6) A special subtype is found in the young man who inherits money and has only one occupation—"to enjoy life." Even the laymen can recognize that this individual lives only his respective neurosis, since the layman often naïvely pronounces that work could "heal" him. Such a neurotic is utterly convinced that he could not earn a dollar; he is very miserly and lives in constant fear of social changes which might endanger or diminish his income.

(7) With but few exceptions the person suffering *objectively* from retirement neurosis does not feel sick *subjectively.* In other words, the presence of the retirement neurosis is not acknowledged consciously; quite the contrary, the objections stemming from the outer world are consciously discarded, in spite of the fact that an *inner* feeling of guilt is present. A patient of this type enters analysis—if at all—because of other symptoms, seemingly not associated with his retirement neurosis.

As can be seen from these conditions, we are not speaking about people who retire for reasons of health or invalidism. Nor do we have in mind old people who, after many years of work, want peace and rest. We have in mind exclusively organically healthy individuals who have the same psychology in *young* years which, when encountered in the sixties, would be considered normal.

Here is a clinical example, analyzed by myself many years ago: A woman of 32 entered psychoanalysis because of "frigidity, depression, sleeplessness and personality difficulties, showing up in always choosing the wrong man," to quote her. She was—at the age of 32!—a retired [43] employee of a Viennese bank, having started her career at the age of 19 and having retired with a small pension on the first day on which that pension could be attained—after ten years of service. All of her life, she claimed, she had wanted to be "independent." She chose her career in a bank, purposely in order to retire after ten years with a pension. She endured the "hell and boredom" of working only with the consolation that one day—at 30—she would be free to do as she pleased. She achieved her goal and retired with a small pension, further bolstered by a small sum which she had managed to save during her "slavery," as she called her 10 years of employment.

To her amazement, the new life did not work out so well. For the first few days she enjoyed the fact that she no longer had to live "under the tyranny of the clock"; she could stay in bed as long as she wanted; she could eat at unconventional hours and sit at the window observing passers-by. She felt superior to her colleagues, who made fun of her retirement, considering them "silly slaves." But very soon she felt depressed; however, she attributed this to difficulties of adjustment. She postponed the expectation of happiness for a few weeks, hoping that the adjustment period would pass. Time went by but her boredom and sense of depression deepened. She was surprised that, in her ten years of work, she had made no definite plans on how to spend her free time. The only thoughts which she always had were purely negative ones; *not* to live according to the clock, *not* to be forced to get up in the morning, *not* to have to rush to the office, *not* to waste time on boring work, etc. There were only two

[43] In pre-Hitler Austria it was possible for an employee of the government or a large corporation to retire with a small pension after at least ten years of service, independent of the state of health.

positive ideas in her plan: to sit in a chair indulging in day dreams and to read as much as she liked. Both bored her now, to her amazement. She enlarged her program and decided to "regulate" her sex life. She had previously had a few sexual experiences always avoiding marriage. According to her, all of her male friends were "pigs, wanting only sex without tenderness." She had retired from sex a few years before her retirement from work, having become disgusted with men. Shortly after her retirement, though, she met a young man who seemed to conform better to her ideals of tenderness. She was hit squarely in the face, however, when this man, too, left her, explaining that she was "frigid and yet sexually sponging." This experience and the complete emptiness of her life were the outward reasons for her feeling of being sick. She consulted the physician of her health insurance company, who consented to pay for psychoanalytic treatment for four months. She was sent to me and started treatment.

Conflicts arose immediately in the analysis with regard to the time of her appointments. Since the appointments started and ended at precise times, it was up to her to be punctual. However, she always came late, though she had no occupation, cutting the appointment in half or sometimes even appearing for only five minutes. She claimed that her coming late was a neurotic symptom in itself and was furious that the analyst refused to make allowances for her tardy arrival, closing the session at the appointed time. Even the fact that the next patient was waiting did not convince her that she suffered no injustice.

From her family history it could be gathered that her autocratic mother was the real head of the family, her father "being a weak and unimportant person." She was conscious of having hated her mother all her life, provoked her mercilessly and lived in constant conflict with her. She had two younger brothers whom she also hated. She accused her mother of playing favorites with the boys; only for a short time did she have the fantasy of wanting to be a boy herself. The typical penis envy developed, leading to aggressive actions toward her brothers. After the birth of the second boy she "retired completely from reality" and became a precocious and omniverous reader at the age of six! There were reasons to assume that the patient regressed orally at this point, activating an early, inwardly not rejected, libidinous-aggressive position. Her incessant reading signified: "I am independent of you, Mother; I am autarchic and 'get' as much as I want." Of course, that spiteful desire to "get," the precursor of her pension-mania, was not the real wish at all. It represented the defense against the masochistic wish of being disappointed. That this interpretation was correct could further be proved by the fact that the patient, in her later life, usually presented her wishes in such a way that she received only disappointments, a technique which she also acted out in the transference. She went through her school years shy, sullen, indignant, often experiencing conscious hatred for everyone. She left home at 19, did not want to see her family again, and lived only for her "retirement" fantasy.

Very little information could be obtained from the patient during her eight weeks of analysis, for she wanted first to "straighten out" the difficulties over her appointment hour. Since the analyst insisted that she come at her appointed time and the patient insisted that she could not, a stalemate ensued, especially when she refused to analyze her attitude. She was shown that she was provoking unconsciously a masochistic situation, that she wanted to be disappointed. By means of the simple device of coming too late with the excuse that she could not help herself, she was utilizing reality for her unconscious desire to be disappointed. It was explained to her furthermore that her outbursts of hatred and indignation were only a covering cloak for masochistic enjoyment. Every attempt to trace this attitude back to experiences and fantasies connected with her mother was blocked by her insistence that the problem at hand was a "real" problem and had nothing to do with the past. The idea that she should seek *displeasure* seemed senseless to her, since she was not "such a fool." To prove that she was definitely a "pleasure seeker," she pointed out that she had spent the last ten years in seeking pleasure—by working toward a pension. The objection that her retirement at 30 was a neurotic action in itself was pooh-poohed by her on the ground that "slaves could not understand the free."

One day she proposed that she should come after the analyst's last appointment (at 7:30 P.M.) and wait. Since the analyst would be eating dinner during the next half hour, he would not be inconvenienced by her late arrival; he could analyze her after dinner. She parried the objection that even the analyst's working day must end somewhere with the furious exclamation: "So you simply don't want to give in!" In the superficial layer, this queer proposal showed megalomania and also that she considered herself an exception, who had to be loved. In a deeper layer, it was intended to interfere with the analyst's pleasure in eating, since even she admitted that only "a person who stood above the situation" could accept such a proposal. Her unconscious desire was basically the wish to be refused. During these discussions she had the peculiar habit of playing with her bankbook. This gesture was interpreted sexual-symbolically and as bribe and refusal, implying ironically: "After four months (the time allotted by the health insurance company) I can continue treatment at my own expense." She accepted this explanation gloatingly. Her "tendency to refuse" appeared not in money matters alone. She refused, for instance, to mention dreams and fantasies or to produce free associations, when the analyst refused to give in concerning the time of the appointments. She had, of course, the fantasy that the analyst was upset over her refusal to come at the appointed time; it was obvious that she identified him with her mother.

After two months she started to look for another, "more understanding" analyst. She consulted approximately eight highly-paid colleagues, offering each a twentieth of his regular fee although she was well informed about the fees usually paid for analytic treatment. Tearfully she asserted that she wanted to sacrifice one-third of her monthly pension for analysis. All of these analysts regretted that they had no time available. After thus having "proved" to herself that nobody could understand her, she retired, full of hatred, from her "analytic experiment."

Only a few details can be added to this sketchy outline. The patient practically refused to give material, being interested only in her "real" problem of arranging the time for her appointments. The idea that she was producing neurotic repetition in the transference seemed silly to her. One could reconstruct, however, that she repeated the "mother situation" in the transference. The mother was conceived by her to be a draining monster. What the patient did not even suspect was that she was masochistically attached to this mother, always wanting, through her provocations to push her mother into the situation of refusing, so that she in turn might indulge in hatred toward her. Her own initial provocation was repressed. Afterward she pitied herself masochistically. To what extent her life was based on this wish to be refused was evidenced by her actions with regard to the other analysts. She made clever use of their relatively high fees for her purpose of being disappointed. She knew that one-twentieth of the regular fee could not pay for an appointment. Unconsciously, she did not want the appointment; she wanted the refusal. Consciously, she wanted the opportunity to complain about the first analyst. Her aggressive front as a defense against deeper masochistic pleasure proved very effective: She never understood what was wish and what was secondary defense.

A few glimpses could be obtained into the genesis of her deep-seated retirement neurosis. In the superficial layer it represented an attempt at self-cure from childhood disappointments, an attempt to be independent of the refusing mother. She built a situation in which she seemingly exchanged the refusing mother for a giving one. But that giving mother—the bank—gave very little, barely covering the minimal necessities of life. Interestingly enough, the patient had no conscious feeling of being unjustly treated by the bank. This was explainable by the fact that she still fought with the bad mother, constructing in defense a good one who, for the sake of contrast, had to be as elevated as the real one had to be demoted. Her acceptance of so little meant also an aggression toward her mother: "You see with how little I could be satisfied." On the other hand, the bad mother was masochistically perpetuated: "She gives me so little, and that only as a reward for ten years of slavery."

The attempted self-cure failed, because it was a conscious and purely narcissistic effort to cope with something over which the patient had no control: her deep masochistic attachment to the pre-oedipal mother. She wanted unconsciously to repeat and enjoy the situation of being refused. That she got.

Her frigidity, too, was orally conditioned. With men also she repeated the game of being refused: Everyone disappointed her. She was insatiable in sex; her last friend had called her "sponging." She demanded continuous intercourse, was full of irony for the man who could not be an "intercourse machine." At the same time she was completely frigid. The pseudo-aggressive formula, covering deeper repressed masochism. was: She was not given; therefore she did not give. She reported having had only once a feeling of pleasure in sexual activity; this was a queer sensation of triumph after having indirectly forced the man to have intercourse for the fifth time during one night. Her thought at that time was: cutting off the penis during intercourse through muscular contraction. Ejaculation of the man gave her special pleasure, since the idea of having drained him was near the psychic surface.

Dr. Knopf and I came to the conclusion on the basis of 6 cases, that *retirement neurosis is a specific form of oral neurosis.* It presupposes unsolved conflicts on the pre-oedipal level. The neurotic sign itself, seeking a pension or another form of economically-secured retirement in younger years, where normally the struggle for achieving specific aims in life is the order of the day, is an unconscious attempt to correct and solve the conflict with the "refusing" mother, as a form of self-cure. The desire "to get" is the covering cloak for the deeper masochistic wish to be disappointed by her or by projected mother images.

11. Writer's Cramp.[44]

In 1933 [45] I published a case of writer's cramp, analyzed in 1928, proving its oral genesis. At that time the symptom had been either considered a simple phallic conversion, or a urethral expression (Jokl). The case had been reported in 1929 in the Technical Seminary of the Vienna Psychoanalytical Society, and I suggested as main problem the unclear connection between the urethral and oral components, without getting any usable answer from the participants of the seminar.

The patient, at the time of his analysis 41 years of age, had been in previous years a minor official in a bank; he was dismissed with a small pension because of his persistent and "incurable" writing cramp. It had started "without reasons" when he had to sign some unimportant paper a few years before in the bank. Subsequently, he underwent various types of treatment, without any change of symptom. The use of the right hand was otherwise not inhibited at all, only when writing,

[44] "Writer's *cramp*" should not be confused with "writer's *block*" (section 7). The first denotes a pseudo-neurological problem, the second sterility in artistic productivity. Writer's block is an occupational disease of professional writers; writer's cramp can befall everyone.

[45] Case II in "The Breast Complex of the Male." Int. Z. f. Psychoan. 1933.

or using the spoon for fluid food, in drinking a glass with water or beer, shaking became very pronounced. Writing with a pencil was less difficult than with ink and pen; the patient tried to learn to write with the left hand, but discovered to his dismay that the left hand was shaky, too.

It turned out that the provoking incident, preceding his writing cramp, was the discovery of his wife's frigidity. The latter was an aggressive, sexually disinterested woman, interested solely in horses. The realization of his wife's a-sexual attitude, started the ball rolling back: he acquired his writing cramp and since a bank employee in those days "had to be capable of writing," he effectively took revenge on his wife, who keenly felt the pinch of diminution of his income.

Behind this superficial layer was hidden a deep oral regression only gradually clarified in analysis. His life history was this: he was the younger son of a minor official in the post office, previously a police officer. That father died when the patient was four years of age. The patient claimed first that he had only one recollection of the father: he sees him dead before the coffin is closed; he feels no emotion at all. Later, he recollected conflicts with the father whom he provoked soundly, getting the punishment he unconsciously expected. A few scenes were remembered: he once tried to open the parental "piggy bank" with a knife though father was in the next room. The main conflict with the father, however, centered around the boy's *bedwetting*, for which the father had no understanding. Once, he was put in the cellar as punishment and decided in his confinement to shoot his children's pistol at night "to scare father." A clear cut oedipal competition (coupled with strong castration fear) became visible; even the primal scene (father died of a sarcoma when the boy was 4) could be recollected with only one point left out. He remembered the father's homecoming (the father worked late hours in the post office), his eating dinner, going to bed, extinguishing the light, mother's using the toilet—here the recollection faded, to be taken up in the morning when the child investigated mother's face for "scars." The reconstruction was possible, that having acquired sadistic misconceptions of parental intimacies, he assumed that father inflicts wounds on the mother which, freely disregarding the time element, were healed overnight.[46]

After the father's death, the mother took up the position of the janitor in the house where they lived and had to part from one of the sons, who was given in the care of an orphanage. She decided to keep the younger (the patient). The older brother left full of fury. The reasons prompting the mother to keep the younger son at home, were twofold: he was a friend of the son of an aristocratic family, living in the building; and the female janitor obviously expected some advantages from that close connection with the influential family. The second reason was the boy's enuresis. The latter persisted till the age of seven, though it was desperately fought by the child. For instance, he attached a long rubber hose to his penis at night, put the other end in a container near his bed, to avoid soiling the linen. Or, suffering from phimosis and blaming the latter for enuresis, he stretched the foreskin with a compass, the sharp ends bandaged in cotton.

The strong passive castration wishes and reactive fears—defensively warded off with a "giant penis," the rubber hose—remained the patient's companion throughout life: he was, e.g., an eager object of operations. During puberty he suffered a rather peculiar accident: though an excellent bicyclist, who had won prizes at competitions, he collided with an oldfashioned two-horse carriage belonging to the postoffice (remember: father had been a post-office employee), came under the horses, and broke his femur and os coxis. Repeated operations followed, the fractures were badly set and a visible deformity resulted, with one leg being shorter than the other. He took all that—operations, poor results, statements of a world-famed authority on orthopedic surgery to the effect that physicians had done a bad job on him—with remarkable stoicism, never complaining and never accusing anyone.

At first, the patient gave the impression of a typical case regressed to the negative Oedipus, the propelling factor being castration fear in connection with the father. Many passively endured "seductions" by homosexual aristocrats seemed to point in the same direction. The

[46] There were other, more "fluid" fantasies of that type: mutual forcing of urine into the mouth or anus. The latter idea, projected upon mother, could be reconstructed from the fact that the child was in the habit of comparing the amounts of his own urine with that of his mother.

seeming passive feminine identification and wish to be overwhelmed was visible in later life: choice of his wife, the horse-lover (see accident!), the fact that after mother's death he took a protective-feminine attitude toward the aggressive brother, cooked for him, etc. His conspicuous lack of genital interests pointed in the same direction. Finally his infantile enuresis could be traced in its different phases to the same source: First, urinating meant in the *active* phase competition with father's sexual activity being perceived as a urinary problem. That active sexual competition was visible also in the elongation of the penis via rubber hose. In a subsequent transitory phase, enuresis was a protest against alleged castration. In a third phase, after regression to the negative Oedipus, enuresis meant also *feminine identification*, the idea behind it being that a girl, since she lacks a penis, urinates "constantly." This connotation (first stressed by H. Deutsch) could be proven from a recollection of the patient: the boy and his friend were caught while looking at the anatomical books of the friend's older brother, a student of medicine. Asked ironically what interested them so much, the boys presented their problem: does the girl control her urination, or "doesn't it flow without interruption?"

Viewed from the oedipal basis, the patient's symptom of writing cramp, had these tributaries:

(1) The symptom represented superficially revenge on his wife—it started after he discovered her frigidity. In letting himself be dismissed with a small pension, he hit her effectively in her standard of living. Unexplained, however, was the deep self-damaging tendency and the specific choice of the symptom.

(2) The symptom also contained superficial, though repressed aggressive murderous impulses directed against his wife. It remained unclear whether this aggression, too, was real or defensive.

(3) After regression, the symptom activated old urethral components, as was visible in his infantile enuresis.

(4) The symptom also activated old and infantile feminine tendencies: many of his "homosexual" passive seductions by the group of aristocrats consisted of masturbating their penes till ejaculation occurred. The sexualization of the arm contributed in the symptom to the disturbance of the normal function.

(5) The symptom was bisexual: the hand had the symbolic meaning

of vagina and anus, the pen that of the penis, the whole procedure constituted symbolically coitus with guilt and resultant inhibition. The hand is cramped, so that the pen (penis) cannot flow (micturition, later ejaculation).

Thus the symptom seemed to have tributaries from urethral, anal, and phallic sources, and at the same time expressed his passive and active tendencies.

So far had his analysis progressed, and these nice and dutiful interpretations were given. Unfortunately three points marred contentment:

First, nothing changed in the patient's symptom, though he had already been eight months in analysis.

Second, a specific recollection, produced earlier, did not fit: during his "cooking period" for his brother, after the mother's death, he was deeply concerned over his brother's over-drinking. He waited up for him and one night, he pushed him to the window, forced his finger into his mouth, in order to make him vomit. The rationalization adduced was that otherwise the brother would soil the carpet.

Third, during the period of stalemate, the patient produced a peculiar symptom in the transference: he had *yawning spells* of considerable duration. These could not be understood only as expressions of disdain, especially since another symptom made its appearance, too: *severe eating disturbances*.

All this, especially the yawning spells and food-rejection, promoted the suspicion of untouched oral material. By pressing that point, finally a recollection came to the fore: In the building which was his childhood home lived a psychopathic Ph.D. who "forced" him to oral-homosexual practices. The scene remembered went back to the fourth year: "Dr. C. took me into his apartment, undressed me and himself, and forced me to take his penis into my mouth. He ejaculated, I felt nauseated and vomited. Dr. C. gave me sour milk to drink."

Now, here was the explanation of the peculiar scene with the brother. He acted in reverse, actively repeating what happened to him *passively* (Freud's "unconscious repetition compulsion"). Hence the yawning cramp in the transference represented an inner defense against the approaching recollection and corresponding wishes.

The scene with Dr. C. had such lasting effect because it activated the unsolved oral-masochistic attachment to mother. First, in his enuresis, later in his writing cramp, he acted at bottom the reversal of the role *giving* mother—*passively fed baby*. This strong masochistic oral passive tendency hurt his narcissism, hence he repeated it *actively*. In his writing cramp, he acted the *refusing* mother! The hand symbolized the mouth, the pen with ink the breast.

That fact elucidated also the provocative factor preceding the symptom: his wife's frigidity was perceived as oral refusal. That refusal was counteracted by the superego reproach which objected that that was exactly what he inwardly wanted. Finally, the *symptom* represents a *defense against that accusation:* he is actively refusing! The symptom had, therefore, a *three* layer structure and could be analytically cured.

Subsequently, I found the identical structure in a series of patients afflicted with the same symptom of writer's cramp.

12–13. Male Homosexuality and Lesbianism

A great deal of confusion is encountered in the analytic literature concerning male homosexuality. The reason is historically explainable: at the time in which the center of analysis gravitated exclusively around the Oedipus Complex, perversion homosexuality was considered the "negative of neurosis," hence a volcanic eruption of something which, under neurotic conditions, would have created neurotic defenses. That theory was later modified,[47] and homosexuality was viewed as the result of regression to the negative Oedipus. Interestingly enough, Freud himself suspected as early as 1910, the oral regression in homosexuality, as proved by his prophetic statement in his study on Leonardo:

"We will for the present leave aside the question as to what connection there is between homosexuality and sucking at the mother's breast." (G.Schr. IX. 309).

Later studies on male homosexuality (Bergler-Eidelberg) and on Lesbians (Jones, H. Deutsch) showed conclusively that an oral regression is the basis, though no agreement exists about the contents of the regression—at this point a difference of opinions ("I want to get"—"I want to be refused") enters the picture.

[47] Review of literature in my paper "Eight Prerequisites for Psychoanalytic Treatment of Homosexuality." The Psa. Rev., 1944.

My present opinion is this: [78]

Perversion homosexuality is characterized by conscious acceptance of sexual gratification derived from a relation with an object of the same sex. Whether feelings of guilt are connected or cynically discarded is immaterial for the diagnosis, though not for the therapeutic prognosis. Homosexuals pretend consciously that they simply imitate the husband-wife relationship. Therefore—in the passive variety—they imitate women, in such things as manner of dressing, movements, talking, walking, and use of perfume and cosmetics. This superficial (consciously desired) impression results in the typical misconception that every "effeminate" man is a homosexual. Nothing is further from the clinical facts. In accepting the superficial camouflage, the naïve observer plays into the hands of the unconscious "alibi" of homosexuals. He is in the situation of a detective who takes at face value all the clues planted by the wrongdoer, to hide his real identity.

What is the unconscious situation of a man suffering from the disease-entity "perversion homosexuality?" He has regressed to the earliest level of psychic development, the "oral stage." Every child has to cope with the fact of weaning from bottle or breast. The normal solution is in itself fantastic: The male child overcomes the trauma of weaning by denying its dependence on the mother and by consoling himself that he has on his own body an organ similar to the withdrawn breast or bottle, that is, the penis. Anatomic differences do not bother the child. His problem is to rescue vestiges of childish megalomania. Hence the ridiculous overvaluation of the "breast substitute," hence the well-marked "penis pride" of the boy.

[48] Reference is made to my work on homosexuality, as reported in: "The Breast Complex in the Male" (with L. Eidelberg) Int. Z. f. Psa., 1933; "The Present Situation in the Genetic Investigation of Homosexuality," Marriage Hygiene, 1937; "The Respective Importance of Reality and Fantasy in Female Homosexuality," J. Crim. Psychopath., 1943; "Eight Prerequisites for the Psychoanalytic Treatment of Homosexuality," Psa. Rev., 1944; "Psychology of Friendship", Med. Rec., 1946; "Unhappy Marriage and Divorce," Int. Univ. Press, New York, 1946; "Differential Diagnosis Between Spurious Homosexuality and Perversion Homosexuality," Psychiatr. Quart., *21*:399–409, 1947; "Facts and Fiction About Lesbianism," Marriage Hygiene, *1*:4, 1948. (Lesbians have the identical conflicts as do male homosexuals, but elaborate them somewhat differently since they do not possess the organ used as compensation.) "The Myth of a New National Disease—Homosexuality and the Kinsey Report," The Psychiatr. Quarterly, *22*:1, 1948.

One of the many abnormal solutions of that early conflict is encountered in homosexuals. These persons are so angry with the disappointing breast or breast-substitutes that they discard the whole disappointing sex: women. They run in life after the "reduplication of their own defense-mechanism"—the penis. Every analysis of homosexuals (the writer has analyzed dozens of them) confirms the fact that behind their frantic chase after the male organ the disappointing breast is hidden. How can this seemingly-fantastic connection be proved clinically? Simply by analyzing without bias the unconscious conflicts of homosexuals. They all labor under the "mechanism of orality," as described repeatedly in previous chapters.

The existence of the "mechanism of orality" which is operative in homosexuals gives a clue to the fact that these people are orally regressed, and that the Oedipus complex is *not* decisive for them. But the mechanism of orality does not make a homosexual. There are many entirely different neuroses in which the mechanism is visible. The existence of this mechanism in a specific person only proves his oral regression. What is characteristic *specifically* of the homosexual is the fact that the narcissistic structure accentuates the mechanism to the *nth degree.* The truly meglomaniacal superciliousness of homosexuals is unique. Precisely because of their narcissistic substructure, the blow caused by incapacity to maintain the infantile fiction of omnipotence hits children who become homosexuals so severely. They recover only partially from the defeat of weaning, and even then only with narcissistic recompense. It is here that the "reduplication of their own defense mehcanisms" comes into play.

Another proof of the oral substructure of homosexuals is a fact first stressed by the writer: In analysis, nearly all of these patients go through, during the end-stages of destruction of the perversion, a period in which they produce the symptom of premature ejaculation with women. And complicated cases of premature ejaculation always show an oral substructure. Such patients refuse the woman pleasure, "they spill the milk before it can reach the mouth." They still live on the basis of their alleged hatred toward the sex, women. So deep is the fright of their own masochistic attachment that pseudo-aggression is their *modus vivendi.*

The amazing degree of unreliability of homosexuals—the combination they show with psychopathic trends—is also one of the end-results of the masochistic elaboration of the oral trauma. Superficially, it refers to the revenge fantasy; basically, under this thinly-veiled palimpsest, deep self-damaging tendencies are hidden. The broad pseudo-aggressive facade covers the self-damage poorly in the majority of homosexuals.

Why do so few homosexuals want to change? The reasons are: Living out the perversion guarantees them pleasure which is felt consciously. This is a very precise distinguishing mark of perversions as contrasted with neuroses, in which the pleasure gain is without exception on an unconscious level. Moreover, the neurotic symptom is always rejected consciously as a foreign body. There are no impotent men, for instance, who are proud of their impotence. In cases of perversion, the situation is quite different: Some homosexuals accept, and are even proud of, "being different." Psychoanalytically, we know today that a complicated inner defense is involved. *Homosexuals approve of their perversion because such acceptance of it—corresponding to a defense mechanism—enables them to hide unconsciously their deepest conflict, oral-masochistic regression.* Since the homosexual who has not been treated has no inkling of the real state of affairs, he clings "proudly" to his defense mechanism. Only in cases in which a portion of inner guilt is not satiated by the real difficulties (hiding, social ostracism, extortion) which every homosexual experiences, does the problem of changing come up.

Characterologically, homosexuals are classical "*injustice collectors,*" resulting from the "mechanism of orality" sketched in the foregoing.

Recently, Dr. Kinsey in his report has tried to establish a "homosexual-heterosexual balance," giving homosexuals a clean bill of health. The psychologic naiveté of the biologist, his unfamiliarity with psychoanalytic findings and lack of genetic differentiation in Kinsey's "taxonomic" approach, resulted in overlooking the fact that homosexuality is not a single entity, but covers many diversified *genetic pictures.*

The only differentiation Kinsey advocates among various forms of homosexuality is a *quantitative* one. He is opposed to calling a man a homosexual in whom the "heterosexual-homosexual balance" is only slightly or temporarily shifted to the homosexual side. Kinsey introduced a "rating scale":

0. Exclusively heterosexual with no homosexual tendencies.

1. Predominantly heterosexual, only incidentally homosexual.
2. Predominantly heterosexual, but more than incidentally homosexual.
3. Equally heterosexual and homosexual.
4. Predominantly homosexual, but more than incidentally heterosexual.
5. Predominantly homosexual, but incidentally heterosexual.
6. Exclusively homosexual.

The *quantitative* approach cannot replace the *genetic* one in medicine. Imagine that someone advanced the idea of subdividing headaches entirely to quantitative principles, rating them from 1 to 6 according to the severity of the headache. Medically speaking, a headache is only a symptom indicating a variety of possibilities: from brain tumor to sinus infection, from migraine attack to uremia, from neurosis to high blood pressure, from epilepsy to suppressed fury. Instead of the genetic viewpoint, we would have in this new order only six types of quantitatively varying degrees of big, middle-sized, and small headaches.

The quantitative viewpoint is *one* of the necessary criteria, but the genetic approach is indispensable. Not only correct diagnosis but therapy depends on it. Using only the quantitative yardstick leads to erroneous conclusions: It omits differentiation of the underlying diseases. Moreover, in the previously mentioned rating of headaches, at a specific moment a headache produced by a sinus attack could be more severe that one produced in certain stages of a brain tumor.

The homosexual "outlet" covers a *multitude of completely different genetic problems.* Hence a genetic yardstick is necessary for the differentiation and cure of the confusing and many-faceted variety of types of the man-to-man relationship. Before arriving at such a differential diagnostic yardstick, let us look at the problem genetically.

1. *Transitory Phase in Adolescence*

The frequent homosexual episode in adolescence does not allow any conclusion as to the future sex life of the boy. The endocrinologically-based sexual "push" revives, in a "second edition," the psychological infantile conflict which was closed at the age of five. Hence pre-Oedipal and Oedipal conflicts arise again. All these conflicts are linked with "castration fears" connected with women of the nursery-days. These fears can, for a time, promote a homosexual intermezzo, which is secondarily rationalized.

The early onset of maturation, stressed by Kinsey as decisive for homosexuality, is but a *somatic* expression of a *psychologic* fact: Inner conflicts influence inner glands no less than inner glands influence inner conflicts. One could assume that *early* puberty is an antedated defense expressed organically. The activity inherent in the sex drive is used as defense against the passivity and *guilt* revolving around reverberations of the infantile conflict. Puberty, in favorable cases, decides the battle of infantile passivity and guilt in favor of activity. Hence people with greater conflicts—such as orally regressed neurotics —try to save themselves with biologic help earlier. Kinsey's statistical revelation of early adolescence in homosexuals speaks, in effect, against his assumption of "heterosexual-homosexual balance."

2. *Perversion Homosexuality*

Perversion homosexuality denotes genetically a stabilization on the unconscious defensive level: "I cannot be masochistically attached to mother; I have nothing in common with her and am not even interested in a woman." He singles out the disappointing organ (breast or breast equivalent), finds on his own body (in his penis) a duplica of it, and throughout his life runs after the copy of the replica—the penis of the other man.

Secondarily, a "philosophy" is created by the homosexual to bolster his unconscious defense. He "approves" of his homosexuality *because* it camouflages well the facts he runs away from: those of oral-masochistic regression.

He cannot escape, though, other reverberations of that conflict: In his personality, he is the classical "injustice collector." Hence he constantly feels "unjustly treated."

Sometimes homosexuals assert that they are completely "happy," the only thing bothering them being the "unreasonable approach" of the environment. That is a convenient blind. There are no happy homosexuals; and there would not be, even if the outer world left them in peace. The reason is an internal one: Unconsciously they want to be disappointed, as does every adherent of the "mechanism of orality." A man who unconsciously runs after disappointment cannot be consciously happy. The amount of conflict, of jealousy for instance, between homosexuals surpasses everything known even in bad heterosexual relationships.

Imagine a baby wanting to prove that its mother is unjust; imagine further a pathologic mother wanting to harm and refuse the baby's demands—there one has in a nutshell the basic conflict of every homosexual relation. *The homosexual is sick inwardly;* and he shifts the blame, in a convenient process of displacement, to the evil outer world. In a roundabout way he gets once more, in his way, his chief diet: psychic masochism.

It takes a homosexual some time—usually until his late 'teens—to discover, and take cognizance of, his perversion. The period of fighting against conscious awareness of his defense mechanism—which he misunderstands as his final destiny—is, under typical conditions, concluded in the late 'teens, or at most, in the early twenties.

Applying these precepts, we can arrive at a *genetic yardstick* for the differential diagnosis: *A male homosexual is a person who predominantly uses the unconsciously-based defense mechanism of man-man relationship to escape his repressed masochistic attachment to the mother*—and *who shows predominantly in his personality the mechanism of the "injustice collector."* Only the combination of the two ingredients constitutes the homosexual.

Paradoxically the homosexual never "escapes mother" although his overdimensional inner fears push him into "another continent" in his frantic flight. His main character trait—"injustice collecting"—belongs genetically and historically to—*mother*. The penis of the partner which he allegedly craves is a disguised breast or breast-equivalent of —*mother*. His quick "turnover" of partners is a pseudo-aggressive defense directed intrapsychically against—*mother*.

3. *Spurious Homosexuality: the Innocent Milquetoast*

In a rather grotesque misunderstanding, a specific type of passive man is constantly accused—*and accuses himself*—of homosexual "tendencies": the Casper Milquetoast type. In a longer essay [49] I have tried to vindicate this innocent victim of a miscarriage of rumors and misconceptions.

The genesis of the passive-feminine man runs as follows: The boy

[49] Differential diagnosis between spurious homosexuality and perversion homosexuality, *loc. cit.*

develops at the age of two and one-half to five a strong attachment to the Oedipal mother, and a strong aggressive rejection of the father. A typical "positive Oedipus complex" is built up. By itself, that development is typical for every child, as Freud proved fifty years ago. Normally these transitory wishes of libidinous-aggressive contents are given up—a road which leads to normality.

Parallel with the "positive" Oedipus, every child develops also (to a quantitatively negligible degree) an attitude called the "negative" or "inverted" Oedipus complex. The boy's relation to his father does not consist merely of rejection. He admires his father's alleged strength and power. He identifies also with the mother and wants to enjoy all the mysterious and "cruel" things father does with mother. Here the father is loved, the mother rejected as competitor. Under normal conditions, these passive trends pass without causing trouble. In hysteric neurotics, fixated on the "negative" Oedipus, this harmless and transitory phase becomes predominant. Expressed analytically: The hysteric neurotic with the unconscious feminine identification is fixated on the level of the "negative" Oedipus.

The result spells troubles without end. The inner conscience (superego) objects constantly to the passive wishes. The inevitable result is that the passive-feminine man is forced to build up unconsciously a series of defenses, to disprove the accusations of conscience. He produces a compensatory he-man attitude, later becomes a woman-chaser, and speaks disparagingly of woman. His potency is weak and full of "whims"; sometimes it works on a record-breaking level—mostly it refuses to "behave."

Not always does the compensatory mechanism embedded in the forced and cramped he-man attitude work so perfectly. In some cases, the defenses are weak—and the outerworld designates this Mr. Milquetoast as an effeminate man, misjudging him as a homosexual.

The resulting two types—super-he-man and Milquetoast—are genetically carved out of the same wood; it is only the strength of the defense which varies.

How did it come to pass that the poor Milquetoast was unjustifiably accused, even in scientific literature, of homosexuality? This is understandable only by reviewing the development of psychoanalytic science. Freud started his discoveries, not from deepest level of regression, but from the highest, as was indicated earlier in this book. He first discovered the Oedipus complex, which plays a decisive role in hysteric and obsessional cases. The oral level was at that time either unknown or neglected. The result was that homosexuals, too, were considered specific aberrations of the Oedipus complex.

The external behavior of homosexuals and that of the homosexually innocent "passive-feminine" men, are not only unreliable indicators, but are completely misleading. The effeminate man is not a homosexual; the markedly effeminate homosexual, on the other hand, shows a camouflage, hiding his real conflict. One must distinguish between two forms of unconscious identification, the "*leading*" and the "*misleading*." The "leading" unconscious identification petrifies, as it were, the representation of the decisive wishes of the personality, crystallized as the end-result of the infantile conflict. The "misleading" identification denotes identification with persons chosen for the purpose of denying and rebuffing the reproaches of the superego, directed against the basic neurotic wishes. The passive-feminine man's "leading" identification pertains to the Oedipal mother; his "misleading" unconscious identification to the he-man type. The "leading" unconscious identification of the homosexual pervert pertains either to the pre-oedipal mother (active variety) or to the baby (passive variety). His "misleading" unconscious identification is either with the oedipal father (active) or the oedipal mother (passive).

A person confusing the two types of identification can blame only himself if the whole problem of homosexuals and "effeminate men" is full of unsolved contradictions for him. He cannot even explain the active variety of homosexual perverts, since he is blinded by the fallacy of the effeminate man. By the same token he classifies every weakling of a man who is mistreated by an aggressive shrew as a homosexual. Further, poor Milquetoast is apt to accuse himself of homosexuality—unjustifiably.

4. *Homosexual "One-timers"*

A very large number of men have one or two homosexual experiences but no more. The group constituted by these men is genetically extremely heterogeneous and comprises a variety of unconscious reasons leading to the homosexual interlude. For the most part these men are not homosexuals.

(a) *Temporary oral aggression in specific situation of stress.* Here belong transitory episodes of inductees in the armed services during the war. Loneliness, danger, fear, provoke the unconscious infantile accusation: "Bad mother is responsible." Masochistic attachment being revived, the latter is warded off with pseudo-aggression leading to the homosexual act as "revenge" and reassurance. The whole process is, of course, unconscious.

(b) *Allurement of the forbidden.* In some cases the homosexual episode is but an expression of the masochistc wish for a short journey into "transgression of the forbidden." In the same way, not all persons who drank during prohibition were drinkers; some were looking for the "adventure of danger" (psychic masochism).

(c) *Shifted guilt.* Frequently guilt pertaining to other inner causes is expressed in single homosexual episodes. This guilt may have its origin in entirely different sources.

(d) *The mirage of lack of heterosexual objects.* One of the pillars of the assumption of shifting and exchangeable "balance" between heterosexuality and homosexuality is the argument that in prisons even previosuly heterosexual men become "homosexuals." But a curious oversight is here involved. Most prison inmates are persons who use the "mechanism of criminosis"—hence an orally-determined solution occurs. The problem cannot be discussed without elaboration of the problems of the genetic factors leading to crime in general.[50]

Using the genetic yardstick advocated in the foregoing a differentiation between true and spurious cases of homosexuality is possible.

5. *Homosexuality as Inner Admission of the "Lesser Crime"*

There are literally dozens of elaborations of the "mechanism of orality" leading to injustice-collecting. As stressed before, the existence of that mechanism proves oral regression. To this is added a specific mechanism explaining why different clinical pictures result.

There exists, however, one type of orally-regressed man who uses a strange defense in his "battle of the conscience." Accused by his superego of masochistic repetition of an infantile conflict with the mother, projected upon a *woman* (he associates regularly with termagants) intrapsychically he denies the attachment by *temporarily* running to the—*man.* These neurotics use transitory homosexual "spells"

[50] See "Battle of the Conscience."

as defenses against another "crime": that of masochistic attachment. They *fortify themselves*, so to speak, *with a dose of homosexuality.* They gain "immunity" toward women by using the homosexual conflict —temporarily. After a short time, they revert to termagants only to repeat the identical procedure. The whole process is, of course, unconscious.

Very likely this type accounts for Kinsey's observation of *sporadic* homosexuality in specific ages in specific individuals. Kinsey, of course, takes it as proof of the shaky "heterosexual-homosexual balance."

6. *Homosexuality in Conscious Fantasy Only*

There are neurotics who never revert to overt homosexuality, though their masturbatory sex life is concentrated on homosexual fantasies.

Using the previously expounded genetic yardstick, we are able to distinguish between homosexuals and pseudo-homosexuals in this group. The fact that only fantasy outlet is used does not, per se, exclude the fact that homosexuality is involved.

7. *The "Bisexuals"*

Some homosexuals are seemingly "bisexual"—that is to say, slight remnants of heterosexuality can be detected. These remnants guarantee, for some time, erective potency in a lustless coitus. Nobody can dance at two weddings at the same time, not even the wizard of a homosexual. Equal distribution of libidinous drives between homo- and heterosexuality does not exist, simply because *homosexuality is not a drive but a defense mechanism.* The so-called "bisexuals" are in reality homosexuals with a slight admixture of potency with unloved women. Frequently they belong in Group 5, the "lesser crimes" type.

Kinsey claims that his statistics prove that "*one male in three* of the persons one may meet as one passes along a city street has had some homosexual experience." I believe, however, that Kinsey became the prey of psychologic mistakes in evaluating his test objects.

Kinsey and his collaborators gathered their conclusions by questioning 12,000 people. I believe that Kinsey's figures are correctly compiled and presented in good faith. Still, his disregard for psychologic factors has very likely played a trick on him; he takes his human guinea pigs for idealists who volunteered only for the purpose of further scientific research.

The chances are that many volunteers who secondarily interested other volunteers, though *consciously* inspired by noble intentions, had some less altruistic *unconscious* motives. Among these, one could suspect, were many homosexuals who gladly used the opportunity of proving, by volunteering, that "everybody" has homosexual tendencies —thus seeking to *diminish their own inner guilt.*

Moreover, the clinical fact remains that the circle of friends of neurotics consists almost exclusively of neurotics. Hence the second and third "crop" of volunteers must have consisted of too many neurotics, too.

I believe that Kinsey's figures about homosexual outlet will be revised downward as the present 12,000 interrogated are increased to 100,000, as Kinsey promises in the next twenty years.

It can be clinically established that the homosexual is but a *frightened fugitive from misconceptions he has unconsciously built around women.* The fact remains that even the later male homosexual had (like every human being) a specific *first* experience in life with his mother. And this very real emotional experience *with a woman* leaves its marks. When later in life he turns to man as sexual object, he does so in a *neurotic elaboration of that first and undigested experience.*

The question of whether or not homosexuality has a biologic substructure, is, though unsettled, doubtful to me. In any case, the therapeutic nihilism consisting of reconciling the homosexual with his "destiny," is therapeutically completely unjustified.

On the other hand, endocrinology has nothing therapeutic to contribute to the problem of homosexuality. This fact is best illustrated in the summary of a witty endocrinologist: "Some psychiatrists claim that the best they can do for a homosexual is to make an unhappy homosexual a 'happy' one. This is little, but still more than endocrinology can do for a homosexual: the latter can only make a prosperous homosexual a less prosperous one."

The most that can be said psychiatrically about the biologic substructure in homosexuality was summarized by P. Schilder:[51]

"It has been repeatedly attempted to apply the results of Goldschmidt's experiments to the problem of homosexuality. His experiments deal with very definite physical characteristics, and to transfer his results to the psychic field has no scientific basis at the present time. As to

[51] "Goals and Desires of Men," Columbia University Press, 1942, p. 159.

the experiments of Steinach, who had feminized male guinea pigs which really behaved like females and were sought as females by males, it must be emphasized that there is no proof that in homosexuals changes in the hormones take place similar to those experimentally produced. I agree therefore with Oswald Schwarz that *no proof exists that homosexuality is due to biologic hermaphroditism. . . .*"

The fact remains that today homosexuality is a curable neurotic disease, requiring specific therapeutic techniques and prerequisites.

This does not mean that one should force homosexuals into psychoanalytic treatment. Far from it, only if specific prerequisites are given, is the prognosis favorable. My "Eight Prerequisites for the Psychoanalytic Treatment of Homosexuality" [52] were arrived at empirically, i.e., along the road of failure and success. Naturally it can be seen that these prerequisites are of quite unequal worth; some are, to my belief, a *condito sine qua non;* others simply have a favorable influence on prognosis without representing an indispensable condition. I have arranged them in order of importance. With the exception of the first three (I will bring forward eight points) they are not prerequisites in the strict sense. I simply don't know any better term and on this point, as of course on others as well, I am open to suggestions.

I. *Inner Guilt Feeling Capable of Being Made Use of Analytically.* We trace the unconscious feeling of guilt of homosexuals back to the oral pre-oedipal conflicts with the phallic mother. It cannot be recalled too emphatically that the pre-oedipal and oedipal mothers represent, according the Freud's conception completely different personalities in the child's unconscious. We know that feeling of guilt is present without exception in homosexuals; yet in many cases it is apparently not visible and, what is more important, even when it is present in a latent state. it cannot be utilized analytically. The question is therefore: where is it typically deposited? The answer is to begin with quite commonplace. It is generally deposited in the social rejection, in the real danger of coming into conflict with society, with the law, with blackmailers. This saturation of the desire for punishment is enough in many cases and such people do not wish to get out of their vicious circle; they therefore do not come for treatment.

The inner feeling of guilt in homosexuals is particularly tricky.

[52] The Psa. Rev., Vol. 31, No. 3, July 1944, quoted previously.

For a long time I believed that a direct conclusion as to the extent of the unsaturated part of the guilt feeling could be drawn from the depression appearing on the surface, from the feeling of aversion and disgust as after-appearance, found in many homosexuals after their perverse behavior. The feeling of warding off an inward compulsion may be included. There is moreover a remark of Freud's that points in the same direction:

> Such a struggle against the compulsion to inversion may offer a favorable condition for treatment. . . . (Drei Abhandlungen zur Sexualtheorie, p.9, note 1, *Ges Schr.* V).[53]

Bitter experience has taught me, however, that no conclusions as to the depth or amount of the unsaturated portion of the guilt feeling can be drawn from depression appearing on the surface or from the feeling of unhappiness. Especially instructive appeared to me the following experience of two analyzed cases by chance occuring simultaneously. Despite the virtual absence of conscious guilt feeling, a homosexual man, who came for treatment because of other neurotic symptoms, was cured of his homosexuality, while with another, despite what appeared to be excessive guilt feeling, little could be accomplished. He did not get beyond ejaculatio praecox with a woman.

We must, therefore, admit that we cannot yet fully grasp the practical estimation of the possibility of making use of this guilt feeling in homosexuals. Without the presence of the wish to get well nothing can be done analytically; on the other hand, we are often deceived into a favorable prognosis by an inflated feeling of guilt which proves to be a mirage. In these cases, one has the feeling that the patients unconsciously inflate and magnify their depressions inwardly precisely in order to be able to prove to their inner conscience: "I am not enjoying myself; I am suffering." Hence in doubtful cases a trial period of two or three months is advisable.

A separate group is composed of patients with mixed symptoms. It sometimes happens that a practising pervert comes to an analyst not on account of his perversion but on account of some neurotic symptoms. Thus, for example, a patient of this kind required of me that I cure him

[53] In another place it is said: "Inversion can be removed through hypnotic suggestion." Freud adduces this as an argument for the acquired character of perversions and denies the "occurrence of innate inversion."

of an ejaculatio praecox within his homosexuality and was quite indignant when I declared that I was unable to do so. Another patient, a good looking woman "from the social register," who was a practicing Lesbian came to analysis because of her furious outbreaks and angry attacks against her woman friend, as well as because of disturbance in her work, which three symptoms were to be eliminated with the express condition that her perversion was not to be touched. Prognosis in such cases is generally unfavorable.

II. *Voluntary Acceptance of Treatment.* Freud states that homosexuals will sometimes come for treatment for the sake of their loved ones, parents or relatives, but he maintains that the power of these libidinous strivings is rarely adequate for success. From my experience it would appear that for homosexuals there is no such thing as beloved parent or relative, that these patients are filled with a savage unconscious hatred against the latter, a hatred that is comparable only to the patient's wild self-damaging tendency. I am of the opinion that willingness to enter treatment is an indispensable prerequisite. Naturally, one may attempt to mobilize the feeling of guilt in a sort of trial treatment, but I have increasingly gotten away from this attempt as futile.

III. *Not Too Extensive An Amount of Self-damaging Tendencies.* Without doubt, the social disgrace as well as the methods of hiding and self-protection to which every homosexual is compelled to resort, contains an element of self-punishment which absorbs a part of the unconscious feeling of guilt stemming from other sources. Nevertheless, it is striking how great is the proportion of psychopathic personalities among homosexuals. Many homosexuals bear the stigma of unreliability, to speak popularly. This unreliability is, psychoanalytically considered, a part of the homosexual's oral character. These people always construct and provoke situations in which they feel themselves unjustly treated. This feeling of injustice suffered and perpetuated through their own behavior gives them inwardly the right to be constantly pseudo-aggressive and grudging in relation to their environment and to pity themselves masochistically. This revenge tendency it is that constitutes what the unpsychological but accurately observing outside world calls the "unreliabilīty" and ingratitude of homosexuals. Naturally, on socially different levels this tendency manifests itself differently.

Yet it is striking how great is the proportion of homosexuals among swindlers, pseudologues, forgers, law-breakers of all sorts, drug purveyors, gamblers, spies, pimps, brothel owners, etc. The above-mentioned "oral mechanism" is at bottom masochistic, though with an admittedly very broad aggressive facade. It undoubtedly depends on the amount of this self-damaging tendency, an amount that for the time is unmeasurable, to what degree this tendency is accessible therapeutically. A quick orientation is possible by judging the amount of other neurotic investments of the patient. In other words: how much did the patient damage himself otherwise? These "impossible and conceited people," as the mother of one of my patients characterized her son and his friends, are frequently good for nothing as patients. A patient of this type informed me after the first four weeks that he would have difficulty in paying next time since his sick-benefit payment had expired and he would have to pay the next month's bill out of his own pocket for the first time. To explain his payment difficulties he said that his chief would this time be present in the city. At first I did not understand and asked if he meant that his salary would not be paid because his chief would be absent. "No," the patient replied, "I mean present." The whole matter became suspicious and I pressed him for an explanation. Hesitating and yet laughing cynically, the patient informed me that in recent months he had been stealing money regularly from his office and that this was possible only in his chief's absence. He had spent the stolen money on his homosexual friend, but now he wanted to make use of it for the analysis, as he graciously added. I explained that I would not make myself into an accomplice of his by permitting myself to be paid with stolen money. Hitherto the treatments had been paid for with the sick-benefit money he was receiving from his organization. If this organization would not continue paying for the treatment and he himself could not manage it out of his regular salary, the treatment would have to be postponed to a later period. In any case, I would break off treatment immediately. The patient was furious and told me it was none of my business where the money for my fee came from; indeed he accused me of hampering his cure. That he had provoked the entire affair himself he refused to see. This is without a doubt a typical example of the previously mentioned oral mechanism.

As another example of difficult patients, a young foreigner studying in Vienna was summarily arrested along with thirty other young people during a raid upon homosexuals in a cafe at a well-frequented summer resort in Austria. There was nothing against him and the young man would surely have been released by the police with ample apologies after he had established the facts of his personal status. The young man, however, when he faced the police officers was seized with a veritable compulsion to confess and began, voluntarily and unasked, to admit all his homosexual relations. As rationalization for this he adduced fear of the "third degree." The result was that the confession was officially reported to the district attorney and he was sentenced to six weeks in prison. After his return to Vienna, he was prevailed upon by one of his friends and a lady who was a friend of the family in the patient's home country, to come to me for treatment. The young man himself had no interest in analysis and had no desire to change. I explained to him that under the circumstances an attempt at analysis would be purposeless. Pressed on by the people around him, he however insisted on some sort of trial treatment, pretending that he had become anxious over his extraordinary, utterly uncalled-for compulsion to confess. Although it was clear that this was a lie—for example, he answered my question as to how he had felt in prison by saying laughingly that he had missed listening to the radio, something made possible for convicts in his own country—I agreed to his proposal. The treatment lasted three months and was complicated by a disconcerting attempt of the patient to act the fool, although in his pretentious, extravagant way he would always report about the intellectual superiority of homosexuals. In addition, it happened that a number of good-for-nothing young male prostitutes began extorting money from him once it was discovered he had some. He was able to arrange it that one of these audacious young men would always follow him to my office and the arguments with the blackmailer would take place on my staircase. One day he had agreed with a friend of his that in case he (the patient) did not phone him by one o'clock it would show that he had been arrested; one o'clock was, of course, the hour when the blackmailer's ultimatum would expire, and according to the blackmailer's threat, the patient would be denounced to the police if he had not by then turned over a definite sum of money. The objection that this was all empty talk, since the blackmailer himself would have to confess to the police that he had had homosexual relations with the patient and thereby would endanger himself; all such objections he naturally brushed aside. He further arranged with his friend that if he did not 'phone the latter should call up the consulate of the patient's country, report that the patient had been arrested and request intervention. As was to be expected it was all bluff and the patient was not arrested. But on the other hand, he "forgot" to ring up his friend who punctually set the entire consulate machinery into motion. A veritable farce resulted with half the Viennese detective force searching in vain for hours for the "distinguished foreigner" in jails, police stations and patrol wagons. They naturally couldn't find him; the idea that the consulate of this dreaded state might have been misled struck no one. The case was finally clarified and that evening at his session with me the young man proudly reported his experience as a good practical joke and acknowledged that the police official, on finally finding him at home reading, had promptly "breathed a deep sigh of relief," which touched the patient very much indeed. This affecting state of affairs was rudely disturbed by a letter from the consul a day or two later, asking him in no uncertain terms to transfer elsewhere the scene of his "miserable tricks." The consul's letter coincided with the beginning of my vacation and I told the patient that I would continue only on condition that he really wished it inwardly. Every attempt to show him the meaning of his provocations naturally failed. In the fall, I heard from the patient's father who was visiting Europe and who in a personal interview made an urgent attempt to persuade me to continue, a request which I was compelled to reject as purposeless. I gave him a list of analysts in his own country and recommended the continuation of the treatment should his son, after a few years, wish to do so.

As a third example of the kind of patient unsuitable for treatment, I present one who came to me with a recommendation from a well-known neurologist. The document was addressed to me and, among other things, it included the letter that the specialist had written to the family doctor who had sent the patient to him. The specialist declared that the patient was suffering from a psychic disturbance of potency which would be easy to get rid of analytically, because the patient desired to get well so eagerly; the neurological findings were negative, he said. On questioning the patient, it appeared that he was a practicing homosexual. That was not mentioned in the letter. I asked him whether he had told that to the two doctors, and he answered hesitantly in the affirmative. Nevertheless, the matter seemed suspicious and I cleared it up with the doctors, which naturally changed the prognosis. The patient presented himself as a minor employee and urgently requested a moderate rate. The family doctor intervened; asserting that he knew the patient well, he gave me over the telephone a lecture on social duties toward minor employees and he practically forced me to take the patient over. The joke of the matter was that after some time it turned out that the patient had consistently deceived all three doctors, one after the other. In the first place, he had given an assumed name to all three of us; secondly, he knew how to conceal his main symptom; thirdly, he prevailed upon the family doctor, who knew him only superficially, to intervene with me with inaccurate information; fourthly, he was not an employee at all but the head of his business. His complicated web of lies, distortions and concealments, that could be unravelled only with great difficulty, came to the surface only when he began to realize that he was hurting himself with them. He did indeed cheat me out of the normal fee for a short time; but on the other hand, his employee, whom in his reports he made out to be the head of the business, had for years been stealing money in small but regular sums that could not be established, and had used his (the patient's) money to set up a competitive business right opposite on the same street. Having been cheated in this way by his employee, the patient realized that because he had concealed and withdrawn this material, he had made it impossible to analyze his masochistic relation to his employee and friend. He regretted what he had done very much, was very penitent, yet declared cynically that he had not cheated me since he could not in any case have paid me more. In this case too the feeling of injustice suffered was decisive for the inner justification of the deception. The patient was born in 1917 in a small locality in Rumania then occupied by German troops who had stripped it of all food. The child, like the rest of the people in that country, literally starved and his later illness reflected the psychic working over of this first oral deprival, which was not fantasied but was in the highest degree real. He held his mother responsible for his starvation. The case is interesting because it is rare today to treat those who have actually starved in earliest childhood, although European analysts at least will hardly find it so rare in the next generation of analytic patients.

IV. *Therapeutic Preferability of Homosexual Reality to Homosexual Fantasy.* It sometimes happens that younger people who feel themselves driven in the direction of homosexuality come under analytic treatment at the very time when they have already decided to take the step from fantasy to reality in homosexuality but still have not been able to find enough courage to do it. The analysis then becomes the alibi, but a different sort of alibi from the one Freud mentions in the "secret plan" of failure so as to prove to oneself that everything is futile and that, therefore, homosexuality may be enjoyed without guilt. The alibi I have in mind consists in the patient's pacifying himself with the fact that he is under treatment, which might even make it possible for him to get well under special conditions. Everything taking place in the meantime is a transitional phase. In this way, this type of patient misuses analysis to live out his perversion. Naturally, the context is more complicated. In taking up homosexual practices for the first time during the analysis, there is unconsciously an element of scornful pseudo-aggression against the analyst, whom the patient, in the transference of the defensive "hate" conflict, reproaches with being against homosexuality as "beastliness," on moral grounds. Every attempt to show these patients that we regard them not as "beasts" but as sick people, is blocked by incredulity. The analyst is thus put to a test, which can be quite unpleasant since the family is apt to insist that it was the analysis that made the patient a practicing homosexual. Should the analyst show the slightest inner opposition or chagrin at the taking up of active homosexual relations on the part of the patient, the treatment is then generally to be regarded as hopeless. As an example of this type, I cite a patient who came to me for treatment for kleptomania, but who was also homosexual. He constantly uttered polemics against me, asserting that inwardly I regarded him as a criminal, although I always told him that I merely looked upon him as a sick person. One day he brought me a present, a book, and he told me precisely where he had stolen it. He was evidently counting on an emotional outburst on my part that would expose me. I thanked him kindly for the book and proposed to analyze what the purpose of his aggressive gift was. It proved possible to convince the patient that at least *this* book should be returned to its original owner.

The test presented by the homosexual who enters into relations during the analysis may last half a year and is, therefore, more difficult to endure than in the case of the kleptomaniac. It exposes the analyst to a heavier burden for which not everyone is a match.

Experience teaches that it is better if the patient has already entered into homosexual relations before the treatment. This is a simple fact of experience, which is not changed whatever the age of the patient or the length of his relations. In other words, even people who have maintained homosexual relationships for many years are often, with due regard to the three conditions *sine quibus non,* easier to change than patients who enter into relationships for the first time during the analysis.

A word now on the transference of homosexuals. It is very different from the libidinous-erotic attachments that might naively be expected. What these patients repeat in essence are pre-oedipal oral pseudo-hate conflicts, constantly projected masochistic feelings of being treated unjustly, etc. Naturally, this does not exclude libidinous wishes being repeated in dreams and fantasies. It is moreover striking that homosexuals frequently select an analyst who does not correspond to their love-type; indeed, they even avoid one of that type, obviously a sort of protective device.

V. *No Real Experience of Complete Psychic Dependence on the Mother.* I am referring to cases in which the mother had been the sole educator; for example, early divorce of the parents, or completely disinterested father. That reality situation can be masochistically misused, and is—in cases of homosexuality—not too favorable.

VI. *No Persistence of Reasons for Maintaining Homosexuality as an Aggressive Weapon Against the Hated Family.* There is a difference whether the pseudo-aggression directed against the family (in being a homosexual) belongs to the "historical past" or can be used as an actual weapon.

VII. *No Authoritative Assertion of Incurability.* I would first like to explain what I mean by an example. A number of years ago in

Vienna I treated a nineteen-year-old man for homosexuality. He had two forms of homosexual relations: one stable with an older man, the other a series of transitory "half-minutes," relations with young fellows, unknown to him, whom he masturbated in public comfort-stations. As a result of a certain special situation (he was very nearly arrested), he grew afraid and opened his heart to his family doctor, who sent him to me for analytic treatment. He was an unfavorable case because there was no genuine wish to get rid of the perversion. He permitted himself to be showered with presents by his old friend (who was a big industrialist) and was thus on the way to becoming a male prostitute. In the analysis ever greater resistance began to develop. For example, he plainly tried to provoke me to get rid of him when he seriously demanded that I should place my bathtub at his disposal before every appointment: it was distressing to him, he said, to give me his hand upon his arrival unless he had washed and bathed, since he often came to his appointments direct from his homosexual escapades in the toilets. He avoided every attempt to analyze this idea. There seemed ground for the supposition that in his wish to bathe in my bathtub he was attempting to repeat an important determinant of his hatred for his mother. As a three-year-old child he had a sore throat and the doctor ordered hot vapor. His mother arranged this in a very primitive manner; a big tub of hot water was put in front of the bed and the child was told to lean out and breathe in the water vapor; while this was going on the mother conversed with a neighbor. The child leaned over too far, fell into the tub on his left side and was badly burned. All his life he carried scars of this accident. Without doubt there was here a real cause for his aversion to his mother. The patient was completely inaccessible and his resistance grew stronger when he told his rich patron that he was under analysis, which he had hitherto very wisely kept silent. That man did something disconcertingly shrewd; instead of simply trying to dissuade the patient from continuing the treatment and exerting pressure upon him by threats and so on—which is what usually happens—he told him he was wasting his time for he had it from the best analytical authority that homosexuality was incurable. He confessed that twenty-five years before he himself had been under treatment by a high analytical authority, who had discharged him after a few months with the statement that he was now reconciled to his homosexuality and that no more could be accomplished. Whether the old man's story was true or false, I do not know. But he gave the young man so many details about his treatment that the latter was actually convinced that the old fellow was speaking the truth. At any rate, I did not succeed in convincing the patient that a continuation of the treatment would make any sense. I also had the impression during the last few days—the entire treatment lasted four weeks—that with his running away he was re-enacting his revenge on the mother as well.

However that may be and whatever weight we may desire to ascribe to the citing of the analytical authority, I believe it would be better if authoritative pessimistic judgments were avoided. The fact remains that some of our colleagues regard homosexuality as incurable and others regard it as curable. There is no reason to conceal all this from the mistrustful patient. But there is also no reason to disturb the optimists in their work; should we be mistaken, our mistake would bring a heavy retribution. I am, therefore, pleading that analysts should express themselves with care in such matters and above all should keep their ex-cathedra pessimism to themselves as private utterances.

VIII. *The Analyst's Knowledge.* As can be seen, I bring up the special knowledge of the analyst as the last, hence relatively unimportant, point. Without wanting to be cynical, I must say that when I read the case histories of homosexual patients published in our journals and see how many different types are differentiated, how the decisive oral material is sometimes even reported but is assigned no central significance and how, although no more than the psychic surface is scratched, the patient is sometimes cured, sometimes regarded as hopeless and sometimes the result is not even announced, I can only wonder how this is possible. Not that I have any objection to a multiplicity of confusion-breeding types; quite the contrary. Yet I sometimes get an impression very much as if scholars were to describe the different forms assumed by the sand of the desert under the influence of the desert wind and yet forget that at bottom they are after all dealing with sand. The forms assumed by the sand may very well be manifold, but if one wants to know the chemical composition of the sand, he will not be made any the wiser if in place of the formula for the sand he is in sober earnest served up with the many descriptive forms of sand as chemical formulas. Every analyst has a deep prejudice in favor of his own experiences acquired through many bitter disappointments. I believe what I have seen, clinically, namely, that the psychic center in male homosexuality is the pre-oedipal mother attachment, the breast complex, and that the fate of the Oedipus complex is of merely secondary importance for these patients. On the other hand, there is no reason for casting doubt upon the bona fide experiences of other colleagues although in my opinion they merely touch the surface layers. I must, therefore, come to the conclusion that, on the one hand, the improper handling of the oral structure of these patients contributes to ill success; on the other, that where a certain modest success is obtained, it occurs despite the failure to penetrate to the essentials. Of course, in many cases, it is not necessary to penetrate very deeply and merely touching upon the essential layers obviously brings danger to those lying deeper still so that, very much as in the pathology of neuroses, success because of unconscious fear ("Angsterfolg") is possible. By this term I mean the fact that in many cases when essential motives are analytically touched upon directly or indirectly, such strong defense reactions are aroused that the patient unconsciously, instead of selecting the radical manner of running away, renounces the symptom without otherwise changing his psychic structure. Unconsciously these patients renounce a symptom in order to save still deeper lying unconscious tendencies of pleasurable kind and to withdraw them from analysis. Freud speaks of the "flight into health." These successes because of unconscious fear may be distinguished from genuine hard-won analytic successes in two essential points. In the first place, genuinely successful results do not come overnight, as do the "successes from fear"; in the latter the month-long vacillation and fluctuation between apparent progress and apparent regress, the typical ebb and flow, is absent. In the second place, in "successes from fear" no connection is to be noted between the working through of the material in transference and the disappearance of the symptom, and quite intelligibly so since it is the purpose of the "*success from fear*" to protect these layers that are to be destroyed. The unfavorable aspect of the "success from fear" is the virtual certainty of a relapse. We must also be very clear as to what we mean by success in homosexual cases. I reject as the aim of analysis the opportunistic idea of reconciling the homosexual to his perversion as something God-given. And I likewise reject any attempt to trumpet it forth as an analytical success when a homosexual occasionally becomes capable of coitus as a matter of mere duty, though quite without interest in it and still retaining his attraction to the same sex. In my opinion, we are dealing with striking failures in both cases. What I mean by success is: (1) Complete lack of sexual interest in the same sex; (2) normal sexual enjoyment; and (3) characterological change.

I am the last to maintain that this is possible in every case. On the contrary, it is possible only with a quite definite and limited group of homosexuals. I have already mentioned the pitfall of therapy: many patients never get beyond ejaculatio praecox with women. It is most difficult to change the oral-envious-masochistic personality of these patients, which may survive the disappearance of the perversion itself. I have listed the conditions which render prognosis possible and have brought forward the prerequisites which make it possible to pick out suitable cases. The ill repute enjoyed by our therapy among homosexuals is to be explained not only by analytical scepticism and the improper application of the analytical instrument. To all this we must add the unselective acceptance of homosexuals with bad prognosis for analysis, as turns out later. These cases then become the worst propagandists against us. The danger can be eliminated by a selection of suitable cases. I believe that the prerequisites I have listed may help in this selection.

Lesbianism

Lesbianism has a structure similar to that of male homosexuality with a specific distinguishing mark: Lesbian girls, not being endowed with a penis, cannot use the boy's outlet of identification of breast and penis. This leads to different defenses.

The peculiar nature of the clinical Lesbian conflict consists of the fact that a three-story structure is unconsciously erected: *masochistic injustice collecting*, warded off by *pseudo-hatred*, secondarily warded off by *exaggerated pseudo-love* towards a representative of the infantile image of the mother.

The narcissistic substructure of Lesbians explains also why the conflict of babyhood with the mother is never outgrown. Normally, the conflict with the mother is solved by the girl by splitting it off: the old "hatred" remains with the mother, the "love"-component is shifted to the father. Instead of the duality "child-mother" (called the pre-oedipal phase), the triangular oedipal situation, "child-mother-father," enters the picture. The future Lesbian attempts the same way out, only to be thrown back ("regression") to the original conflict.

The definite proof for the relative unimportance of the oedipal "solution" for homosexuals (which in itself is a transitory phase, given up by the child in the process of his normal development) is the fact that Lesbians use the man-wife (father-mother) disguise as a covering *defensive* cloak.

Real life is less obliging than are textbooks which subdivide complicated phenomena into chapters. Real life "mixes up" and impertinently combines different chapters. Here is an example of a "quadrangular" hetero-homosexual love-affair.

Mrs. M. married and the mother of two children, attached herself to Mr. N., a promiscuous man. She was soon tortured by violent jealousy and general "injustice collecting." The jealousy pertained first to the near-certainty of N's different "affairs", and secondly to the "strange relation" to his friend, Mr. O. Messrs. N. and O. shared everything: apartment, car, office, profession; all of N's possessions, including his life insurance, were written in O's name, without any obvious reasons. They were just friends; the very early suspicion of Mrs. M. that N. and O. were homosexuals was dispelled by the fact that both N. and O. had many, though quickly changing heterosexual affairs. These relations, though, were strange: they were not exactly on the sharing basis, but openly quadrangular. All four (N. and O. plus the changing girl friends of both) were drinking together, teasing together, using obscene words, and constantly alluding to their sexual intimacies.

After some time, Mrs. M. introduced her best friend, Mrs. P. to Mr. O. The official reason given was that since Mrs. M. and P. were friends and lived in the same building, "covering up" before the respective husbands was thus made easier. The introduction of Mrs. P. had a disturbing effect on the relation between Mrs. M. and Mr. N.: the latter paid more attention to his friend O.'s advances than to Mrs. M. Mr. O. fell in love with Mrs. P.—and this fact disturbed the shaky balance between the half-homosexual duo Messrs. N. and O. As long as both merely had "alibi-coitus" with indifferent women, to prove to themselves that they were not homosexuals, everything went well. The moment O. showed real interest in a woman, N. became moody and jealous. Mrs. M. discovered this to her dismay, and "suffered hell." It went so far that at times when Mrs. P. was menstruating, N. refused to have intimacies with Mrs. M.: "He was just watching them and didn't want to leave them alone," complained Mrs. M. indignantly.

To complicate matters, Mrs. P. was not at all interested in O. and was homosexually attached to Mrs. M. She admitted freely that she started and continued the affair with O. only to be "near" to Mrs. M.

From the strange quartet, only Mrs. M. was analyzed. She entered treatment under peculiar circumstances. Her sister, a journalist with a vivid imagination, in whom she confided, convinced her that N. and O. were homosexuals and predicted the outbreak of jealousy paranoia with subsequent murder. Afraid of the possible scandal, Mrs. M. was nearly in panic and consulted me.

It soon turned out that unconsciously Mrs. M. was an exquisite seeker after disappointments: her choice of Mr. N. was made not despite but because of N.'s unfaithfulness. Moreover, Mrs. M. was half-concious of her own homosexuality, though at times she denied violently, in analysis, the very same attachment. Two sets of facts convinced her: her dreams, and the fact that Mrs. P.—"just a friend"—surprised her as she claimed, with the decision to give up Mr. O. "whom I tolerated only to be near to you." The next sentence of Mrs. P. was a direct confession of homosexuality: "You seem not to realize how deeply I love you."

These four people obviously represented two homosexual pairs, who, instead of living together, fought a defensive battle of half-conscious alibis with bisexual weapons. The "difficulties" arose because these four homosexuals were not fully synchronized in their defensive efforts: some were nearer, some farther, from conscious acceptance of their perversion.

Homosexuality is frequently combined with psychopathic trends.

Homosexuality per se has nothing to do with psychopathy; the combination arises because of the common oral regression.

Superficially, the psychopathic actions refer to the revenge fantasy; behind that thinly veiled palimpsest, deep self-damaging tendencies are hidden. As already stated, the broad pseudo-aggressive façade covers poorly the self-damage of the great percentage of homosexuals of both sexes among swindlers, pseudologues, forgers, drug purveyors, gamblers, brothel owners, procurers, etc.

What cleverly fantastic results the combination of homosexuality and psychopathy can produce is visible in the following case.

A homosexual woman had a relation with a man of higher social and financial position and wanted to marry him. The man half promised to divorce his wife, a wealthy schizophrenic who spent the greater part of every year in a psychiatric sanitarium, the remainder at home. Some time later, the man retracted his steps and broke his promise, which led to violent scenes with his girl friend. She demanded that he introduce her to his wife. He refused, foreseeing conflicts even were he to introduce her as the widow of a deceased friend. (The patient was in reality divorced). One day my patient decided to out-smart him. Without his knowledge she visited his wife and introduced herself as "an angel sent by God" to discuss her marital situation. The angel idea was very cleverly concocted, since in the woman's delusions angels were constantly present, as my patient knew from her friend's reports. With this fantastic but intuitively well chosen approach she won the psychotic woman's confidence. They became good friends, and she admitted that she really liked her. One day my patient suggested that all three of them should live together. The weakling of a husband fumbling with rage, as he said, was helpless, and accepted this grotesque proposition. For three months they had a "*menage à trois,*" the sex life "improving a good deal," as she ironically stated. The husband was impotent with his wife. The typical sequence of events was that the patient played sexually with him in her room until he achieved an erection, but refused intercourse and sent him to his wife's room to have intercourse. "Everything went well" in this strange cure of his potency disturbance until the psychotic woman became suspicious of the angel, whom she now classed as a female devil. Violent conflicts of jealousy followed, with the result that the wife had to be confined to an institution once more. The wife related her strange experience to the physicians, who took it as a "typical delusion." After the wife's latest confinement the patient became completely unmanageable, and the result was the commencement of her analysis.

A precise differentiation has to made between "masculine identification" in hysterical women and perversion Lesbianism. The outer world in its ignorance considers Lesbians masculine women. Blinded by that scotoma, which is fostered by Lesbians, these people cannot explain the "passive" Lesbian; nor can they account for the fact that the sexual practices of Lesbians centre chiefly around cunnilingus, and breast-sucking, both pointing in the infantile direction; mutual masturbation with penis-games are centered around the clitoris, unconsciously identified with the nipple.

The simple facts are that the pre-oedipal child-mother situation is repeated with baby (passive) and mother (active) connotations with occasional reversal of the roles. Let me repeat that the *external behavior of homosexuals and that of the homosexually innocent hysterical "masculine" woman are not only unreliable indicators but are completely misleading.* The masculine woman is not a homosexual; the markedly masculine Lesbian, on the other hand, shows a camouflage, hiding her real conflict. One must *distinguish between two forms of unconscious identification,* the "leading" and the "misleading" one. The "leading" unconscious identification petrified, as it were, the representation of the decisive wishes of the personality, crystallized as the end-result of the infantile conflict. The "misleading" identification denotes identification with persons chosen for the purpose of denying and rebuffing the reproaches of the inner conscience, directed against the basic neurotic wishes. The masculine, hysterical woman's "leading" identification pertains to the oedipal mother, her "misleading" unconscious identification pertains to the oedipal father.

The "leading" identification of the Lesbian pervert pertains either to the pre-oedipal mother (active variety) or to the baby (passive variety). Her "misleading" unconscious identification is either with the oedipal father (active) or the oedipal mother (passive).

A Lesbian is a neurotic with a *triad of unconscious concealment,* leading to a rather tragi-comic *quid pro quo*, the joke being on the naïve observer.

First, Lesbianism is, paradoxically, not an erotic but an aggressive conflict: the basis of psychic masochism is an undigested aggressive conflict which boomerangs because of guilt, and is only secondarily libidinized.

Secondly, under the disguise of a husband-wife relationship, a neurotically charged child-mother relation is hidden.

Thirdly, Lesbianism gives the impression of a biologic fact; the naïve observer is blinded by the conscious pleasure-gain, whereas a curable neurosis lies here concealed.

The problem of male homosexuality and Lesbianism has recently acquired greater importance through the popularity of the Kinsey report. If his statements are at least statistically correct, homosexuality in both sexes is *the* national disease.[54]

If Kinsey's opinion corresponds to the facts that every third adult had some homosexual experiences after maturation, then the figure reaches 18 million males. Add to this figure the vast army of Lesbians, and the total becomes even more fantastic. What matters most is the biologic orientation, propagandized by Kinsey to the effect that homosexuality is an unchangeable fact. In clearcut contradiction, I believe that homosexuality in both sexes is a curable disease with excellent prognosis.

14. Alcohol Addiction

The analytic elucidation of alcoholism has been clouded for decades by the repeatedly stressed tragic fallacy: orality = I want to get. To complicate matters, alcoholism has been considered a technique of "narcotizing the superego," thus releasing directly repressed drives, e.g., homosexual tendencies. The wit who claimed that the superego is the "alcohol-soluble part of the personality," showed more conferencier-talent, than psychological insight.

The homosexual theory is easy to explode: homosexuality is not a drive, but a complicated defense mechanism (See preceding section).

[54] "The Myth of a New National Disease," The Psychiatric Quarterly, Vol. 22, pp. 66–88, Jan., 1948.

Hence, a person under the influence of alcoholism cannot bring to the surface a non-existing drive. What he can do, is to use that defense mechanism in his alibi in the battle with his inner conscience. Since every orally regressed person fights his losing battle with the image of the pre-oedipal mother, one of his techniques in denying that conflict can be the formula: "How can I be accused of masochistic submission to mother, if I'm really interested in the man?"

Nearest to the clinical facts came K. Menninger who specifically stressed one facet of the alcoholic riddle: the self-destructive tendencies:

> "Alcohol-addiction . . . can be considered a form of self-destruction used to avert a greater self-destruction deriving from elements of aggressiveness, excited by thwarting ungratified eroticism, and the feeling of need for punishment from a sense of guilt related to aggressiveness. Its further quality is that in a practical sense the self-destruction is accomplished in spite of, and at the same time by means of, the very device used by the sufferer to relieve his pain and avert this feared destruction.

The fact that severe cases of alcohol addiction are suicidal candidates *in dosi refracta* is undoubtedly clinically correct. A great poet knew this intuitively 100 years ago. In his *Mémoires,* Heinrich Heine says of the end of the alcoholic poet Grabbe:

> First poverty and later on domestic affliction pushed the unfortunate Grabbe to seek cheer and oblivion in inebriation, and at last he may have grasped the bottle as others the pistol to put an end to his own wretchedness. "Believe me," a naive compatriot of Grabbe once told me, "he could stand a good deal, and he did not die because he drank but he drank because he wished to die; he died of self-drink." [55]

As important as the self-destructive tendency in alcoholics may be, it does not explain the specificity of alcohol. One could perhaps stress, as is done repeatedly, the fact that there are connecting links between compulsive drinking and depressive psychosis, as described by Freud: identification of the suicide candidate with the hated object. That explanation would coordinate with the fact of identification with the mother, as emphasized later.

Important is R. P. Knight's classification of "essential," "reactive" and

[53] For details see Chapter 4 of my book, "Talleyrand-Napoleon-Stendhal-Grabbe." Vienna; Psychoanal. Verlag, 1935.

"symptomatic" inebriates. Knight believes that "alcohol is used as a pacifier for disappointment and rage, as potent means of carrying out hostile impulses to spite his parents and friends, as a method of securing masochistic debasement and as a symbolic gratification of the need for affection."[56]

It is obvious that all studies of the psychological reasons for alcohol addiction stress only *one* aspect—the psychological one. They do not overlook the pharmacodynamic effects of alcohol; they simply have little to contribute toward knowledge of it. Compulsive drinking is a complicated problem with many facets. From the psychiatric viewpoint, only the genetic reasons and the psychic superstructure can be described. The problem of alcohol addiction cannot be solved from this viewpoint alone, however.

The most sensible thought ever uttered about alcohol, in my opinion, was that of the English jurist, John Selden (1584–1654): "'Tis not the drinking that is to be blamed, but the excess."[57] Undoubtedly a banality, but a banality which expresses in a nutshell the difference between the normal person, who "takes a drink," and the compulsive drinker, in whose case "the drink takes the man."[58]

In studying alcoholic addicts,[59] we find, first, the "mechanism of orality."

An alcoholic patient was full of hatred for his wife. He upbraided her constantly for her lack of understanding concerning his drinking. True, he came home only too often in a drunken state, to quarrel with her and abuse her. True, he neglected his business and gave his wife practically no money, forcing her to ask for financial help from her stingy family. True, in his drunken state he visited prostitutes, paying them with money acquired by pawning his wife's valuables. "All of this

[56] Summarized in Jellinek's book "Alcohol Addiction and Chronic Alcoholism," Yale Univ. Press, 1942, p. 13.

[57] "Table Talk."

[58] Edward Rowland Sill: "First the man takes a drink—Then the drink takes a drink—Then the drink takes the man." (An Adage from the Orient).

[59] My studies are published in Chapter 4 of "Talleyrand-Napoleon-Stendhal-Grabbe."—"The Psychological Interrelation between Alcoholism and Genital Sexuality," Journal of Criminal Psychopath., *4*:1–13, 1942. "Contributions to the Psychogenesis of Alcohol Addiction," Quart. Journal for Studies on Alcohol, *5*:434–449, 1944. "Personality Traits of Alcohol Addicts," ibid. *7*:356–359, 1946.

is true," the patient said, "yet if she loved me she would understand." It was difficult to show this man that the initial provocation was his. He denied that he saw only his wife's "injustice," and reacted to it with the greatest fury, only to pity himself afterward because nobody loved him.

Another patient had an arrangement with a cab driver to look for him after 2 A.M. in different bars, and to deposit him safely at his home. He dared not use his own car, having learned through a previous "disagreeable experience" the danger of harming someone through drunken driving. The taxi driver, an elderly, robust man, fulfilled his duties correctly, starting his rounds at 1 A.M. However, constant quarrels sprang up between the two men since the driver insisted on being paid not alone for the journey home but for the preliminary search as well. Since he could never predict at which bar his customer would be, he often had to look in several places, often distant from one another. Needless to say, the taxi meter showed considerable amounts. The patient understood consciously that the man was justified in being paid for the whole time; still he was furious paying "under protest" only. He called the driver an extortionist but was unwilling to change the arrangement. The money itself was not the important point, since the patient was a man of means. We see here the same mechanism; first, provocation; then repression of it and aggression, seemingly in self-defense; and finally, masochistic complaints of being taken advantage of ("nobody loves me").

A third example of this mechanism is an alcoholic patient who was completely uninterested sexually in his wife. She complained always of sexual neglect. Only occasionally, when he was under the influence of liquor, would he have intercourse with her. Then, however, he called her by another woman's name, thus provoking her jealousy. The man did not see that he provoked the conflicts with his sexual refusal and teasing. His constant refrain to her was, "You wanted intercourse; you got it, didn't you?" That he "gave" under impossible conditions was beyond his comprehension. He indulged, however, in constant self-pity and accusations of his wife.

These examples could be continued. They all add up to the fact that the alcoholic unconsciously provokes refusal from others, is aggressive apparently in self-defense, and revels in masochistic self-pity. He is inwardly a chronic disappointer. Even if he gives, he does so in circumstances reversing the conscious aim of the giving. His conscious story does not correspond to facts. He claims that he cannot help disappointing his beloved family; quite the reverse is true. He wants unconsciously to disappoint them and therefore does so.

The "mechanism of orality" proves the oral regression. The *specificity* of alcohol addiction is based on the fact that it "says it with liquid"—meaning, a specific sector of defenses and counter-defenses in the "fight of alibis" with the inner conscience. That sector is further *specifically* characterized by a peculiar pseudo-aggressive poisoning-technique directed against the interjected image of the "cruel mother."

An old popular saying describes the results of drinking in witty terms as follows: *Jocose, morose, bellicose, comatose.* Let us examine the four elements of this entity. The "jocose" part springs from the attempt to repair the original oral trauma by establishing an autarchy and state of independence from the allegedly refusing mother, and also from the attempt to retaliate against the mother in unconscious identification with her.

If our assumption is correct, that the alcohol addict repeats unconsciously the situation of the bad mother refusing and orally frustrating him, why, then, does he allow himself to be served drinks? Why not repeat the situation of scarcity and refusal directly? To understand his reasoning, we must take into account two facts: first, drinking in itself is at first an attempt at self-cure and reparation, based on the idea, "Mother refused me; now I will give myself everything she refused. I am independent and autarchic." That element of reparation accounts for the initial happiness when drinking. In other words, drinking is at first a triumph over the refusing mother. The second fact to be taken into account is even more complicated. It refers to the inner identification of the drinker with his mother.[60] I might mention an incident which happened to a patient of mine years before he entered analysis because of compulsive drinking. This man once had a violent conflict with his mother, whom he accused of being responsible for his obtaining what he considered an unfair share of his father's estate. His mother defended herself against these—by the way,

[60] Similar conclusions were reached, although through a different trend of reasoning, by British analysts.

unjustified—accusations. During their argument the man drank one brandy after another. His mother asked him reproachfully: "Why do you drink so heavily?" "What's that to you?" was the son's brusque retort. His mother objected with the sober and rather melancholy statement: "Everything which harms you harms me, too." The patient responded by taking *two* brandies at once. In evaluating this scene, we have to assume that the man, in identification with his mother, wanted to harm *her*. He was filling her, so to speak, with poison. Actually he harmed himself; in doing this his self-damaging or psychic masochistic tendencies had their expression.

This jocose phase also reflects irony achieved through making fun of authority in general, and, at the same time, kindness toward the environment. Everyone is familiar with the transitory initial mood of the drinker: "You are my friend; everyone is my friend." This mood shows the ambivalence of the conflict: pseudo-aggression toward the intrapsychic mother-image, coupled with denial of loss of love. It also expresses propaganda for one's own kindness, based on the theme: "You see how good I am although mother was so bad to me."

The tendency toward logorrhea, often observable in drinkers in the jocose phase, gives us an indirect hint concerning the genetic basis of the illness. The superabundance of words—giving of words—is an indirect reproach toward the denying mother. It is a "magic gesture," that is, an unconscious device of pseudo-aggression designed to pillory the mother by giving freely the very thing which she denied, the formula being: "I shall show you through my behavior how I wanted to be treated originally by you." The potus-logorrhea demonstrates in an unconscious innuendo that the child in the drinker allegedly wants to be given kindness (words = milk, love) by the mother. Magic gestures must always be scrutinized for the unconscious pseudo-aggression hidden behind their apparently gracious façade. They must also be scrutinized always for the defense mechanism they represent. The drinker makes use of magic gestures to give an exaggerated impression of his defensive desire to be "given", and thereby disguises his real aim to be unjustly treated. The masochistic enjoyment of being refused, not pleasure in being given, is his real purpose in life.

An example of the magic gesture is offered in the conduct of a well-to-do patient who, in the initial stages of inebriation, would promise people who happened to be at his table his aid in getting jobs. Seemingly full of kindness, a trait really foreign to him, he would promise them recommendations to various important acquaintances. Confronted by the applicants on the following day, he always denied having made such promises. Only once did he keep his word; on this occasion, however, he wrote the promised introduction in such ambiguous terms that it gave the man to whom it was addressed the impression that its bearer was an impostor.

Drinkers of a special group substitute sentimentality for hilarity in the "jocose" phase. These tearful neurotics exercise their lachrymal glands without being able to explain why they are sorry. Alcohol just has that effect on them, they claim. Analysis of these people proves that they are even more masochistic than those of the jocose variety. They are not even capable of furnishing the harmless defense of autarchy in fighting the mother-image. In other words, these individuals go immediately into *medias res* of masochistic complaints and self-commiseration.

The solitary drinker represents another subtype. He is even more neurotic than the drinker in company. He reaches the mechanism of reparation, described previously, only partially, and uses specifically ideas of grandeur in the form of narcissistically fantasied achievements. He resembles the day-dreamer in certain respects; however, he is capable of his day-dreaming only under the influence of alcohol. The drinker of this type is often a schizoid personality. I have twice observed the following facts in regard to solitary drinkers: First, the change from drinking in company to solitary drinking; this represented the outward sign of the increase in severity of the neurosis. Second, the permeation of masochistically tinged insecurity even in the narcissistic fantasies: achievement of the desired goal in the fantasies, but only with trembling and after long moments of insecurity.

The second stage of drinking, according to the witty and accurate slogan quoted before, the "morose" one, is de facto the stage of depression. The first attempt at reparation and denial of the maternal dependence via pseudo-aggression in its different disguises seemingly exhausts itself. Let us adduce a statement of a woman patient: "Whenever I drink, I am happy at first, *then feel a deep depression coming on.* I keep on drinking in order to recapture my initial happiness. Unfortunately, in vain." Her experience seems to indicate that the defensive power of the unconscious ego spends its ammunition, leaving the old depression, which is to be warded off, again at the fore. This stage of depression is characterized either by morose silence or by pessimistic remarks about the senselessness of life. "Cheer up," the husband of the woman just mentioned would say, "what you need is a drink!" She got her drinks (it is not a *pluralis majestatis*), and remained sullen. The technique which is so successful in the first, jocose phase fails in its repetition.

The third stage in the course of a drinking spree is not hilarity but bellicosity. Verbal or actual attacks on persons and objects by drinkers in this stage are not a rarity. Quarrelsomeness is frequent, although the single instance is easily forgotten. This is the stage in which various sexual acts take place. The question arises as to the relation between alcohol and genital sexuality. According to the testimony of the alcoholic himself, alcohol is sexually stimulating up to a certain point, then becomes sexually debilitating. This fact is stated succinctly by Porter in *Macbeth* (Act II, Sc.3): "Lechery, sir, it /drink/ provokes and unprovokes; it provokes the desire but takes away the performance."

The most superficial explanation of the alcoholic's sexuality, itself also a rationalization, is that alcohol serves as a "narcotic of the conscience."[61] According to this theory, alcoholics have stored up in them powerful sexual impulses (of a normal or perverse kind); under pressure of the nonalcoholized conscience, these impulses are kept down, but once the restrictions of conscience are lifted, the sexual desire is allowed expression. To this view it may be objected that the connection between impulse and defense against impulse appears analytically to be rather more complicated. Between the impulse and its inhibition there intervenes the particular defense mechanism. Thus what appears on the surface is not simply the impulse—even when the defense against it has partly fallen away—but primarily the defense against the impulse in the form of defense mechanism.

The chief objection to the "narcotic theory" is that if it were correct it should be possible to point out in the lives of these people

61 Many people, indeed, deliberately use drink to remove inhibitions. The efficacy, however, lies rather in suggestion than in pharmacological effect, as appears from the fact that very small quantities of alcohol are "effective."

elements of a strong, though suppressed genital-sexual life. Nothing of the sort is to be found. On the contrary, it can be precisely established from clinical evidence that the typical alcohol addict exhibits in general a rather weak and restricted genital-sexual life. This becomes easily intelligible if we bear in mind that the instinctual tendencies expressed by the alcoholic in drinking are of a pregenital, oral character, and not genital.

A third objection to this theory lies in the layman's habitual confusion of aggression with sex. Thus, to take an example, the layman considers a pathological sexual act, which in reality serves to discharge aggression under the disguise of sex, to be a veritable expression of sexuality. This assumption is quite mistaken; at best, it might be possible to speak of this act as sadism, which is unquestionably a mechanism foreign to normal sexuality, since in normal sexuality tender feelings toward the object are dominant. Apart from that, alcohol arouses nothing but aggression in the case of many people. It is worth noting that so significant a portrayer of human beings as Frank Norris, in his *McTeague*, refers plainly to the aggressive component without so much as mentioning the genital component, and this is due far less to delicacy of feeling or poetical embellishment than to naturalistic observation of facts:

> "The alcohol had its effect for all that. It roused the man, or rather the brute in the man, and now not only roused it but goaded it to evil. . . . McTeague disliked Trina /his wife/. She was a perpetual irritation to him.
>
> He drank no more whiskey than at first, but his dislike for Trina increased with every day of their poverty, with every day of Trina's persistent stinginess. At times he was more than ever brutal to her. He would box her ears or hit her a great blow with the back of a hairbrush, or even with his closed fist. His old-time affection for his "little woman," unable to stand the test of privation, had lapsed by degrees, and what little of it was left was changed, distorted, and made monstrous by the alcohol. The people about the house and the clerks at the provision store often remarked that Trina's fingertips were swollen and the nails as purple as though they had been shut in a door. Indeed, this was the explanation he gave. The fact of the matter was that McTeague, when he had been drinking, used to bite them, crunching and grinding them with his immense teeth, always ingenious enough to remember which were the sorest. Some-

times he extorted money from her by this means, but as often as not he did it for his own satisfaction."

I therefore doubt that the psychic structure of the alcoholic is really simple enough to be reduced to the formula of the "narcotization of the conscience," alcohol permitting "suppressed desires" to break through to the surface directly and volcanically without experiencing complicated transformations in the form of defense mechanisms.

Let us take clinical examples as a starting point. An alcoholic patient lived on his wife's money. Sexually he was completely uninterested in her; otherwise, too, his genital sexuality seemed to play a subordinate rôle. Only occasionally did he treat himself, using his wife's money, to the "luxury" of hunting up a prostitute, with whom he would get drunk and have intercourse. It was clear that the decisive point was revenge on his wife—he used her money to pay for the prostitute and the alcohol! He could not, however, explain why he was pursuing his wife with such hatred; the reason was an unconscious one, the identification of her with the "denying" mother of his babyhood.

Another patient was very gay and adventurous while drunk, and in that situation would attempt to seduce her sexually uninterested husband, usually without success. She herself was entirely frigid, but she experienced—as she herself put it—a "perverse satisfaction in draining him against his will."

A third patient when intoxicated was first in a pleasant humor, then deeply depressed. In this stage she would oscillate between weeping and aggressive reproaches of her husband, whom she accused of showing lack of love and of sexual neglect. But if he attempted to satisfy her sexually she proved frigid—and insatiable.

A fourth patient when drunk was first aggressive toward the people around him, whom he would provoke and insult. Alone with his wife in this alcoholic condition, he would tell her that he was completely "through" with her and would revile her for her alleged stinginess toward him and extravagance on her own behalf. He was seldom capable of coitus with his wife, and when he did engage in it, he did so full of contempt toward her.

A fifth patient denied that he was an alcoholic. He explained his frequent excesses in drinking as an attempt to "drink in courage" in order to demand urolagnistic practices from a prostitute. In truth, he never ventured to express this wish; he was in part impotent and unsatisfied.

This revenge motive creates justified scepticism about the genitality of the alcoholic. But the actual state of affairs is even more complicated. Grotesquely, genital coitus is employed by these sick people as a "moral alibi" for the even more dangerous oral aggression. Let us not forget that the basis of neurotic oral aggression is murderous revenge, which in turn is a defense against deeper repressed masochistic traits. Even in pathological conditions (with the exception of lust murder), genitality requires an affirmative and let-live attitude toward the object. Accordingly, these people unconsciously employ genitality as a device to save themselves from defensive oral murderous fantasies on the one hand and from self-destructive masochism on the other. These aggressive fantasies are, however, a desperate inner defense against the masochistic attachment. It is therefore possible to say that alcohol does not in any way enhance genital sexuality but, on the contrary, reduces it. What alcohol does provoke among oral neurotics is oral revenge fantasies, or, rather, murderous fantasies, against the mother or women unconsciously identified with her, as a primary defense against deep psychic masochism. As a secondary defense against these murderous revenge fantasies, genitality is produced as a life-affirming defense mechanism. How poorly this defense mechanism works in most cases may be seen from the fact that the coitus of these people is permeated with aggression or else, in the later stages of drunkenness, no longer succeeds at all.

This utilization of "alcoholic" coitus as a "*moral alibi*" is one of the most fantastic facts in the unconscious psychology of alcoholics. It turns upside down, so to speak, all customary and recognized moral notions. Let one but think of the widely current concept that alcohol is dangerous because it is sexually exciting. The phrase current in all languages, "Wine, Woman and Song," reflects this notion. And yet wine and woman have a very different significance in the unconscious psychology of the alcoholic.[62]

[62] I have deliberately quoted such writers as Frank Norris because they instinctively and in a somewhat exaggerated way express thoughts that are normally deeply repressed. Thus, for instance, Trina's pathological stinginess, which leads her to show her hungry husband the door, is simply an unconscious

About the last (fourth) stage of drunkenness, popularly called the "comatose," there is little to say. It is the stage of sleep and, later, of the hang-over. The dreams which follow drinking excesses, as far as they can be ascertained from patients, seem to deal habitually with situations of being refused. The hang-over, as far as psychological facts are concerned, is characterized by the feeling of guilt and sacred resolutions to abstain in the future, which are forgotten only too soon, when the whole vicious circle is renewed.

An interesting objection to the use of the self-destructive tendency as the explanation for alcohol addiction has been raised by Schilder:

> ". . . To stress the self-destructive tendencies of alcoholism, as Menninger does, overlooks the deep striving of the alcoholic to be loved and appreciated by society, which would grant to him the integrity of his body and his sex parts. He merely feels that without alcohol he will also be exposed to criticism and destruction. It is true, however, that in the deeper layers the alcoholic experiences the striving for prestige as a struggle for life and death."

In my opinion the alcoholic's "wish to be loved and appreciated by society" and his "striving for prestige" are not in themselves the reasons for his inebriety but merely unconscious defense mechanisms created for the purpose of negating the repetition of the basic mas-

representation of the child's fantasy that the mother is letting it "starve," or is indeed devouring it, as fairy tales, for instance, "Hansel and Gretel," show. In reality, mothers are neither cannibalistic nor always refusing; on the contrary, they are loving and devoted. In these stories and in the unconscious fantasies of oral patients is to be found a projection of the aggressive desires of the child himself, who reacts with hate-laden, biting aggression to the withdrawal of the breast (M. Klein). Thus, for example, McTeague murders his wife in revenge, after he had in drunkenness often bitten her fingers; these digits obviously have a symbolic meaning. In the case of another writer, the dipsomaniac Grabbe (discussed in my book of psychoanalytic biographic essays), these biting-fantasies found clear expression in a number of his dramas and satires. Especially significant is his fairy-tale play *Cinderella.* In this the fairy queen places at the disposal of the heroine, Olympia, an extraordinary domestic staff: The coachman is a metamorphosed rat; the lady's maid is a bewitched cat. The maid wants to seduce the coachman, but the latter is afraid of being devoured:

"Fairy Queen: The beautiful maiden frightens you? You will yet one day take her to wife."

"Coachman: So that on the morning of the wedding night I will lie not beside her but in her belly . . ."

ochistic situation, "nobody loves me." The wish to be loved in alcoholics is one of the inner defenses proving that the child in the alcoholic did not want to be disappointed; another defense is the "magic gesture," described previously. In its deepest layers the alcoholic's whole life is dedicated to the unconscious repetition of recreating the masochistic pleasure of being refused. The same holds true with regard to Schilder's statement that "It seems more or less accidental that the alcoholic ingests the alcohol by mouth, and the satisfaction received from drinking has no deeper relation to the oral gratification of eating." Insofar as Schilder refers to eating in itself, he is undoubtedly correct. I have shown that in compulsive drinking there is no direct repetition of the oral pleasure; quite the contrary, the alcoholic repeats the wish to be orally refused. Like Schilder, I do not believe in Rado's "alimentary orgasm" in drinkers. Another argument for this doubt is the fact that the alcoholic turns to alcohol and not to milk. Besides the pharmacodynamic effects, it is the self-damaging tendency that is responsible for this fact; he is filling his mother with poison. His unconscious reasoning runs as follows: "What can you expect of a bad mother *but* poison (= spoiled milk)." Another factor in his choice is his desire to do something forbidden. To a much less degree the same mechanism was manifested during prohibition, when the unconscious reason why many people turned to drink was because it was officially forbidden. Let us not overlook the fact that the alcoholic desperately strives, unconsciously, to prove his aggression as a defense against his masochistic regression.

15. Gambling [63]

The popular opinion concerning gamblers boils down to the naive assumption that they want to obtain the maximum amount of money in a minimum amount of time and without hard work. The unconscious reaction of the unpsychological spectator is a mixture of admiration, if the gambler seems to win, and gloating, if he loses, gloating based on the thought, "Why should he achieve what the average person cannot?" The question of whether or not the gambler wants to win is,

[63] First published in Journal of Criminal Psychopathology IV, No. 3, pp. 379–393, 1943, under the title, "The Gambler—A Misunderstood Neurotic." The original paper is more extensive.

of course, never asked, since popular opinion regards the purpose of gambling as a rational one, though one dangerous and difficult to achieve.

Other groups sincerely object to gambling on moral, religious or social grounds.

Observation of the psychology of the gambler with the analytic microscope shows that the basic question concerns just that which seems self-evident to the naive observer—the aim of the gambler. I submit that the gambler is not simply a rational though "weak" person who wants to gain money by means of a short cut, taking the risk of failure and of moral reproach from his environment, but *a neurotic with the unconscious wish to lose.* I will substantiate that seemingly paradoxical formulation clinically.

An explanation of terminology is at first necessary. What is a gambler? What are his signs and symptoms? Six characteristics must be considered:

1. *The gambler habitually takes chances.* Is the movie-goer who sometimes plays "Screeno" or "Bingo" by accident or chance a gambler? Is the man who risks a dollar betting that Dewey or Bennett will be elected governor of New York State a gambler? Or the reader of the *Times* who bets in a joking mood that the editorial page in the next edition will be page 16 or 24? One would doubt it. The stress rests first on the word "sometimes." The man in our example does not go to the movie every evening to play Screeno; he chooses a feature which he likes, though the fact that Screeno is offered may be for him a pleasant additional factor. The second man has a chance every four years to place his gubernatorial bet. And the *Times* reader is not in the mood every day to wager on such nonsense as the sequence of pages. The whole picture changes if, instead of "sometimes," "typically" is substituted; and if the primary objective of our movie fan is Screeno and not the feature itself, and he visits the same boring picture for the third time only because it is offered with Screeno; or if a person places his bets habitually, whenever he has a few dollars, using any opportunity, ridiculous though it may be. The quantitative factor is indispensable for differentiation. In like manner, we don't call a person a drunkard if he takes a cocktail before dinner.

2. *The game precludes all other interests.* A further descriptive

characteristic of the pathologic gambler is that his entire interest is concentrated constantly on gambling, its "chances" and prognostications. All of his fantasies and day dreams are centered in it. That pathologic concentration overshadows everything else—vocation, love, hobbies.

3. *The gambler is full of optimism and never learns from defeat.* The gambler is seemingly the last optimist, one who is totally uninfluenced by experience. That queer surety of success cannot be shattered, especially by financial losses. He did not win today? So what? Tomorrow will be lucky. He lost once more? Doesn't prove anything. Some day he simply must win. There is nothing more tragic than the gambler who has lost his last dollar and is still absolutely convinced that if only he had the money to overcome the string of bad luck he would "surely" win a fortune. Every gambler conveys the impression of a man who has signed a contract with Fate stipulating that persistence must be rewarded. With that imaginary contract in his pocket, he is above all objections and logical arguments.

4. *The gambler never stops when winning.* As a result of his pathological optimism, the gambler never stops when winning, since he is convinced that he will win more and more. The result is that in the long run he always loses. He does not look at the money he has won as a result of chance but as a down payment on his contract with Fate to win permanently. This inability to stop is, by the way, an argument against the earnest assumption of all gamblers that one can get rich through gambling. One can imagine that a man may win a certain amount of money in a game of chance. Were he able to stop gambling immediately, his bank account could conceivably increase. However, in the great majority of cases, the game is continued until the gambler proves to be exactly what some people call him—a "sucker." The fact that he doesn't stop when winning is one of the reasons that gambling houses always win. One of my gambling patients visited a fashionable French gambling resort and paid a social call on the manager of the casino, to whom he had a letter of introduction. The specialist in gambling asked him whether he had visited the casino. "Of course," was the answer, "I have even won a few thousand francs." At this his host became serious and gave him the advice to leave town immediately. "If you don't, you will continue to gamble and lose

everything. We make money because the gambler cannot stop when he loses and especially when he wins."

5. *Despite initial caution, the gambler eventually risks too large sums.* For the gambler, every game of chance is associated with either conscious or unconscious feeling of guilt; consequently, he uses certain mechanisms to appease his conscience. The most typical one is the small stake: "It doesn't matter if I lose that sum; I can afford it." Gradually, though, his stakes increase, with or without scruples regarding their size. At this point the pathologic optimism described above enters the picture as an excuse. The next step is that the source of the money is disregarded. The family man who bets with the money expected to feed the family is a well-known tragic figure. Nearer the abyss is the man who defrauds his clients or his employer to gamble, using the eternal excuse that he was convinced that this time he must win. Every gambler is familiar with the situation of "losing his head" and despite "good intentions" risking everything on one card—and losing. The fact that in these situations the behavior of the gambler is unexplainable logically (it is senseless to risk everything at once) proves the decisive importance of unconscious motives in gambling.

6. *"Pleasurable-painful tension" (thrill) is experienced between the time of betting and the outcome of the game.* The "rational" motives offered by gamblers for gambling are making money, pastime or both. Obviously, both reasons are excuses and rationalizations. Gamblers, who are not too hypocritical admit freely that they are looking for the strange tension experienced in the game. The understanding of that mysterious tension is one of the pivotal factors in deciphering the psychology of gambling, and that "thrill" is impossible to understand from the descriptive plane. It is very likely not by chance that that sensation, well known to everyone who gambles, is not correctly described in either scientific literature or belles-lettres. This is because it is impossible to understand without knowledge of unconscious factors. The tension is a mixture of pleasurable and painful sensations not comparable to other known sensations. The formulation itself, "pleasurable-painful tension" (I am quoting an observing patient of mine) shows the alogical element involved. That the expectation of an event whose outcome is uncertain should be pleasurable is in itself enigmatic. Many persons do everything possible to avoid uncertainty, but uncertainty

is exactly what the gambler looks for. One might rationalize by stating that the gambler expects success and is therefore in an elated mood. Even were this true, the painful element of the tension of gambling would remain unexplained. Should someone object that the painful component of the feeling arises from the uncertainty of winning, we would have a vicious circle and wonder why the gambler plays for stakes in the first place.

I repeat that the tension of gambling is logically unexplainable. It is erroneous to assume that it springs from the interim which the gambler must endure between the placing of his bet and the finish of the game. He looks forward to that interval and the accompanying tension. It is of no consequence whether he realizes it or not, whether it is conscious or unconscious.

The thrill of that "tension" is recognized by the man who wrote the best literary dramatization of a gambler, Dostojevsky, in "The Gambler." In one of his letters the famous Russian, who was himself a pathologic gambler confesses in self-defense: "The main point is the game itself. On my oath, it is not greed for money, despite the fact that I need money badly."

How far that "thrill" overshadows greed for money is proven by the fact that even professional card sharps are sometimes victims of it and gamble for gambling's sake and lose. That is reported, for instance, of Casanova. Another evidence of the predominance of the thrill-component was offered by a patient of mine, treated for pathologic gambling. He told of a game played with 15 matches by two persons, in which each person had the right to take in his turn one, two or three matches. The loser was the person who, because it was his turn, had to take the last match. The initiated always won if he started by taking two matches and was careful to leave an unequal number of matches each time to his opponent. This cat-and-mouse play was financially agreeable to my patient, since even an intelligent but uninitiated opponent would not learn the trick before ten or fifteen games had been played; but he told me that after some time he would become bored—"There was no thrill to it." In other words, if you take away the tension, you destroy the pleasure of gambling. The element of "insecurity," regardless of winning or losing, seems to be of prime importance and one of the prerequisites of that strange thrill.

The best approach to the *unconscious* problem of the gambler's psychology is to be found in his astonishing, logically senseless conviction that he will win. A literary example of this is provided by a passage from the diary of a victim of her husband's gambling, Mrs. Dostojevsky:

> "Fedja (F. M. Dostojevsky) took eighty gulden, gambled and lost. He took once more the same sum and lost. . . . He fetched the last forty gulden and promised me *unconditionally* that he would bring home my earrings and my ring which he pawned for 170 francs. He said that in a *tone of complete conviction, as if it depended only on him whether or not he would win.* Of course, that conviction did not help him and he lost that sum also." (August 22, 1867).

When we ask ourselves whether we could recall an example of such conviction on the part of an average person in real life, we have difficulty, since such a phenomenon is to be seen only among pathologic fanatics. We have to go back to the fiction of omnipotence of the child. The child lives for a long time in a sort of megalomania (as Freud and Ferenczi have shown), knowing only one yardstick, his over-inflated ego. His misconception of reality is fostered by the conduct of adults, who attempt automatically to fulfill his every wish concerning nourishment, sleep and attention. The child misconceives causality and sees in these wish fulfilments, not the results of kindness and love of his mother or mother representatives, but simply the result of his own omnipotence. That fiction is destroyed gradually by real experience, and its destruction is very likely the deepest disappointment of childhood. An excellent example of this megalomania of childhood is found in a passage of "Jean Christophe" by the French writer of genius, Romain Rolland. The poet describes his character as a little boy:

> "He is a magician, too. . . . He commands the clouds. He wants them to go more to the right. But they continue their way to the left. He scolds them and repeats his command more urgently. He observes with high pulses whether at least one little cloud obeys him. But they continue to run to the left. He stamps with his foot, menaces them with his little stick and changes his command. He now wants them to go to the left, and this time the clouds obey. He is happy and proud of his power. . . ."

The poet as if it were a clinical case in transitory phase: The child acknowledges that he is not an omnipotent magician any longer but wants to save through post facto sanction at least a little part of his fiction of omnipotence. It is as if someone, looking at his watch at one minute before six, should command the watch to point to six o'clock in one minute, and the watch "obeys."

How does education bring about the transition from the "pleasure principle" (Freud) to the "reality principle"? By love, persuasion and threats. The clinical fact remains that only with great difficulty is the child forced to give up that phantasy. We all still possess unconsciously the old wish of paradisiac omnipotence, even if we are very "grown-up." Further life experience convinces the child that certain facts are unchangeable. He learns that it does not pay to run his head against the wall after trying it a few times and finding that the wall remains stationary in spite of his command from the arsenal of childlike omnipotence that it give in. Secondarily, he learns to avoid by a form of protective mechanism, so to speak, certain fights with predictable defeats. He becomes smart, but he does so without enthusiasm. Deep inside the old fiction of omnipotence is buried and can, in certain circumstances, as could Homer's dead heroes in Hades when they drank blood, be resuscitated.

The power of the "reality principle" is based on the fact that by accepting it the child, and later the adult, avoids many escapable defeats. *There is, however, one exceptional situation in life in which following the "reality principle" brings not the slightest advantage compared to following the "pleasure principle"; that is gambling.* There, blind chance is dominant, chance which, in pure games of luck, cannot be influenced by logic, cleverness, and the attitude of being a "good boy." An old anecdote quoted by one of my patients illustrates this. A college student won $10,000 betting on a "dark horse" at the races. He met his professor of mathematics, who, full of curiosity, asked him how he figured out the winner. "Very simply," was the reply, "I dreamt about the figures 2 and 3 and thought that 2 x 3 equaled 12; therefore I placed my money on number 12." "But 2 x 3 is not 12!" objected the professor. The pupil became excited. "You want to teach me how much 2 x 3 equals? I won!" The humor of the situation lies in the fact that the boy won using his "private," alogical system of mathematics, and in this action reduced logic to absurdity.

Gambling activates, therefore, unconsciously, the old, childish phantasy of grandeur and megalomania. More important, it activates the *latent rebellion* against logic, cleverness, moderation, morals and renunciation. That latent rebellion, based on the inwardly never-relinquished "pleasure principle," scoffs ironically at all rules of education. Heavy inner retaliation is the result. Since all educational rules are given to the child by his mother and father and their representatives (teachers, priests, superiors, etc.), that rebellion activates a deep unconscious feeling of guilt.

How typical that aggression toward the childhood authority is in gamblers is described with the fine intuition of a genius by Dostojevsky in "The Gambler:" ". . . In five minutes I accumulated 400 gold pieces in roulette. I should have left at that moment, but a strange feeling came over me—to challenge Fate. It was the wish to give Fate a punch in the nose and show her my tongue."

We have only to substitute for Fate the parental representation of it for the child and we have in a nutshell the psychic situation of the gambler. Priority in all discoveries goes to the poet and dreamer: science describes more precisely, using clinical proofs, and in different terms. In general, scientific discoveries are re-discoveries of truths felt intuitively by poets hundreds of years before.

The psychic situation of the gambler, therefore, is, first *unconscious aggression,* and second, unconscious tendency toward *self-punishment* because of that aggression. That childlike, unconscious, neurotic misunderstanding of the whole process of gambling results in a vicious circle without end. If one thinks through that fact, which I found confirmed in all of my analyses of gamblers, one comes to the conclusion that unconsciously the gambler wants to lose. His losing is simply the price he pays for the neurotic aggression he expresses in attacking unconsciously the educational authority of his childhood. Long analytic experience teaches us that in neurosis no aggression is possible without self-punishment. The whole conception of the neurosis is based on the knowledge that neurotics unconsciously transfer conflicts experienced with their mother and father to innocent persons whom they unconsciously identify with their parents. Since aggression toward their parents was forbidden, every aggression toward the substitutes is inwardly forbidden, too, and if executed, expiated by severe self-punishment. We see here, by the way, the difference between normal and pathological aggression. In the former the enmity is directed toward the real person only and not toward the imaginary one; in the former too, no inner feeling of guilt is present, since normally our aggression is aroused only in self-defense and, since the enemy is not identified unconsciously with persons associated with childhood, the righteous indignation justifies itself without feeling of guilt.

Hence my conviction that the gambler cannot win in the long run because losing is needed for his psychic equilibrium—it is the price he pays for his neurotic aggression, and at the same time makes possible the continuation of gambling.

The unconscious driving force which gives rise to the phenomenon "gambler" springs from unconscious resuscitation of the childish megalomania, with all of its neurotic results. In other words, the gambler is a "naughty" child who expects punishment after performing his forbidden, aggressive deal. Basically, the *pleasant* component of the tension which the gambler feels is derived from the pleasure of aggressively-used childish megalomania; the *painful* component of this tension arises from expectation of punishment for his crime. The whole psychic problem is complicated, however, by a *masochistic* substructure. A prototype of the situation described above would be the "bad" boy expecting a spanking for his "naughtiness." Between aggressive deed and punishment is interposed a period of expectation of punishment which varies in length. A patient whom I was treating because of gambling told me that the interim between staking and the outcome of the game reminded him of an experience he had had in school. During a written examination he was tortured by the thought that because of insufficient time and inadaquate preparation he would fail the examination. In that moment his fear changed into sexual excitement. "Is it possible to experience sexual pleasure in a situation of anxiety?" asked my naive patient. My patient's comparison was only partly correct. The tension felt in gambling is of shorter duration; sexual excitement in itself is repressed and above all, is not at all of the genital type; the pleasure experienced is unconscious only and is made up partly of "psychic masochism." The sequence of events in the tension of gambling is, in other words, aggression toward mother and father, expectation of punishment, rebound of the aggression like a boomerang toward the gambler himself because of feeling of guilt, and *sexualization of that punishment as psychic masochism.* Anyone who denies that fear can be sexualized unconsciously should simply observe people enjoying a mystery thriller in a movie house. These fans identify deeply with the victims and enjoy thereby the "thrill of being overwhelmed." Another example of this sexualization of suffering is found in neurotic children who remain unchanged by punishment. Having provoked punishment, they continue the deeds for which they are punished. A permissible deduction is that they "like" it unconsciously.

That "masochistic component" proves, from the standpoint of the possibility of winning, very dangerous. Since the gambler wants, unconsciously, masochistic pleasure, he can achieve a maximum of it only by losing. Of course, that he consciously has the wish to win is undeniable, but that wish is dynamically not at all effective.

Still, the fact that the gambler experiences psychic masochistic pleasure unconsciously does not answer the problem entirely. Why should the gambler choose that means of obtaining this pleasure when there are thousands of ways of obtaining it? That masochistic enjoyment contributes something to his thrill is to be accepted. But it does not explain the *specificity* of the problem of gambling.[64] This is to be found elsewhere.

[64] The analytic literature does not give us any definite clues concerning gamblers; the whole problem is, with but a few exceptions, still terra incognita. When analytic authors do speak about gamblers they do so only in a tangential manner. Freud mentions the fact that gambling may be, in certain cases, unconscious substitutes for masturbation with self-punishment. ("Dostojevski und die Vatertoetung," Ges. Schr., XII). Simmel believes that gamblers regress to the anal level of libido development ("Zur Psychoanalyse der Spielers," Int. Z. f. Psychoan., 1920). Hattingberg assumes that the gambler looks for a pleasure in fear (Analerotik, Angstlust, Eigensinn," Int. Z. f. Psychoan., 1912). Laforgue stresses the same point of erotization of fear in gamblers ("Ueber Erotisierung der Angst," Int. Z. f. Psychoan., 1930). Ernest Jones describes the "Case of Paul Murphy" (Psychoan. Bewegung, 1931) and believes that Murphy's chess talent was based on a sublimation of the son's oedipal aggression toward his father. Similar conclusions are drawn by Pfister ("Ein Hamlet am Schachbrett," Psychoan. Bewegung, 1931).

First, the vicious circle described above between constant rebellion against all educational rules, based on reduction to absurdity, with subsequent self-punishment as a factor. Not everyone feels the need of that constant rebellion against authority and of resuscitation of infantile megalomania. The constant proof of the futility of every attempt to destroy the childlike omnipotence through the "reality principle" is pathognomic for the gambler.

Second, only a specific subgroup of a specific group of neurotics makes up gamblers. These people are orally regressed and consistently use the "mechanism of orality." Not all neurotics who use the "mechanism of orality" are gamblers; on the other hand, all gamblers use that mechanism. In other words, gamblers represent a specific subgroup of "oral" neurotics. The significant fact in the "oral mechanism" is that it gives masochistic pleasure behind a facade of pseudo-aggression. But whereas other oral neurotics are content to push by various means the mother of the pre-oedipal period and her successive representatives into the situation of refusal, the gambler uses a *specific* device for that purpose—the derisive one described above, of proving how senseless are all the parental rules and moral principles since in gambling chance is decisive.

From that viewpoint we understand why the gambler is 100% convinced that he must win. His surety derives from the unconscious certainty of reducing his mother to absurdity as a giving person, shifted upon optimism of winning.

One might object that, even if that theory of gambling were correct, it would be applicable only to games of pure chance (for instance, roulette, dice, etc.), not to games combining chance and "reasoning" (for instance, races, bridge, stock exchange, etc.), where judgment, ability to bluff, etc. *also* play a part. Strangely enough, genetically and psychologically there is no essential difference between these games. The original form of childlike omnipotence is always repressed. How-

---

The only existing psycho-analytic paper covering the whole problem of gambling with an attempt to explain, not details, but the underlying problem is that of the present writer, "On the Psychology of the Gambler," Imago, 1936. The study presented in that preliminary publication had been later enlarged in "The Gambler—A Misunderstood Neurotic," J. of Criminal Psychopathology, 1943.

ever, since this omnipotence remains dynamically effective in the unconscious, the adult is always on the look-out for a situation in which he can continue his aggressively-meant omnipotence in a compromise. That concession to the "principle of reality" gives some people the opportunity to continue their childish drive. Ratio intervenes as a connecting link between the original omnipotence of thoughts—the vehicle of childish megalomania—and reality. Behind the mask of ratio, of intellectual achievements, the old sacrifice before the alter of the pagan god, omnipotence of thoughts, is tolerated by the "principle of reality." For instance, in the book mentioned earlier, the boy Jean Christophe, who so desperately wanted to direct the clouds, later becomes an orchestra conductor. In other words, the amount of disguise required determines to what degree a pure game of chance is chosen or some intellectual substitute. In this respect, it is interesting to note that even in the "queen" of all games of intellect, chess, the development described above can be proven. Every student of chess knows that in its oldest form, in the "Tschaturanga" of old India, both partners had to throw dice to decide what the next move should be. One should not be deceived by the fact that so many gamblers lay such a preponderance on reasoning, "tips," experience and "intellectual" evaluation of chances; they attempt thereby to deny that they gamble, that is apply childish megalomania. The best proof of that mechanism of negation is the constant attempt to find "systems" in pure games of chance, for instance, roulette. That is of course impossible. The only advantage this attempt provides is that of saving the gambler the pain of ambivalence—of deciding what his next move should be. The same interpretation holds for the gambler's superstition—it is reminiscent of the horror-chamber of obsessional neurotics, based, as Freud has shown of superstition in general, on the idea of omnipotence of repressed aggressive wishes.

Gambling is a curable neurosis. It happens rarely that a gambler understands that a disease is involved. Sometimes, the family insists on treatment. Nothing can be done without the patient's insight—he simply does not consult the psychiatrist. If he consults him out of his own despair, the chances of cure are good.[65]

[65] For a typology of gamblers, see "The Gambler—A Misunderstood Neurotic," *loc. cit.*

PSYCHOPATHIC TRENDS

16. Impostors [66]

The psychoanalytic literature on impostors [67] (Abraham,[68] Deutsch, Alexander,[69] Alexander-Staug, Zulliger, Meng, Bally, Kielholz, Pfister, Wittels, Keiser-Bromberg) contributed a series of interesting facets, viewing the impostor mainly as a hysterical individual plus X (psychopathy), without solving the problem. The main reason seems to be lack of analyzed material. The best case history of an impostor, that of K. Abraham, is of a patient whom the analyst saw in a field hospital while he was in military service, without having the opportunity to analyze him.

Another general difficulty in the psychologic evaluation of impostors is the lack of clarity in terminology. Specialists of forgery, swindling, bankruptcy, extortion, impersonation of officials—all of these "criminotics" (Foxe) are in some papers mentioned as representing separate entities, in other papers all included under the heading of impostors [70] or, more often, "psychopaths." In other words, not even the problem of terminology with regard to impostors has been fully solved.

The impostor has specific *descriptive* characteristics which, as far as I can determine from my cases and from the literature, comprise the following:

1. *Social climbing.* The impostor is "one who imposes upon others

[66] First published in Journal for Psychopath., V. 2, pp. 695–715, 1944 under the title "Psychopathology of Impostors." A cross-section if the analytic literature on that topic is included.

[67] I refer to papers by Freudians exclusively.

[68] "History of an Impostor," Imago, I, 1925. An attempt at evaluation of this work is found on p. 270 ff. of the present section.

[69] "Der Neurotische Charakter," Int. Zeitschr. f. Psychoan., XIV, 1928, p. 32.

[70] Ben Karpman in his impressive monograph, "The Individual Criminal" (Nerv. & Mental Disease Monographs 59), describes in great detail 5 "criminal insane" cases, at least 2 of which (Cases IV and V) show a connection to impostors. One of these persons impersonated a U. S. officer and attempted to extort money; the other was under sentence for forgery of government checks and impersonation of a U. S. officer. The terminus technicus "impostor" is not used; however, Karpman gives an instructive description of Babelian confusion of terms concerning "psychopaths," pointing out the inherent contradictions (pp. 181 ff., *loc cit.*)

by an assumed character or false pretentions" (Webster). Interestingly enough, the term applies only to persons pretending to be more socially than they really are; it never includes persons who pretend the opposite. Kalif Harun-al-Raschid in the disguise of a merchant would not be called an impostor by the admiring crowd if discovered. In German the word "Hochstapler" expresses exactly that social-climbing: "hoch" means "high," and the old "stapfen" means "to walk;" in other words, "a crook pretending to be of higher social circles" (Meyer). What the phrase basically refers to is the swindling of money or of social acknowledgment or both through the pretense of being "somebody" by someone whom—to quote an impostor—the "snobbish outerworld" would consider a "nobody."

2. *Charming, disarming behavior* inspiring confidence by firmness and self-assurance and winning everyone's friendship. Women, especially, are charmed by the occasional feminine trends in these men, finding narcissistically some unconscious similarity to themselves. There are cases on record where a man of this type has married three women, has been sent to jail because of his trigamy, and still has not incurred the anger of his wives "because he was so charming."

3. *Sense of humor of specific type.* Among the bag of tricks of the impostor is always a peculiar ironic twist which makes fun of social institutions or prejudices, reducing them to absurdity for his own inner purposes. A classical example is the cause célébre of the "Captain from Koepenick." In 1906 a shoemaker, disguised in the uniform of a Prussian captain, confiscated the municipal money in a suburb of Berlin. He was able to steal this money only because nobody doubted the right of a Prussian officer to do what he pleased; no one was suspicious, since respect for the uniform in the Kaiser's militaristic state was universal. Cleverly capitalizing on that prejudice, the "Captain" even mobilized a whole company of soldiers for his purpose. Ironically enough, the ironic twist in his action brought about his pardon later. On hearing the report of his conduct, the Kaiser laughed and considered it a compliment on his successful education of the populace in militaristic respect. The same ironic twist has been psychologically correctly represented in Sascha Guitry's "History of a Cheat." In it a boy is punished for some puerile cheating by being sent to bed without supper. The

next morning the remainder of his family die of poisoned mushrooms eaten the evening before. The irony in this story is that the punishment for good morals is death; the reward for bad morals is survival.

4. *Pseudo-identification-mimicry.* The impostor plays the role he has designated for himself with utmost confidence, as if he really *were* the person he would personify. His identification is that of an actor. On the other hand, he is always aware of his faking, inwardly making fun of the disguise and the people who are taken in by it.

5. *Bombastic braggadocio.* Every impostor presents his fake-story convincingly, with or without false modesty; his sureness is the prerequisite of his success. His feigned conviction reminds one superficially of certain childhood lies. However, the fact remains that the impostor never believes his own story; he is full of conscious irony toward the people who believe him, and derives a great pleasure from "pulling their legs."

6. *Infantile approach toward time.* The impostor does not have the normal person's consideration for the future. His yardstick is today and today's hour only. This tendency is visible, for instance, when he is discovered in his cheating. He maintains appearances until the last second. In one case a young girl patient was caught, years before entering analysis, attempting to swindle in a store, having given her name as that of a wealthy acquaintance. The store manager faintly remembered the woman whose name she was assuming, and called that woman by phone. Until the last the second girl pretended to be that woman. The manager, and later the judge, were completely at a loss to understand what advantage lay in the continuation of the pretence for a few minutes more, especially since it could serve only as an aggravating circumstance to consider in passing judgment.

7. *Pose of "having a good time" covering depression.* The impostor gives the impression of being an everlasting optimist, and often pretends to himself that he is happy.[71] He derives, to be sure, a good deal of conscious satisfaction from ridiculing his environment through his successful fake. Below this thin layer of pleasure in irony, deep depres-

[71] Meng suggests that the impostor regresses "to the time of *satisfied* narcissism." I cannot subscribe to that view.

sion is hidden, somtimes directly visible in the cheater when he is seemingly unobserved.[72]

8. *Inability to enjoy self-created success.* Contrary to popular assumption that the impostor uses cheating for rational purposes, clinical facts prove that he acts irrationally: He neither enjoys nor makes use of his self-created success for any length of time. One can imagine that a person may use incorrect means for the purpose of achieving success; usually once success is gained in this manner, it is clung to. The impostor, however, overdoes his triumph, seems to get "bored" with it, and unconsciously provokes his own downfall. He either leaves the place of his temporary success, partly through fear of being exposed, and renews his pattern in another spot, or goes temporarily to jail because of self-provoked dénouement.

9. *"Cynical" and remorseless attitude.* The cynical and pseudo-conscienceless philosophy embodied in "So what?" is consciously predominant in the impostor. More, he constantly tries to appear "tough," especially when caught. "I married three wives? So what? They were in different places." "I cheated people out of money? So what? Suckers ask for it." "I told fantastic lies about my noble descent? So what? Why were these idiots gullible enough to believe me?" And so on.

10. *Stabilization of type of law-breaking on the cheating-level.* It is interesting that in *typical* cases of cheating no further development in crime is observable; crimes of a more serious character, such as murder, are not committed. The cheater remains a lifelong cheater, repeating his pattern in different disguises over and over.

11. *Pathologic approach toward work.* The impostor works only in transitory periods, usually chiefly to gain the confidence of the people he hopes to cheat. He considers work, not as a necessary means of obtaining a livelihood, but as a prerequisite for his schemes of cheating. Consciously he feels superior to "slaves" who accept work as the natural way of making a living.

12. *Incorrigibility.* The records of typical impostors show that

[72] Impostors conceal their depression well, even before psychologic observers. Bally states: "We also call the narcissistic psychopath sick *not* because *he* suffers, but because *we* are suffering under him." (Italics are mine.)

neither prison nor good advice nor help of any kind changes their behavior.

It is obvious that even the most minute *description* cannot suffice in itself to explain impostors, and can only give clues for a *genetic* understanding of them.

Let's start with Abraham's "History of an Impostor." The patient therein described spent many years following one pattern. He would win the confidence of people, then make them pay for it by involving them in fraudulent debts. He wandered from one prison to another. During his military career in the War, he stole identification blanks and played the role of an officer. After the War he married a wealthy widow and became for 4 years a substantial citizen. Abraham explains this change in his behavior as an exceptional "cure through love," and reconstructs the psychogenesis of the case as follows: The boy did not develop the normal oedipus complex, he felt unloved by parents and siblings. Afterward he felt compelled to disappoint people who liked him, to repeat the revenge on his parents. An overdimensional repetition compulsion forced him always to become a pariah exactly at the moment when he found himself loved or admired. All of his transitory successes were counteracted by unconscious guilt feeling, destroying his own success. He lacked motherly tenderness in his early childhood and could not build up his father as ego-ideal. The well-to-do widow who took interest in him gave him for the first time the possibility to transfer his libido to a mother-type. His feeling of guilt was missing, since the competitor (father—husband of the widow) no longer existed and had died through no fault of his. Abraham explains this change which lasted for four years as an exceptional one, and stresses the incompleteness of analytic knowledge of the problem of criminality in general and of impostors in particular.

I cannot subscribe to Abraham's explanation of the case. My experience has taught me that all impostors or impostor-like persons are, *not* oedipally, but orally regressed. Since Abraham's case was not analyzed, it is impossible to prove or disprove Abraham's belief specifically. Abraham's deductions, however, seem to me fallacious. The oedipus complex fits too well into the *superficial* pattern of the case; hence is overrated without consideration that in oral cases it represents a defense against the deeper oral "danger." I do not believe in "cure through love" even in exceptional cases of *adult* impostors and I do not believe that the patient in question would die peacefully in old age as a substantial citizen in the arms of his loving wife. He would rather rot in prison. Abraham's optimism seems premature to me. He was too much impressed by the four peaceful years.

I personally believe that impostors represent a special group of those people who use the "mechanism of criminosis." To avoid repetition of a longer paper,[73] I shall summarize only the essentials of the mechanism: The criminotic represents a specific case of failure to overcome the oral disappointment and one unique in its specific "solution." The feeling of pre-oedipal disappointment in the mother and absolute helplessness to take a revenge on her for this disappointment force the criminal unconsciously to his herostratic act. His situation is that of a dwarf fighting a giant who refuses to take cognizance of his fight. The only way he can force the giant to recognize his intention is by using dynamite, so to speak, which also destroys him. That tendency to take revenge for oral disappointments in the pre-oedipal mother is projected upon society and is coupled with unconsciously self-intended punishment. *Only unconscious anticipation and acceptance of punishment makes crime possible for the criminal,* since it appeases his inner conscience. The criminal not only has a conscience; he has a very severe one. He uses a specific device to "appease" it—severe self-imposed punishment. In every criminal action two factors are involved, a constant one and a variable one. The *constant* factor ("mechanism of criminosis") explains the motor act, the real riddle in crime. It is based on the masochistic attempt to overcome the inner feeling of helplessness stemming from pre-oedipal oral conflicts, mentioned above.[74] The *variable* factor pertains to the psychologic contents of the specific crime; it must be determined in every specific case and is as multitudinous as unconscious motivations in general. In my opinion, the social factors in crime play a relatively subordinate role; in the majority of cases they are rationalizations for hidden unconscious motives or the hitching-post for masochistic repeti-

[73] "Suppositions about the Mechanism of Criminosis," *loc. cit.* See also Ch. XV "The Neurotic Who Unconsciously Bargains for the Electric Chair—The Criminal," in "The Battle of the Conscience."

[74] For details, see section 27, this chapter.

tion of injustices experienced in reality or fantasy in the child-mother-father relationship, afterward projected and perpetuated masochistically upon society or the social order in general.

Still, the special group of impostors, in itself a subgroup of "narcissistic psychopaths" (formerly sometimes called "moral insanity") has features characteristic of this group alone. Here they are in the order of importance:

1. The narcissism of these sick people is out of proportion, or, more often, cannot overcome its early oral disappointment. To restore that lesion in self-esteem, the *inner, unconscious necessity arises to prove consistently the capacity to inspire love and admiration.* This defense mechanism accounts for the charming and disarming behavior of impostors. But, since that proof is only a narcissistic face-saving device, the masochistic "mechanism of criminosis" comes to the fore immediately afterward and leads to self-provoked, masochistic defeats. The notion often advanced that the narcissistic impostor wants nothing but the admiration which was refused him in childhood, can be easily disproved. Should it be true, he would try to achieve such a situation and enjoy it. Nothing of the sort happens; after achieving love, he throws it away.

2. Impostors avoid success not only because they want psychic masochistic pleasure but also because they want to offend and *pseudo-aggressively take revenge upon people whom they identify with the mother of the pre-oedipal period.* They want to arouse love and admiration, but having aroused them, throw them away in order to offend the mother-substitute. It is as if they would say: "I wanted only to prove to you that I could get your love—but I don't care to have it." [75]

3. The guilty feeling of impostors stems, not—as Abraham assumes—from oedipal wishes; it refers to masochistic wishes to reduce the mother to absurdity as a giving person and to enjoy unconsciously her refusal. The throwing away of love achieved in later repetitions is in itself a *defense mechanism of pseudo-aggression against these deep-seated masochistic wishes* and not simply the result of feeling of guilt because of that pseudo-aggression or oedipal repetition.

4. That unconscious *pseudo-aggressive defense* mechanism is visible

[75] It is known that a similar tendency may be observed in dosi refracta in different narcissistic neurotics.

also in the strange "*sense of humor*" which impostors use to attack venerable institutions or time-honored prejudices of the environment.

5. The "lack of feelings" and "lack of conscience" belong in the same category. *Both are futile attempts to escape psychic masochism.* The wish for punishment finds its expression in a jail term or in the expectation of jail. The impostor's "humor" represents his frantic attempt to deny that he is narcissistically wounded and therefore depressed. Bally's naive opinion that the impostor has "no conscience" proves only that "every absurdity has a champion to defend it" (Goldsmith) and is the result of mistaking surface reverberations for the subterranean conflict they cover.

6. To sum up: The impostor is an oral-parasitic sufferer of criminosis—as are all other criminotics. What distinguishes him from criminotics of other types is an inflated specific mechanism to restore his narcissism—the proof that he can be loved. After achieving that proof, he has no use for it and throws it away out of pseudo-aggression. Since the inner conflict continues, he must prove to himself once more that he can be loved—and so the vicious circle continues ad infinitum. The interruptions of his career by jail are unconsciously self-provoked and self-intended. Whereas the habitual criminal works with intimidation and murderous weapons, the impostor—"the laughing and charming criminal"—works with irony and hurting feelings. Impostors use a specific device of "self-cure": restoration of their narcissism through being loved and admired. That "self-cure" turns out to be only a "self-cure" in—narcissistic degradation.

There is in the impostor a strange contradiction to his psychopathic personality: his charm and amiability, inspiring confidence. Wittels speaks correctly of the "impostor's demoniacal and uncannily successful wish to please." Let's compare that tendency with the typical psychopathic personality, as described, for instance, by Ben Karpman in "The Individual Criminal" (loc. cit.). The psychopath is characterized in it as follows: "Inconsiderate and indifferent to the suffering of others . . . he is prone to use even his own family to further his selfish interests . . . is unscrupulous and dishonest. . . . The desire of the moment is his only goal. His behavior is impulsive and lacking in persistence. He is a chronic borrower and spendthrift . . . often lives by his wits as a professional idler . . . is audacious and shortsighted, whose aim in antisocial behavior is personal gain." In other words, the psychopath is exactly the opposite of a "charming personality." Still, the charming and pleasing personality is the impostor's greatest asset; more, it represents a prerequisite for "success" in his career. Then, we would conclude, he fakes and pretends to *be* the pleasing personality. The fact is that his charm is real because he needs it unconsciously not less than consciously. The impostor unconsciously fights constantly his depression over being unloved or not loved enough or no longer loved [76]—love always pertaining to the pre-oedipal childhood situation. In reality the question seems to be not at all whether or not the child was loved enough. The real problem is *whether the child could "take" the disappointment to his megalomania* of real or alleged lack of love. Expressed differently: The amount of love which he actually received in childhood is not the factor which determines his feeling of oral disappointment. The real cause of his oral fixation is his inability to overcome the disappointment to his megalomania which everyone must experience. This explains the confusing but well-known fact that the psychopath sometimes springs from families in which he was pampered and sometimes from families in which he really did not receive motherly love and tenderness. The impostor, specifically, has been hurt, as have been all neurotics, criminotics, and psychotics, but *uses a specific technique in attempting to overcome his disappointment.* He denies that he was not loved or was "not worth loving" (Abraham) by creating, *first,* situations in which everyone loves and trusts him. This defense accounts for his charm and ability to inspire confidence. *Second,* he cheats exactly the people who were charmed by him. *Third,* he seeks punishment unconsciously (jail). The question arises as to the unconscious significance of that triad. More specifically, why does the impostor not take advantage of the trust he inspires? The second part of the triad—the cheating of those who trust him—is the most amazing element. It has been suggested, especially by Abraham, that his feeling of guilt prevents his making of permanent value the confidence he wins. I doubt this, and believe that another factor is involved. What the impostor really wants is not love at all; *he wants proof that he can*

[76] Interestingly enough, Karpman states: "Criminality may sometimes arise through sheer loss of sympathetic emotions where the individual has previously been conditioned on such" (*loc. cit.,* p. 192, Case IV).

inspire love and confidence, to restore his narcissism. After having given himself that proof, he throws it away and starts again somewhere else his unconscious game. One of the reasons for that behavior is also the constant inner necessity of using *pseudo-aggression* to ward off the superego reproach of masochistic pleasure. The feeling of guilt is taken care of by his unconscious seeking of punishment, which society metes out to him with regularity.[77]

Why does the impostor cheat people of money precisely? Why not of women, power, influence, or other valuables? The reason is over-determined:

1. Unconsciously, he continues irony on a childlike level: "You don't love me; you love only money." As countermove, he takes away exactly that commodity.

2. Cheating people of money is the surest way to make of them irreconcilable enemies. Even the psychic masochist, who unconsciously wants to be mistreated, when cheated of money uses pseudo-aggression as a defense and clamors for the sheriff. The impostor takes a sure bet on a jail ticket when he uses precisely money as the tool for his tricks.

3. The moral odium of cheating others of money is greater than that of any other offense on a similar level. People forgive almost everything but being cheated of money. Consequently, the "negative moral odium" is a part of the masochistically-aggravating technique of self-damagement.

Impostors seem so inaccessible even to psychologic understanding that a round-about approach to this understanding has been tried—through their tendency to pseudologia fantastica. This approach is, in my opinion, fallacious. I do not believe that impostors simply live out, in a distorted way, their unconscious fantasies of grandeur, but are trying to produce the defense mechanism, "self-cure in narcissism", mentioned above. Using that approach, we could imagine, for instance, that Abraham's patient acted the role of an officer because to be an officer was one of his unconscious wishes, symbolically disguised. However, there is also the possibility that he pretended to be an officer

[77] It is noteworthy that the law is very specific concerning the field covered by impostors. Foxe states: "It is interesting to note that, whereas the penal law is very brief and succinct in its definition of crimes that come under criminosis in action, it is quite detailed with respect to crimes that come under criminosis in reaction and unusually detailed with respect to border violations of legitimate business transactions."

in particular only because in wartime an officer enjoys the most influence and because he had access to officers' identification papers. In other words, it is perfectly possible that the "self-cure" comes first, the paraphernalia used for that purpose being more or less opportunistic. A patient of mine collected money for advertisements, posing as the representative of a Zionist organ of Palestine. The idea occurred to him when a friend who was employed in an advertising concern mentioned to him the relative ease of procuring ads. As it happened, his friend was collecting ads for a liberal newspaper. The patient's family was ardently Zionistic; his ironic twist is obvious in his choice of Zionists as prey; it accounts for his selection of a Zionist paper. At the same time, the Zionist paper in Palestine was far away and exposure of his pose therefore difficult. Thus, conscious self-protection was involved, too, in his choice. In some cases specific determining factors can be found for the *specific* choice; in other cases the *opportunistic* and accidental factors are more predominant.

Freud stated long ago [78] that many an hysteric lie starts from repressed memories of infantile traumas. H. Deutsch corroborated this assumption,[79] expressing the opinion that the content of pseudologia refers to cover memories for true facts. She believes that in pseudologia a distorted eruption of repressed memories can be discerned. Fenichel [79a] assumed that, not only does such an eruption take place, but these fantasies have the purpose of continuing repression by pretending that the fantasies are real, despite the knowledge that they are not. According to Fenichel, these lies are built upon the formula: "If it is possible to make someone believe that untrue things are true, then it is also possible that true things, the memory of which threatens me, are untrue."

Genital sex plays a relatively unimportant role in the make-up of impostors. This fact has been repeatedly observed and described by various authors. Why is this so? First, because the impostor's sex life is immature, full of inner pseudo-aggression, pre-genital. Consequently, it never reaches the genital level. Second, because it is subordinated to the one and only driving force of these people—their

[78] Kl. Schr. z. Neurosenlehre, 2 Af., Bd. 1, p. 113, footnote.

[79] "Uber die pathologische Lüge," Int. Z. f. Psychoan., VIII, 1922.

[79a] "Zur Oekonomie der Pseudologia phantastica". Int. Zeitschrift f. Psychoan. XXIV, 1939.

narcissistic reparation, "I can be loved." Third, because it is subordinated to that narcissistic reparation also insofar as it is "scheming", to use a patient's word. It is used as a weapon for neurotic cheating ideas. For details, consult the original publication.

The impostor is a typical victim of the "mechanism of criminosis" with one specific distinguishing characteristic: the attempt to restore in his defense mechanism a lesion of his narcissism. Everything else is subordinated to the goal of providing in defense to himself that he can make people love him. The real, dynamically-effective masochistic wish is repressed. The moment he has achieved this "proof," the love itself becomes unimportant and the chase for narcissistic reparation, interrupted by jail sentences, starts anew.

Wittels sums up very precisely the psychoanalytic opinions concerning the thereapy of impostors: "We are not as yet very efficient in the treatment and 'cure' of the criminal psychopath. Regular psychoanalysis can be of some help, but rarely, because the transference necessary in this work is unreliable and desultory with these patients."

In addition to the difficulty of achieving a workable transference, other factors complicate the problem of therapy of impostors. First, these men never enter analysis of their own volition. Second, if they come at all, they do so under pressure of their desperate and well-to-do family, who pays and pays (for instance, for forged checks, debts illegally contracted, etc.) to keep the criminotic out of trouble and who tries analysis as a last resort. Third, every analysis "made to order" (Freud) has a bad prognosis to start with. It is, of course, theoretically possible to mobilize the latent and "misplaced" unconscious feeling of guilt for therapeutic purposes; practically, however, the chances are very slim, indeed. With stoicism, cynicism, or hypocrisy the criminotic accepts all of the statements concerning threatening jail sentences, social disgrace, family grief, etc., without changing his course. Fourth, it happens, though relatively seldom, that a patient of this type enters treatment because of some other neurotic symptom, for instance, impotence, neurotic headache, hypochondriacal symptoms, etc. Indirectly we are thus given the possibility to analyze his whole personality. However, he brings forth the greatest objections to "dragging in things which are nobody else's business", to quote such a patient. Fifth, the cases we see are never clearcut; in general, they are mixed cases. A combination of impostor features with gambling, alcoholism, drug-addiction, kleptomania, homosexuality are common. The patient singles out one pat symptom and refuses to analyze anything else. Sixth, the general instability of psychopaths results, even among those who enter analysis voluntarily, in their treating the whole procedure as a joke and often running away the moment they understand, even for a short time, the seriousness of their situation. "I understood yesterday for the first time what you really are after," said a kleptomaniac patient. "You want to make a good citizen of me. There is no fun in that for me. Goodby!"

After having had repeatedly the same experience as many of my colleagues that it is nearly impossible to mobilize the guilt feelings of impostors through the channels of transference, I no longer try to mobilize these feelings in the *beginning* of analysis. I now start immediately to point out how *ridiculous* their constant attempt to restore their narcissism is as it manifests itself in their specific defense mechanism, "I can achieve love," covering their deep masochistic attachment. The result is that it is possible to keep these patients in analysis at least for some time. Furious and ironic objections at once begin; these patients are vulnerable in one point only—fear of appearing ridiculous. *There* their narcissism comes into play, and whereas previously *all* of my analyses of impostors ended more or less without any success, in general being terminated by the patient's refusal to continue treatment, now my experience is more favorable. In a series of cases patients have been helped, a few even to a degree which one could, euphemistically, call something like a cure. There is, however, in general no reason at all to be over-optimistic about the results of treatment of impostors; quite the contrary. Still, I believe that the mechanism described above gives us, not only some clues to the understanding of the impostor's unconscious, but also the beginning of a therapy of his queer disease.

17. Kleptomania

Kleptomania denotes stealing not for the stolen object's sake but for the sake of an "emotional" reward exclusive of the benefit of the loot. If an unemployed person steals bread, the law calls it stealing; if a lady of means steals an article which she could well afford to buy, the emotional and compulsive act is called a "kleptomanic" manifestation. The result has been the popular assumption that kleptomania is the well-to-do's excuse for his stealing.

The confusion results from bringing in social and economic values into a purely psychiatric problem. The differentiation between "simple" stealing and "kleptomanic" stealing rests on a rational consideration: the advantage derived from the act of stealing. What blinds "rational" people, is their fantasy that a seemingly rational act has exclusively rational reasons. We know that this is not so, and that many "rational" crimes have a purely emotional basis.

In cases of kleptomania, the unconscious reason sought for has been the symbolic connotation of the stolen object. Phallic symbolism predominated, and every kleptomanic woman became suspect of stealing a symbolic penis. Since every woman has in her make-up also phallic castration resentment, the proof could be easily adduced. The trouble is, that the motoric act was not explained—that troubled the explainers very little. But another difficulty troubled them even less; the kleptomanic man; here the excuse was that there are more kleptomanic women than men.

Later, the oral genesis was understood by some authors; but here the trouble consisted of an erroneous explanation of what orality meant—the term being used as denoting an aggressive taking away.

As in every criminal action, one has to distinguish between the *psychologic contents* and the *motoric* act. Gratuitously overlooking the latter one falls into hopeless contradictions. Why an "overt" act instead of a neurotic symptom? More about it under "criminosis" (see Section 27).

In my opinion, kleptomania belongs with the criminoses. The motivations of the *psychologic* aspect of it are *not* directly related to the wish to "get," but with the typical defense against the masochistic wish to be "refused." As inner defense, the getting desire is acted out.

18. Coprophemia

Coprophemia denotes a perversion consisting of "the pleasure of embarrassing moralistic people with obscene words."

The problem of obscenity is, as usual, complicated and has been repeatedly analytically attacked (Freud, Ferenczi, Jones, Reik, etc.). In continuation of these papers, I wrote my study on "Obscene Words" [80] and came to these conclusions:

The papers on obscene words so far published date from the early days of psychoanalysis (Freud, 1905; Ferenczi, 1911). This makes it plain that four problems have not been given consideration: 1. Information is lacking regarding the conditions under which the ego condones obscene words. 2. One fails to find any reference to the mitigating of the sense of guilt to which the employment of such words gives rise. 3. Emphasis was placed too much on the anal, and too little on the oral. 4. Obscene words were treated solely from the standpoint of the man uttering them, while nothing was said with regard to the passive desire to hear obscene words on the part of both men and women.

On the basis of a number of case histories of orally fixated or regressed patients, I showed that in the oral stage the giving forth of words on the part of the child corresponds originally to a proof of love towards the mother, much as the stool represents a gift in the anal phase (Freud). Secondarily there may be observed a complete interruption of this giving forth in consequence of alleged disappointment with the mother—"oral obstipation." All these individuals go through a period of obstinate silence during their childhood, and only as a tertiary development is the giving forth reëstablished at a phallic level with negative manifestations, possessing now, however, in the form of obscene words the meaning of abuse and disparagement, in form of pseudo-aggression. Nevertheless, in this *active* uttering of obscene words the old-time pleasure is again smuggled in. These words represent a reproach addressed to the mother: "See what you have made of me."

In orally fixated or regressed men who want passively to hear obscenity spoken by women, these words are built into the total pathological attitude which results from the subject's being shipwrecked, so to speak, on the "mammary complex." They belong in the symptom complex of allegedly wishing only passively to receive. What is really involved is an ironic innuendo: "See, what I can get from Mother, only dirt!" At the same time pseudo-aggression is displayed—Mother is forced to use exactly the words which she did forbid in childhood. In this

[80] The Psan. Quart., V. 2, 1936.

way guilt feeling is allayed, since the woman is made responsible for the sexual transaction and at the same time vengeance is exacted, since the mother image who originally forbade these words is now forced to utter them.

These words derive a pleasure-giving quality also from the economy of inhibition and suppression described by Freud in connection with wit. If in orally fixated or regressed individuals obscene words are important only in relation to the *mother*, in compulsion neurotics there occurs a secondary displacement upon the loved and hated *father* in the form of blasphemies. Normally, however, obscene words play a variable rôle among healthy people too, as an act of forepleasure, so much so that often the uttering of these words on the part of the man is expected by the woman as part of her sexual subjection.

On the clinical side, individual cases, together with the frequently noted combination of masochistic-passive and voyeuristic tendencies, are demonstrated, and referred to the living out of infantile megalomania in coprophemia. Finally, the very variable means of disposition of the guilt feeling resulting from the utterance of these words (that is, the fantasies concealed behind them) are reviewed, and as a common example of this, that of the cynic is emphasized. The cynic makes use of the so-called "cynical mechanism" which is itself a means of mitigating the sense of guilt.[81]

I here present a clinical example:

A kleptomaniac of twenty-six entered analysis because of his uncle's insistence. The uncle, incidentally, also paid the initial fees. The young man regarded his stealing rather as a practical joke and was "tickled to death that that old hypocrite of an uncle was socially embarrassed." It was revealed very shortly that the patient was a check forger, a pathologic gambler, suffered from a potency disturbance and a specific type of perversion called "coprophemia." The latter manifested itself in his picking out well-dressed women on the street and whispering obscene words to them.

"It is really superb," mused the patient, "how I am able to embarrass such a high-class lady with one well-chosen word or short epigrammatic sentence. These women either blush, pretend not to hear, or are silently furious. It is enough for me to see their faces redden in

[81] See sec. 8 "Pseudo-bluffers and Hucksters."

embarrassment or fury. *I feel like an omnipotent sorcerer with inexhaustible power.*"

Asked whether any of his victims ever denounced him to a police officer, he laughed and said that only a very few out of "hundreds of these women" ever threatened to do so and even they were too embarrassed to go any farther. Once a "bitch" had denonuced him, but his uncle's lawyer was able to convince the investigating officers that the lady must have misunderstood "something." In any case, no prosecution followed.

The patient presented superficially the picture of a constantly amused psychopath. He ridiculed accepted moral standards, claimed that "bourgeois values" were good only for "idiots," and considered himself a "superior person." He quoted Napoleon: "The usual moral laws do not apply to me."

I asked him whether he was aware of the risk he was running with his check forging, kleptomania and coprophemia. He shrugged his shoulders and replied: "Until now, nothing has happened. For his own protection, my uncle covers me up." Pressed further, he said: "One has to take chances. Take for example my gambling. . . ." This was the way his gambling was brought into the discussion, tangentially and accidentally. The patient did not consider his gambling a pathologic phenomenon and was rather amused that I was of a different opinion. He used gambling as a "moral alibi." His argument was: gambling, compared to kleptomania, is a socially acceptable way of getting money. What's wrong with that? If, as I claimed, both his gambling and coprohemia were based on the fantasy of childlike omnipotence, masochistically colored, why not tolerate gambling which society tolerates?

The next day he reversed the argument: "Isn't gambling 'morally' inferior to coprophemia since the former is more 'materialistic'?" Thus, shifting his argument illogically, he proved one day that gambling was "moral" and the next day that coprophemia was "moral." The common denominator was the old trick of reducing bourgeois standards to absurdity.

The patient was the only and posthumous child of a short-lived marriage; the father drowned before the child was born. His mother was an obstinate, illiterate, aggressive and "half-wild" person. She owned a canteen near an army camp and promiscuously changed lovers every few weeks. The child was frequently present during intercourse. One scene he remembered especially clearly during analysis: an "enormous" soldier forced the mother to have intercourse by squeezing her breast until she nearly fainted from pain. That incident was repressed and came to consciousness in connection with the analysis of a queer habit the patient had developed during puberty: he believed that squeezing girls' buttocks was the surest technique for seducing them. It became apparent that this "squeezing technique" represented the precursor of his coprophemia. The reason was twofold. The progress of his neurosis necessitated stronger repression (in squeezing he repeated the soldier's technique but shifted from the forbidden breast to the more harmless buttocks); and, at the same time, coprophemia represented a megalomaniacal "improvement." The soldier had to resort to an action, but he could get the same results with a word. This explains the previously quoted boast: "It is really superb how I can embarass a lady [82] with *one single word* . . . I feel like an *omnipotent* sorcerer. . . ."

The next step was the shift from coprophemia to kleptomania. The patient began stealing electric light bulbs, which he stole for no apparent practical purpose. He did not sell them but destroyed them in the lavatory. Later, when he began to steal other things, he sold his loot and lost the money gambling. A series of dreams proved that, in the symbolism of the patient's unconscious vocabulary, the bulbs represented breasts.

We see that the patient went through a series of pseudo-aggressive acts aimed against the consciously hated mother: the "squeezing-technique"—projected later upon women in general—coprophemia, and kleptomania. When his mother reproached him, he stated that all his actions were for the purpose of "taking revenge on her." This conscious hatred was then shifted to the family; he embarrassed his uncle socially by stealing and forging the latter's signature.

[82] Once more: unconscious ironization of bourgeois values. Since he did not consider his mother a "lady," he even debased those on a higher social level. Considering his mother a "low grade type," he demonstrated his superiority and megalomania by "seducing" upper-class women. The neurosis manifested itself in exhibitionism and peeping-Tom activities, too.

This pseudo-aggression was only a cover, however, for psychic masochism. The erotic and "sadistic" elements served as a defense against the more deeply embedded masochistic tendency. This became clear the moment this question was put to the patient: "Don't you see that you are damaging yourself more seriously than your mother and uncle?"

One could argue that all these self-damaging acts were only belated revenge-aggressions, carried out under self-damaging conditions because of inner guilt. But this was not true, as proved by the fact that he sought, at least later, these self-damaging conditions because they satisfied his desire for psychic masochistic pleasure. The perfect proof of this was his attitude toward gambling. He stated very precisely that during gambling he experienced a thrill "not comparable to any other sensation known to me. Only once, when a lady whom I'd insulted with an obscene word called the police, did I experience anything similar to that thrill. Why, an orgasm in sex is nothing compared to it. After all, sex is not forbidden. . . ."

DEFENSIVE USE OF THE ORAL ZONE

19. Logorrhea

Logorrhea is a phenomenon encountered on all levels of the libidinous-aggressive development. I have published an investigation,[83] subdividing the symptom according to oral, anal, and phallic manifestations. I am reproducing here only conclusions of the oral sections of the study.

One of the most typical complaints of husbands against neurotic wives—and vice versa—is: "She (He) talks too much." The first impression is that the quantity of words itself is the objectionable feature to these martyrs of abnormal talkativeness, chatter, garrulity and loquacity. A more careful observation shows, however, that they refer to the combination of the following three components:

1. Incessant talking.

2. Inconsistent talking, without regard to transition of even a second's pause or to visible connection.

3. Preponderance of unimportant details chosen aggressively, without perception of the problem as a whole.

[83] "Logorrhoea." The Psychiatric Quarterly *18*:26–42, 1944.

Occasionally it is possible to observe such neurotic[84] logorrhoeic patients of both sexes (there are no fewer among men than among women) afflicted with that triad of signs. What are the unconscious mechanisms used by persons of this type, and why are they used?

Logorrhoea must be distinguished from the usual urge to communicate with others found in the so-called cultural human being. That urge sometimes gives the impression of garrulity. Of course, the distinction must be made by a typical human being and not by one of the "silent" variety of neurotics. The following anecdote about the Swiss poet, Gottfried Keller,[85] illustrates why. Keller used to drink in the evening in the company of friends without speaking a word. One evening one of his friends introduced his grown son. After hours of drinking in silence, Keller dropped his handkerchief. Picking it up, the intimidated young man said: "Here, Mr. Keller." Those were the only words the young man spoke during the many hours. On the way home Keller's friend asked the poet his impression of his son. Keller replied, "A nice young man, but he talks too much."

The usual urge to communicate gives at first the impression that many persons have the tendency to speak solely for the purpose of speaking. Listening more closely, one finds that specific tendencies appear behind the urge. For instance, some persons create small, transitory "garrulity societies"—which disintegrate quickly—and which have the purpose of ranting against a specific group, institution or person. Hatred binds many individuals closer than love. As a subgroup of this type of activity, one might mention "teasing," that superficial, pseudo-witty form of making fun at the expense of someone else.

On the other hand, there seem to be "garrulity centers" whose sole purpose is the friendly exchange of "ideas." These are built upon the narcissistic basis: "I'll let you play the rôle of the 'big shot' on condition that you do the same for me." That reciprocal giving of "medals of genius," based on the idea of acceptance in order to be accepted, is clearly narcissistic. "We give each other the clues so well—one calls that friendship," says one of Arthur Schnitzlers *dramatis personae.* "Mutual admiration societies" is a generally accepted term for these

[84] The writer deals in this section exclusively with neurotic, not with psychotic, logorrhoea.

[85] See Hitschmann's well-known paper on Keller, Imago, 1915.

groups. It is known, of course, that other elements beside narcissism are involved in such gatherings; for instance, unconscious homosexuality, unconscious defense against passive wishes, etc.

Other garrulity societies are based on mutual self-pity. Hypochondriacal chatter of old women of both sexes is found in these groups.

Generally speaking, chronic gossipers in society impress one as being inwardly still children, who would enjoy gossiping perpetually—in the absence of a severe educator.[86] In addition to his garrulity, another element in the behavior of the logorrhoeic person seems to indicate the transgression of a prohibition—the divulging of secrets in the course of gossiping. Knowledge of human nature in general confirms the old aphorism: "Don't let your *friends* know what could be of help to your *enemies*." In typical gatherings of gossipers, many facts are divulged which, after dissolution of the transitory groups, would be recalled if it were possible. The gossiper, therefore, must feel some unconscious tendency toward self-punishment as direct consequence of his transgressed prohibition.

Also indicative of feeling of guilt is another characteristic of the logorrhoeic—his stubborn refusal to acknowledge that he makes himself a laughing-stock with his incessant garrulity. Often he has the reputation of being "simply dumb." This assumption is incorrect, although it cannot be denied that coexistence of both tendencies—logorrhoea and low I.Q.—is possible. The underlying explanation of logorrhoea is more complex than that often given—stupidity.[87] The outer world's ironic

[86] Talking seems to the child one of the prerogatives of adults. This misleading impression is enforced upon him, since the persons in authority are honored with silence and spoken to only at their request. That other elements enter the picture is clear; for instance, child-like ideas of omnipotence, words being used "magically," or as symbolic representation in those cases where words are substituted for phallic exhibitionism.

[87] How mistaken it is to apply the term "stupid" schematically to logorrhoeic persons is shown in the following instance: Some individuals are very fond of the expression, "If you know what I mean." Such an introduction would seem to be preparatory to a deep revelation. However, experience proves that the famous phrase is instead always associated with a banality. That pompous cloaking of a banality conveys at first glance the impression of stupidity and a futile attempt to appear important. In reality, its use is an insult to the intelligence of the listener and serves the unconscious purpose of aggression.

reaction toward, and rejection of, the logorrhoeic is, so to speak, part of his unconsciously calculated and sought punishment for his prohibited deed. The situation is similar to that which the author previously has described elsewhere as being operative in plagiarism. The plagiarist steals often so cynically, stupidly and seemingly without regard for consequences because he expects unconsciously to be discovered.[88]

The logorrhoeic person is blind also in another respect. Not only does he not see that he is ridiculous, but he is insensitive to the fact that he irritates his environment. That scotomy and oversight is reducible to the aggressive core of gossiping.

We see that the logorrhoeic is seemingly full of a queer optimism; [89] exactly the opposite can be observed in the mistrustful hyper-silent person. To quote the joke of a patient, when two sympathetic logorrhoeics meet, the cubic contents of each merge and are doubled. The logorrhoeic is, so to speak, the last optimist. That he receives in return for his optimism a "kick in the pants" is a result included unconsciously as an integral part of his life plan.

It is analytically known that the urge to communicate can serve other neurotic tendencies as well—such as the urge to confess (Reik), an unconscious invitation to participate in joint sexual pleasure, as described by D. Burlingham. The often-encountered opinion that gossiping is simply a display of exhibitionism is, however, in the writer's opinion erroneous; the explanation is far more complicated. Also erroneous is the view that the problem of logorrhoea can be dismissed simply by pointing out the phallic significance of the tongue, whether or not in conjunction with exhibitionism.

It is difficult either to prove or to disprove that language was originally a means of expressing human needs, a theory often advanced. In any case, the present use of the language is a long way from those nebulous beginnings. Consider, for instance, the cynical statement of Talleyrand, that words have the purpose of disguising, not expressing, thoughts. On the other hand, let us not forget that words are the chief weapon of malice and aggression in cultural societies after direct killing

88 "Das Plagiat" ("Plagiarism"), Psychoan. Bewegung, 1932.

89 One form of garrulity is not discussed here—that of couples in love. See "Transference and Love," by L. Jekels and the author, Imago, 1934.

has been renounced. The formula "intolerant, malicious and gossipy" is applicable to many communities all over the globe.

Furthermore, logorrhoea must be distinguished from the *conscious* use of hyper-talkativeness; for instance, to confuse the enemy by unclear and ambiguous words, to throw him off the track. In this case, garrulity is simply a weapon from the arsenal of "war of nerves." Another example is the old formula, "The best way to say nothing is to talk a great deal," a trick used in politics. That conscious trick is based on the wish to please everyone and to avoid losing votes.

To psychoanalysts, logorrhoea has a special interest because analysts —unjustly, to be sure—are accused by nearly every patient of creating a sort of "artificial logorrhoea" in asking him to use "free associations" during his analytic appointment. The more silent and reticent patients, especially, fight this basic analytic rule, objecting to being transformed into "talkative old women." The real reasons for the resistance to using free association are, of course completely different. The interesting fact remains that, in analysis, the therapist is torn by the patient's behavior between the Scylla of loquacity, which he mistakenly offers as "free association" when, in reality, it is simply his usual garrulity used as resistance, and the Charybdis of silence, which is a form of resistance not too simple to overcome.[90]

One of the writer's patients received the following valentine from her husband:

"The rose is red
Viol*ence* is blue.
You talk too much
But—I love you."

The patient was a woman with oral regression, who unconsciously repeated consistently in life the situation of the innocently tantalized child whose mother was refusing her everything. Her behavior was a typical example of the "mechanism of orality." That basically masochistic-pleasure-giving mechanism consists of three parts: unconscious provocation of a refusal, with no conscious knowledge of provoking it; a feeling of being unjustly treated coupled with desire for revenge;

[90] I have described the latter form of resistance in the paper, "On the Resistance Situation: The Patient is Silent." Psychoanalyt. Rev., 1938.

self-pity based on the theme, "Nobody loves me." Of that triad only the feelings of righteous indignation and self-pity are conscious; the provocation and masochistic pleasure are unconscious.

This patient had severe conflicts in her marriage. She treated her husband as a malicious governess would treat a naughty child. On the other hand, the fact that, despite all his protests, her husband enjoyed that kind of behavior unconsciously was proved by his endurance of that marriage for 15 years. The neuroses of the marriage partners were complementary. She treated him aggressively, and he reacted consciously with counter-aggression. First he had the feeling of being unjustly treated; then she enjoyed the same sensation, since, from her point of view, she acted in self-defense against her husband's "malice." Her own initial provocation was repressed. Unconsciously, both marriage partners enjoyed that self-provoked masochistic vicious circle, often changing rôles of being the initial "aggressor." Consciously, of course, her husband was unhappy over her coldness and constant nagging. He expressed this feeling in his pun, "Violence" (for "Violets") "is blue" ("Your violence makes me unhappy.") Had the husband written "I love you because you make me unhappy," he would have expressed his unconscious state of affairs. Consciously, of course, he meant: "I love you despite your making me unhappy."

The husband stressed specifically, "You talk too much." Asked to elaborate upon his statement, he made it evident that he did not allude simply to the quantity of words but rather to their application. His wife possessed the never-failing ability of choosing from a general situation a detail which she could use maliciously. For example: She forced her husband to spend every Sunday with her mother, though she herself hated her. The poor victim had to drive the whole family to the country, miss his rest, swallow his fury, and above all, pretend to be very happy. Driving back once with his wife and mother-in-law in the back seat, he used the brakes too forcefully when stopping for a red light, with the result that both mother-in-law and wife received a disagreeable jolt. Instantly, his wife disparaged his driving ability. At home she continued the attack. Her husband was furious, though incapable of formulating precisely the reason for his fury, simply complaining that she made a great story of a triviality. What he really meant was that, instead of appreciating his sacrifice of the day and his endurance of her mother's company, she scolded him for harmlessly slamming his brakes.[91]

Had the man been capable of formulating what he meant precisely, he would have said, "I mean by the objection, 'You talk too much,' the way in which you maliciously pick out of a situation a detail and magnify it in many offensive words. You are not benevolent. I have a loquacious, malicious, criticizing enemy in my house whose specialty is enlarging harmless details to prove a case against me."

The conclusion so far is: Loquacity contains a pseudo-aggressive element in addition to the superficial urge to communicate. Someone might object here that for many persons garrulity is a pleasure in itself, even without the aggressive element. A more precise analysis shows, however, that the aggressive basis is always present.

What is the genesis of that type of logorrhoea? No satisfactory answer is offered based on the unconscious reasons for talking.[92] If we consider the well-known statement of W. Wundt that animals do not talk because they have nothing to say, we might come to the conclusion that human beings talk because they have important things to relate. But observation would not confirm that viewpoint, especially observation of logorrhoeics. The very few facts concerning talking clinically observed and verified are these: Words are first a gift given via imitation, and later identification, by the child to the mother—even as stool is, in the anal stage, in the child's conception, a gift to the mother (Freud). To verify that fact, one has only to watch a mother praying for every word from her infant. The child denies this gift when he comes to grief with his parent. Analysis of neurotics of the "silent" type proves this fact conclusively.[93] It becomes even more evident in the analysis of the use of obscene words.[94]

The problem is complicated by voyeuristic-exhibitionistic elements: one can be used as defense against the other.[95]

[91] That his overforceful use of the brakes constituted in itself an unconscious aggression against his wife was not conscious to him.

[92] See the unsatisfactory explanation offered in Sperber's theory.

[93] See the writer's paper, "On the Resistance Situation: The Patient Is Silent." *loc. cit.*

[94] See section 18.

[95] See section 6 of this chapter.

Let us apply the assumption that both parts of the scopophiliac instinct can be used in defense against each other to the specific problem of logorrhoea. We see immediately that the simple explanation that the garrulous person exhibits is insufficient. Garrulity is not only exhibition; it transforms the listener into a voyeur through whom the exhibiting, loquacious person can look at himself (self-voyeurism via identification). Furthermore, garrulity extends the invitation to the listener to exchange confidence for confidence, in other words to perform his verbal exhibitionistic act. Therefore, it offers also the opportunity of voyeurism of the other person. The problem becomes clearer if we focus our attention on the element of curiosity. Garrulous persons collect material, discuss and try to decipher endlessly the secrets of others. They are in a sense "Peeping Toms."

20–21. Overeating and Gourmanderie

The child starts his gustatory life with *one* not too spicy food—milk. It winds up as adult as gourmet or at least a lover of a *variety* of food: everyone considers his taste, rightly or wrongly, as exquisite. He smacks (at least mentally) his lips and "enjoys good food," whatever that means.

How and why is that transition accomplished? Besides the obvious role of the taste nerves, a psychologic factor enters the picture: exactly *because* milk was "tasteless" (at least more or less neutral in taste), the overvariety of tasty food is cultivated later. Once more a demotion of what mother had to offer is accomplished. That bit of pseudo-aggression helps the culinary industry, besides making for "delicious cooking."

That this is so, can be best studied in cases in which a neurotic culinary "simplicity" is encountered. To name three neurotic cases:

A wealthy young man had for years been eating only one dish: tuna-fish salad. "It is nourishing and inexpensive," he said. His whole life, however, had also been unconsciously devoted to the proof of the belief "mother starves me."

Another man went through a series of food fadisms only to end up with the following routine: he lived for 3 days on black coffee exclusively ("I'm not hungry") and waited for "real appetite." After three days, he became "really hungry," overate and found that the food "did not agree with me." Then, the same cycle repeated itself. He, too, acted out: "bad mother starves me."

A young girl from a wealthy Western family, living in New York to study violin, received her semi-monthly checks at the 1st and 15th of every month. She spent the money foolishly in the first 2 days, to "starve" for the remaining 26 days of the month, living on cottage cheese and milk. In this simple way, she could prove how "unjust" the family (mother) really was.

The opposite extreme is represented by people with "exquisite" culinary tastes: they prepare their own food (especially pronounced in men who are "good cooks"), thus "proving" that they are "autarchic."

But the masochistic pseudoaggressive refinement does not always go so far; some of these neurotics are simply "overeaters" ("He eats like a pig," complained the wife of such a patient). They counteract preventively the expected starvation allegedly imposed by mother. This appears in small details: they cannot wait till their portion is meted out, they eat from the salad-bowl and the meat-platter.

A special subdivision of that group are vegetarians and food-fadists in general. With some foolish rationalization, they concoct a list of foods to be excluded, mostly meat. They are opposed to the slaughter of animals,—via unconscious identification they are the slaughtered animals. Accused by their inner conscience of overdimensional psychic masochism, they defend themselves with cannibalistic fantasies, secondarily warded off with humanitarian ideas.[96]

Other neurotics restrict their food intake according to hypochondriacal principles—the results are identical: "someone" refuses them their favorite dishes. Whether this "someone" is an organ of their body "practiced by some freak of nature (mother) inside," or the basis for restraint is "ideological" (food fadists), the point is that "bad mother" is denying and not the poor masochist is masochistic. A perfect alibi!

[96] It is quite possible that the respect for the sacred cow in India and the Jewish orthodox precept of division of china for meat and milk-like dishes, has its affective basis in these unconscious ideas. Superficially it means: you have the right to drink milk as long as you dont bite the breast. The problem seems to be one of restricting aggression. At bottom, masochism is found, warded off with that pseudo-aggression.

22. Oversmoking

In a longer study,[97] I have tried to prove the interconnection between oversmoking and neurotic orality. The topic is especially apt for the deduction, because oversmoking is generally regarded as "oral greed" —pure and simple. The question arises: is the symptom a *direct* repetition of baby-greed, or does it go through masochistic channels? I believe the latter.

Limited smoking (10 to 15 cigarettes or four to five cigars a day) is considered in our culture—rightly or wrongly—as normal, and millions of persons live in accordance with this empirical rule.

The problem of smoking becomes clinically important on the following conditions: (1) when the quantity of cigarettes or cigars consumed is exorbitant; (2) when smoking becomes a compulsion; (3) when craving for even limited smoking cannot be fulfilled, because other medical indications ask, "Stop smoking."

The medical problem concerning the harmlessness or danger of nicotine is not fully clarified. The latest investigations even deny that tobacco itself is the dangerous agent, blaming the protein of tobacco as the malefactor.

The pharmacodynamic factor—as is typical for all addictions—is combined with an unconscious psychologic problem. The combination of both—and *only* the combination of both—can clarify the issue. My study is a contribution to the psychologic superstructure without the slightest intention of minimizing the importance of the pharmacodynamic factor. Only a combination of both approaches can solve the problem. It is understood, however, that the psychiatrist can contribute to only one part of the investigation: the psychologic aspect.

Clinical psychiatric-psychoanalytic experience has confronted me with a series of cases in which smoking was quantitatively increased and was, at the same time, a compulsion.

Mr. V., a successful chemical engineer, was from the age of 25 to 40 a compulsive and incessant smoker (40 to 60 cigarettes a day). He acquired a leucoplakia of the tongue and suspected cancer. A famous cancer specialist diagnosed leucoplakia and ordered discontinua-

97 "Psychopathology of Compulsive Smoking." The Psychiatric Quarterly *20*:297–321, 1946.

tion of smoking. Thereupon Mr. V.—"scared to death"—stopped smoking, seemingly without too great difficulty, for five years. Only recently—parallel with a severe psychic conflict starting in the middle 40's—did he take up smoking once more. He described his "craving for a cigarette" as follows: "Every time I am nervous, discontented or jumpy, I light a cigarette. It is like a reflex." Asked whether the cigarette alleviated his "nervousness," he stated: "Temporarily, yes. After a few minutes, however, the same story repeats itself." "What are you jumpy about?" He could not answer that question precisely. He said that his financial success did not make him happy. Being a "born bachelor," he never married and has been having a series of transitory "affairs." His latest girl friend made his life miserable. "How?" "Well, that is difficult to say. She makes me unhappy by being unreliable. Sometimes she provokes my jealousy; sometimes she even makes fun of me." These vague answers were typical of the man.

After a while the following transpired: His present girl friend originally wanted him to marry her, but, seeing the "hopelessness" of the situation, married somebody else without giving up the relation with Mr. V. In other words, she imitated Mr. V.'s behavior, since he, too, played off one woman against another, having at the same time relations with two women and not concealing this fact from "number 2." In the case of Ruth, the latest girl friend, however, the story boomeranged against Mr. V. Every time she promised to call up without doing so, or doing so only after a few days, V. kept brooding over the injustice done to him. "How can she be so mean to me?" During these complaints, he smoked incessantly. Even in analysis, it took a good deal of time to convince him that his relation to Ruth was more complicated than a "simple affair," as he claimed.

It was obvious that the patient misused the whole relationship for the repetition of something irrational and deeply repressed. This could be proved to Mr. V. only after his "logic" was discounted as faulty. He said that all he *wanted* from Ruth was "peace, quite, and a pleasant companion in bed." What he *got* was: constant irritation, self-created jealousy and a severe potency disturbance. On the one hand, Mr. V. asserted that he was glad Ruth had married "a harmless nobody," thus freeing him of her marital demands; on the other hand, every remark of Ruth to the effect that the marriage "though banal seemed to work out along conventional lines" infuriated and depressed him. Asked how he could be jealous when he was not interested in Ruth, he replied, "Everybody wants to be loved." This rationalization satisfied him, even to the extent that he discarded his potency disturbance with Ruth. "I just want to show her that I am better than her husband," was his irrational conclusion. To the question of how he could win this *a priori* senseless sexual competition since he had a potency disturbance, he answered, "That's exactly the trouble." When asked for an explanation as to why he needed two girl friends, since he had potency troubles especially with Ruth, Mr. V. replied evasively. Cornered, forced to realize that his story, "that all he wanted from Ruth was 'a convenient companion in bed,'" was bunk, Mr. V. admitted: "If I behaved rationally I wouldn't have consulted you."

What was Mr. V. really acting out under the pressure of *unconscious* forces? He was a specific—orally regressed—neurotic. Such people act —without knowing it—the triad of the mechanism of orality. What he unconsciously *really* wanted from Ruth—in repetition of his childhood-conflict—was not love, companionship, a quiet life, and what not, but one thing only: disappointment and *refusal,* to be enjoyed masochistically. The deepest *psychic-masochistic* wish was: I want to be disappointed. He himself was the engineer of his defeats: knowing that Ruth was "unreliable," he still asked her constantly to call up at specific times. She never did; it was a sure bet that a call promised for Monday, 3 P.M., would come through, if at all, not before Wednesday evening. The interim between Monday afternoon and Wednesday evening, Mr. V. spent in "depression and fury." The "depression" was the covering cloak for his psychic masochism, self-provoked, to be sure (Layer 1). The "fury" corresponded to a pseudo-aggressive defense mechanism—the alibi presented to his inner conscience, denying his *inner* masochistic enjoyment (Layer 2). The end effect was conscious self-pity—"This can happen only to me"—without understanding though, that this self-pity was once more masochistically enjoyed (Layer 3).

Layer 2 (pseudo-aggression) was responsible for two other peculiarities in the case of Mr. V.: playing off one girl against the other and his potency disturbance. In both he was seemingly aggressive against the two girls (refusal of love and sexual pleasure). In a roundabout way the psychic masochism enters the picture, since the troubles he had in having two relations and the humiliation of being "unmanly" were more than consciously disagreeable, which means in this neurotic mechanism, unconsciously pleasurable.

Where does compulsive smoking come in here? It is a part of Layer 2: an alibi presented to his inner conscience. His "hell within," as Milton prophetically called the inner part of conscience, constantly objected to the psychic masochism, the basis of the whole neurotic mechanism described. As an inner defense and alibi—to disprove the accusation that he wanted to be *refused*—Mr. V. substituted the wish to *get*. Therefore, he reached for a cigarette!

Let us not forget that getting something orally is the first great libidinous experience in life: breast, milk-bottle, pacifier, food. The smoker reassures himself by getting something into his mouth, too. Therefore, smoking "helps" against "nervousness," which, with popular connotations, means situations of refusal or uncertainty. The *compulsive* smoker tries the same technique but achieves it only by the circuitous way of an inner defense mechanism.

This psychologic basis of smoking does not disprove the well-known fact that nicotine may be the basis of an addiction. The psychic *super*structure is present in addictions, too, without contradicting the pharmacodynamic *sub*structure. Substructure and superstructure are interrelated.

Mr. W. was a pathologic gambler.[98] He was a man of 30 whom his friends called a "gambler by profession and lawyer by hobby." Which meant that he lost the money he earned in his learned profession by playing poker. Mr. W., who smoked 15 to 20 Havana cigars during three to four hours of gambling every night, came into analytic treatment neither because of gambling nor smoking. He fell into the hands of a lady who tried to rescue him from his "vices" through marriage, only to discover that the object of her savior-fantasy was completely impotent. "Pushed" by his wife, he ungraciously consented to psychiatric treatment.

We are interested here in one aspect of Mr. W.'s personality only, his pathologic smoking. He describes it as follows: "Every time I

[98] See section 15 of this chapter.

guess wrong, am out-bluffed or lose, I light up a cigar. It helps for a moment." He suffered a few times from serious nicotine "poisoning," had heart troubles; nothing, however, changed his habit.

Asked whether he also felt the impulse to light a cigar when he outsmarted the other gamblers, he replied: "Definitely not. Smoking means I lost. When I have a winning period, I smoke two cigars. At the beginning of the evening, before it is clear whether I shall win or lose, and at the end—I call it my cigar of triumph." In other words, when winning, Mr. W. smoked during the same time (three to four hours) two; when losing, 15 to 20, cigars.

Mr. W.'s unconscious reasons were very similar to those of Mr. V. Both tried—when disappointed—to prove to their "inner district attorney" (inner conscience, superego) that they wanted to *get* and not to be *refused.* In both cases compulsive smoking was a defense mechanism against a reproach of the unconscious part of the conscience.

Summarizing we can state: In all these cases, a similar neurotic substructure was found: These patients represented a specific type of psychic masochists who *unconsciously* wanted constantly to be *refused.* To counteract the inner reproach stemming from their inner consciences, which objected to the wish to be refused, they "proved" that they wanted the opposite—to get. The outward sign was getting a cigarette, an oral "pacifier," symbolically reminding the individual of his first reassurance in life.

All these patients were unconsciously "injustice-collectors," therefore exquisite enjoyers of self-constructed defeats.

The psychologic superstructure does not conflict with the pharmacodynamics of tobacco or tobacco-proteins. Only the combination of both explains the addiction.

Sometimes, oversmoking is combined with overeating and overdrinking—that tripartite "oral" syndrome points in the direction of an attempt at refutation of an inner reproach, "You want to be refused," with the secondary defense, "I want to get."

The person addicted to tobacco behaves in a specific way when forced by medical necessities to restrict or give up smoking completely. He acts like a child to whom mother refuses oral gratification. He immediately feels unjustly treated and reacts with pseudo-aggression—perhaps toward his wife, and later the environment in general.

Pathologic smoking presents a problem which can be solved—the pathologic smoker can be cured psychoanalytically.

23–24. Fellatio and Cunnilinguus

Freud characterized the difference between a sexual perversion and a sexual preparatory act thus: if the action leads to coitus—it is a preparatory act; if the identical act is a sexual end in itself—it is a perversion. One could add, that these preparatory acts must be of a nature which do not endanger the bodily integrity of the partner. Among many such acts are *fellatio* and *cunnilinguus.* It had been early analytically understood that *fellatio* represents a distorted suckling situation dating back to early infancy. It remained, however, unclarified as to why man should reverse the roles: suckling mother—sucking baby.

Here, one of the deductions from the "breast complex" clarified the issue. If it is true that the male achieves his psychic maturity by typically and unconsciously reversing the roles of *giving* mother-*receiving* baby, then there was nothing to marvel about that remnants of this attitude should show up also in the rather universal, though frequently shamefully suppressed, wish for fellatio. Closer analysis proved that additional factors enter the picture.

First, a pseudo-aggressive disparaging attitude of the fellationist toward women. He acts as if he would debase the woman. This *defensive* pseudo-aggression hints at deeper repressed psychic masochism.

Second, analysis of men "despising" fellatio, proved that they are frantically frightened of being bitten at the penis. True, the projection of the baby's own biting wishes onto the suckling woman could also be found. But *not* so simply and directly; these fantasies had later gone through masochistic channels.

Third, the emotional coldness of fellationists, pointed in the direction of warded off fears. One of these sick people gave this strange explanation for his predilection: "Fellatio is the only form of sex where one can—without technical disturbance—read one's newspaper in peace . . ." Superfluous to state, that that man was inwardly scared of the female sex, and impotent to boot.

Fourth, some (even a good-sized percentage) of fellationists derive their excitement from a half-conscious masochistic expectation of fears of being bitten. Hence, under the pseudo-aggressive palimpsest thinly veiled masochistic perverted wishes are hidden.

Fifth, the idea of "being sucked out" is frequently encountered, pointing to the identification: penis-breast. The fellationist acts unconsciously the "masochistically drained" mother.[99]

Cunnilinguus, on the other hand, is even more grotesquely connected with the baby situation. The grotesque admixture pertains to suckling at a non-existent organ in the genital region—the supposed penis (breast) of the woman. Here the suckling baby situation is quite clear and shows the predominance of unconscious fantasies in sex.

Cunnilinguus denotes, however, more. It is also the proof of being disappointed: no breast, no life-giving milk—nothing but a frightening "wound!" To prove his feeling of being refused, the man performing cunnilinguus, "humiliates" himself. At the same time, inner fears are alleviated: the "dangerous" organ (breast, penis) is missing!

25. Inability to Reduce

Every reducing cure, whether recommended by physicians because of esthetic or cardiac reasons, puts the patient's "willpower" to a severe test. With great regularity the candidate for reducing finds that he must abstain exactly from the type of food he likes best. He is constantly tempted by the "forbidden" food and thus fights a never-ending battle.

In studying patients who are losing the battle "on the reducing front" as a witty patient expressed it, one can observe that these people do not consider abstinence from specific food as a rational measure during reducing but as a deep "injustice." They act in a superficial description like children to whom candy is forbidden or denied. Unconsciously they concoct an infantile neurotic situation of denial and react with fury or trespass the prescribed dietetic rules.

[99] If one turns the tables and asks for the reaction of women performing fellatio from predilection, one finds a variety of reasons: pleasure of doing the "morally objectionable" ("Angstlust"), reassurance of not being "castrated" in unconscious identification with the breast (penis). At bottom, once more the masochistic *wish to be refused* is found: "mother" gives but—"poison." Hence the disgust for sperm. Only in exceptional hyper-masochistic cases the sperm is swallowed, frequently with ideas of impregnation or some other "damage."

A woman of 38, stated in analytic treatment, that she never could muster enough "willpower" to carry-on a reducing cure. "I have a marked tendency towards obesity and must reduce. I tried at least twenty times—always in vain. I first get depressed, then furious and the end result is that after a few days I eat more than before. I seem to be incapable of carrying out my decision though I am rather concerned with my appearance."

Another woman of 26, observed that when reducing, she became deeply depressed. "I avoid reducing, since at such times life seems void of pleasure and I am really a candidate for a suicide. Not only is everything colorless but I start thinking about all my defeats in life, all the lost possibilities. The only way out is—eating."

A man of 46, complained that diet makes him "cranky, ill-tempered and hopeless. That stupid food does something to one's self-respect. At such times I smoke constantly, am jumpy and, to improve my situation, go back to normal eating. My doctor recommended thyroid preparations, I really lost a few pounds but became very depressed though I could eat properly. I had to give up my attempts at reducing."

A young man of 24 made repeatedly "hopeless attempts" to reduce. He succeeded only once for a few weeks under extraordinary circumstances. His wife was in treatment because of vaginism and came so far that she became interested in normal sexual relations. The husband, notified of the initial success of her treatment, made first excuses (he was too "tired"), declared afterwards that he wanted to take a "second honeymoon" with his wife. He really took the trip, without touching her. Confronted with the statement that he was impotent, he denied that, stating that he was undertaking a reducing cure and could not do "acrobatic stunts when living on grapes and oranges."

It became clear in his subsequent analysis that his inner battle against "starvation," as he called his diet during reducing, was undertaken only because he wanted to avoid a greater "danger"—acknowledgement of his impotence. In reducing, he unconsciously acted out the fantasy "Bad mother starves me."

In all these, and a long series of other cases, I observed that orally regressed neurotics are incapable of reducing exactly because they are still unconsciously confusing the *rational* and consciously approved act of reducing with the *irrational* equation: lack of food = starvation imposed by the cruel, pre-oedipal mother. Eating has for these neurotics the unconscious meaning of a new "slave rebellion" defense: "I'm independent of mother and don't want to be masochistically refused."

The grotesque fact emerges that some neurotics are incapable of reducing without having analytically "straightened out" their unsettled infantile accounts—with the first provider of food: mother.

TANGENTIAL APPLICATIONS OF THE MECHANISM OF ORALITY

26. "Magic Gestures"

A magic gesture—as I understand it [100]—denotes a specific "public relations operation" of the unconscious ego fighting the "*battle of alibis*" with its own inner conscience. The different steps are, seen in slow motion, these:

"I want to be masochistically mistreated by mother (father)."

"Forbidden," vetoes the inner conscience.

"My client," interposes the inner lawyer (unconscious ego), "is not guilty of psychic masochism, as the indictment claims. Quite the contrary, he *hates* his upbringers, having so many justified grievances against them."

"Forbidden, too," vetoes the inner conscience.

"My client," retorts the lawyer, "is the most misunderstood person in the world. Neither does he wish to be masochistically mistreated nor does he want to take revenge. He just wants to be loved. He will *dramatize* in his behavior how he wanted to be treated in childhood: *kindly and lovingly.*"

The unconscious dramatization of the last alibi is called a "magic gesture." It leads to the amazing fact that an *unimportant* outsider is chosen as beneficiary for these "good deeds." The more unimportant the beneficiary is, the deeper the masochistic inner "injustice collecting": "You bad mother (father) did not care for your own child. I care even for strangers!" It is exactly that discrepancy which makes for the choice of outsiders.

Here is a typical example from an analysis of an orally regressed

[100] For historic development of the term and different connotations, see "The Problem of Magic Gestures," The Psychiatric Quarterly *19*:295–310, 1945.

woman: She lived in constant feud with her family domiciled in a north western state. She constantly complained about their cruelty and neglect, though she, too, provoked soundly. Both parties got a goodsized masochistic kick out of it. One day, the patient's mother informed her that a bookkeeper from their business would visit New York, asking her to be nice to her. The patient reacted paradoxically: she did not complain of the "stinking imposition," which would have been her typical reaction, but devoted the next 10 days exclusively to being a guide for the guest. She invited the girl out, showered her with gifts, went out of her way to be nice and helpful, a trait other wise foreign to her. The unconscious meaning of her action was a reproachful innuendo against her mother.

The synthetic structure of the "magic gesture" can be demonstrated. The beneficiary never feels secure in his new glory. There comes a moment in which the outsider temporarily elevated to the position of the "white haired boy," is dropped—without reason, more—becomes the object of his previous benefactor's wrath. What happens is that the inner conscience objects to the unconscious trick, forcing the poor benefactor to a new alibi. The latter is promptly furnished: he denies his own inner masochistic tendencies by reversing the roles. He now acts the "cruel" parent, reducing the previous beneficiary to the image of the mistreated self! Thus, a "*positive*" magic gesture changes into a "*negative*" one. The latter demonstrates in a caricature, how cruel the educator really was!

Bitterness—over alleged neglect in childhood, the masochistic misuse being tactfully overlooked!—sometimes goes so far that the demonstration cannot be performed on living people, so animals, or inanimate objects are chosen.

A schizoid patient suffered from, among other things, reckless spending. This brought him into serious conflict with his penurious mother, toward whom he used this method of showing aggression. In addition to unconscious motives of revenge, self-injury, and "mechanism of orality," a further curious incapacity to make a decision in the selection of objects for purchase came into play. Wishing to order three shirts, the patient went to an expensive shop, where he saw hundreds of samples. Very definitely and without hesitation, he narrowed down the choice, selecting perhaps 30 samples. Although he could readily separate the ones he liked from those he considered in bad taste, he was incapable of making a further choice among those which appealed to him, and, according to his statement, there was no way out of his indecision but to order the entire 30. On another occasion, he went to a book store to buy a certain recently published book. The salesman showed him several dozen publications which had appeared within recent months. The patient rejected a number on the ground that they did not interest him. About 15 remained, and the patient, unable to come to a decision, bought all 15.

From the history of this patient one could learn that his mother preferred some of her six children to others, neglecting the others. The patient felt that he had been discriminated against. By means of his extravagance and indecision, he acted out a "magic gesture." Unconsciously he performed a symbolic act, clearly, in the superficial layer, an act of aggression toward his mother and one designed to show her how he would have liked to have been treated. His unconscious formula was: "You, Mother, have discriminated against some of your own children; at any rate, you have played favorites. I, however, cannot even choose between indifferent objects—shirts, books, etc. How much less would I be capable of doing so among my own children!" Behind this tearful aggression, deep masochism was hidden. That defense-aggression was not the real reason for his actions was also proved by the fact that, by being a spendthrift, he also showed conscious aggression toward his mother, who paid the bills. His pseudo-aggression was a palimpsest only, covering his deep masochistic attachment to his mother.

In place of inanimate objects, some neurotics choose animals as the recipients of their magic gestures. One of my schizoid patients was an enthustiastic "pigeon feeder." He collected crumbs incessantly and spent hours watching the pigeons eat from his hand, with tears in his eyes the while. He did not wish to be put in the same category as "ordinary animal-loving humanitarians riding their ridiculous pigeon-horse," as he, strangely enough, called his competitors, paraphrasing Lawrence Sterne's "hobby-horse" ("Tristram Shandy"). Correctly enough, he placed the emphasis, not on the pigeons, but on his tears, although he was incapable of explaining their cause. Unconsciously, his tears meant: "You treated me badly, bad Mother. Look how I wanted to be treated—kindly." The previously-described, five-layer structure was fully visible under the analytic microscope, as was the specific determining factor in the symbolic use of pigeons.

Whether the neurotic uses the mechanism of magic gestures on living persons, inanimate objects, or animals, the fact remains that he always expresses in it an aggressive reproach, hidden behind the disguise of the superficial layer: unconscious identification with the "beneficiary" and idealized mother (father).[101] Hidden still further, behind this reproach, is the real, dynamically-effective, psychic masochism, which it warded off by pseudo-aggression.

27. Criminosis

An extensive literature on the problem of criminosis so far has yielded an extensive amount of confusion; criminosis and neurosis have been constantly identified.[102] This has gone so far that Ben Karpmann, one of the pioneers in that field, sounded the justified warning: ". . . the psychoanalytic approach has as yet failed to contribute significantly to the solution of the problem because it gratuitously went on the assumption that the same mechanisms operated in criminals as in neurotics. . . . The great majority of the professional and habitual criminals must be approached by a method different from that used for neurotics." [103]

Without going into the tragi-comedy of errors and misconceptions, I shall summarize briefly my personal opinions on criminotics,[104] whom

[101] There is double identification in every magic gesture. The patient acts both parts.

[102] For a review of the literature, see my study "Suppositions about the 'Mechanism of Criminosis'." Journal of Criminal Psychopathology, V. 2, 1943.

[103] Karpman, Ben, The Individual Criminal. Foreword, p. vii, Nervous and Mental Disease Monograph Series, No. 59, 1933.

[104] For more extensive treatment of the subject, see ch. XV of "The Battle of the Conscience,' entitled "The Neurotic Who Unconsciously Bargains for the Electric Chair—The Criminal." Furthermore: "Suppositions about the Mechanism of Criminosis," J. Crim. Psychopathol., V. 2, 1943. "Psychopathology of Impostors," Ibid., V. 4, 1944; "Eight Prerequisites for Psychoanalytic Treatment of Homosexuality," Psychoan. Rev., *31*:3, 1944; "The Respective Importance of Reality and Phantasy in the Genesis of Female Homosexuality," J. Crim. Psychopathol., V. 1, 1943; "Hypocrisy—Its Implications in Neurosis and Criminal Psychopathology," Ibid., IV, 4, 1943; "The Psychology of Gambling," Imago, 1936; "The Gambler—

I consider propelled by a specific modification of the "mechanism of orality," which I have named "*mechanism of criminosis.*"

The primary difficulty with criminotics lies in the fact that *they act unconsciously under the influence of a pre-Oedipal, and not of an Oedipal conflict.*

I conceive of the criminotic as the *most passive person in this world,* helpless as a baby in his motorically-inexpressible fury. The giant of a mother is not even impressed with that fact that the helpless child wants to take revenge for alleged injustices. *The motor act in criminosis is based on the inner feeling of being incapable of making the mother even feel that the child seeks revenge on her. The situation is that of a dwarf trying to annoy a giant who superciliously refuses to see these attempts.* There is a direct relationship between the "herostratic" tendency in criminosis and the feeling of helplessness in making that revenge evident. *Because of his inner feeling of being a dwarf, the criminotic uses, so to speak, dynamite.* Of that the giant must take cognizance. True, the "revenge" harms the avenger. He may be legally executed. However, the primary inner aim of forcing the giant to acknowledge the dwarf's fury, is fulfilled.

Every criminal action has something "herostratic" about it. Herostrates was the individual who, in 356 B.C., burned the famous Temple of Artemis in Ephesus in order to become "renowned." Our "herostratic" criminals unconsciously perform similar deeds with another purpose: unconsciously to force the image of the mother of their earliest childhood to acknowledge that they are at least capable of taking revenge upon her. The deepest and dynamically most effective core in the unconscious conflict of the criminotic is the compensatory, concealed helplessness, expressed originally toward the mother and only later shifted toward society.

The conception of crime outlined here differs specifically from the usual schematic applications of analytic knowledge, gained from the therapy of neuroses. The usual misconception is that an Oedipus

---

A Misunderstood Neurotic," J. Crim. Psychopathol., IV, 3, 1943; "Problems of Suicide." The Psychiat. Quart, Suppl., *20*:2, 1946; and "Applications of the Mechanism of Orality in Neurosis and Criminosis," in: Handbook of Correctional Psychology, edited by Lindner and Seliger, "The Philosophical Library," New York, 1947; "Crime and Punishment," The Psychiat. Quart. Suppl. *21*:2, 1947.

complex is "discovered" in criminals. The proud but naïve authors of certain treatises flatter themselves on being very "modern," and assume at the same time that they "discovered" the "reason" for crimes. Unfortunately for these "pseudo-discoveries," the Oedipus complex can be found in every human being. Unfortunately for these pseudo-discoverers, not everybody burdened with this complex commits crimes.

Schematic application of neurosis to criminosis leads to another fallacy, too. That fallacy consists of the fact that the findings of unconscious motivations in a specific criminotic are used for explanation of the motor act. *Psychologic motivations* and *Motor act,* i.e., the execution of the specific crime are two distinct and different things. Hence the confusion is further increased.

In my opinion the major confusion in criminal psychopathology is the failure to differentiate between a *variable* and a *constant* factor in every criminal action. The variable factor is made up of the *psychologic contents,* and is multitudinous in form, differing in every case. The variety of motives for a crime is as great as the variety of unconscious motives in general. The constant factor in crime is the now known "X" which explains the *motor act* of executing the criminal move itself. This constant and pathognomonic factor I have proposed to call the "mechanism of criminosis." These two factors must be determined in every criminal action.

The differential diagnosis between these two factors is accomplished by keeping in mind the following: The variable factor explains the unconscious contents of a criminal action. To explain these, we must use all of the knowledge of unconscious mechanisms which Freud has discovered and so successfully applied to the explanation of human conduct in general—unconscious wishes, defense mechanisms, projections, identifications, atonement of unconscious guilt feelings, etc. The constant factor, the mechanism of criminosis, refers not to the variable psychologic contents of a specific crime, but to the motor act executing the results of the variable factor. I repeat, the real riddle in crime is the motor act. It borrows from the inexhaustible source of aggression, using it as the most primitive of human trends without revealing whether that aggression is primary or secondary (pseudo-aggression, that is, aggression used as an unconscious defense mechanism).

What happens if these two decisive factors are not differentiated? The answer is simple, confusion is rampant. That confusion is based mainly on naïveté, sometimes on malice. As an example of the latter, the *cause célèbre* of Halsmann can be cited. The reactionary medical faculty of the University of Innsbruck in pre-Hitler Austria was asked by the court to express its opinion of the reason why a young Latvian Jew killed his father, a crime which the defendant denied and which could only be "proved" by more than doubtful circumstantial evidence. The Nazi-infested faculty decided that Halsmann had an Oedipus complex which was "operative." Freud objected to this biased nonsense, pointing out the universality of the Oedipus complex. Said he: "Even if the conflict between father and son could be proved, one must say that there is a great distance between this conflict and the causative factors of such a crime." Freud illustrated his point by a joke: A man was sentenced for robbery on the ground of circumstantial evidence, having been arrested near the robbed apartment with a skeleton key in his pocket. Asked if he had anything to add when his sentence was passed, he replied that he wanted to be sentenced also for adultery, having that "key," too, in his pocket. . . . The "great" distance mentioned by Freud is exactly the distance between present ignorance and the finding of the "specific factor" in crime.

Obviously the eradication of a misconception is a considerable job, since it involves overcoming the human reluctance to think, or the preference to think along lines of prefabricated patterns. Examples of the naïve variety of the same fallacy are to be found in numerous scientific journals and books. The basis is regularly the same: confusion between neurosis and criminosis.

The criminotic aggression is in my opinion exclusively pseudo-aggression of a specific type. It is differentiated from neurotic aggression in these points:

1. It represents a subdivision of neurotic pseudo-aggression. Proof positive is the fact that the alleged aggression damages the person executing the criminal act by his being caught or being in constant danger of being punished.

2. It is differentiated from neurotic aggression by the greater risk the alleged avenger takes: Whereas the neurotic bargains only for individual, consciously experienced unhappiness as punishment, the criminotic risks jail or capital punishment.

3. Social ostracism is involved in criminotic aggression, and not in neurotic self-damage.

4. In contradistinction to neurotic aggression exhibitionism plays an indispensable part in criminotic aggression. The majority of criminals are caught because of some "little mistakes" perpetrated by themselves. That unconsciously self-intended betrayal not only serves the inner guilt, it also is under the pressure of the exhibitionistic tendency to show the mother-image—shifted to society—that the child was capable of taking "revenge."

5. Childlike megalomania is more strongly represented in criminotic aggression than in neurotic. That is responsible for the criminal's attitude of considering himself as a unique exception as far as the danger of being detected is concerned. That megalomania, coupled with the unconscious wish to be punished, accounts for the incomplete thinking-through of the possibilities of detection and explains why a "perfect crime" cannot be committed.

6. The criminotic accepts inwardly the fact that he will be punished. Therefore one finds phenomenologically, so frequently, criminals seemingly without remorse and guilt.

So far, one may conclude that criminosis represents a specific "solution" of a repressed infantile conflict going back to the earliest months of life. The criminotic act is composed of two parts: a constant one (mechanism of criminosis), explaining the motor act, and a variable one, accounting for differences in psychological content. This psychological content is specific for the specific crime alone.

What about the *conscience of the criminotic?* Why does it not prevent the dangerous act? Does the criminotic have a conscience at all?

To begin with, a person without a conscience cannot and does not exist. Recent investigations prove conclusively that conscience is not at all a photographic copy of the environment, as previously assumed, but an inner institution having an intimate relation with the person's aggression. A part of this aggression is unconsciously curbed and redirected against the person himself.

To state that a person has no conscience, simply means that the investigator who made such a statement was incapable of finding out what hidden inner "deals" the "conscienceless" person made with his conscience to appease his conscience.

For clinical material, the reader is referred to my book, "The Battle of the Conscience."

I am convinced that these 27 clinical pictures of oral neurosis do *not* exhaust the repertory.[105] Nobody claims that we have at last fully explored orality. Quite the opposite, we have only scratched the surface. Future generations of psychoanalytically oriented psychiatrists will have no justification for complaining that the "older generation" did not leave them anything to discover.

[105] To name but one group not included: passive "beating fantasies." See: "Preliminary Phases of the Masculine Beating Fantasy," Psa. Quart., 1938, No. 4, and the continuation: "Further Contributions to the Masculine Beating Fantasy," The Psychiatric Quarterly, Supplement, 1948: *Perverted* masochists accept their defeats only on condition that these are unconsciously self-created; a fact first stated by L. Eidelberg in "Studies on Masochism," Int. Z. f. Psychoan. 1934. Eidelberg's study pertains to *perversion* masochism exclusively, and assumes a specific mechanism of exchangeability in *perverted* masochists: external frustrations are nullified by actively creating those themselves, instead of enduring them passively.

7

Differential Diagnosis, Technique of Treatment, Specific Resistances in Oral Neuroses

THE CONFUSING fact confronting every analyst in every patient is basically this: lack of congruity between textbook and life. In the texbook, there are neat subdivisions; the living patient, unfortunately, is impertinent enough to present a composite picture. Not every patient with hysteric symptoms suffers from hysteria, not every obsession points conclusively in the direction of obsessional neurosis, hypochondriacal complaints and hypochondria are by no means identical. Not every gourmet and gourmand is oral, nor every smoker or fellatio-lover. Confusion—your name is patient!

Everybody talks big about taking the "whole clinical picture" into consideration, few do it. It is easier to stick to symptoms and signs—and classify accordingly. The trouble with that simplification is that symptoms and signs are cruelly misleading.

Every patient has "everything of everything"; the analyst's business is to find out what is unconsciously being magnified to cover up the "real" thing. The moment one is familiar with the fact that every neurosis is but a desperate rescue station from the oral danger, the question of traditional nosologic entities loses much of its importance.

"Let the material the patient presents be the guide." That rule is a commonplace; and like all commonplaces meaningless if not properly applied. Every human being has gone through the phase of the Oedipus complex. Hence one can find that complex in every patient. Whereas, however, the Oedipus repetition in the transference means the "real" thing in hysterical neurotics, it may be a dangerous camouflage in oral cases. Nobody can save the analyst the trouble of finding out the *dynamically decisive spot*—and making him act accordingly.

Otherwise, an analysis becomes a series of dead ends, the analyst is led like a blindfolded man by the patient's undiscovered resistance, and the patient remains uncured. There is no substitute for correct analytic thinking.

If one believes, as I do, that there is only one basic neurosis—the oral—the only yardstick is the question: how much oral "remnants" does the specific patient carry around? The analytic technique gives to the analyst a short respite from acting: we hear the patient's life history in the first four to eight appointments.[1] That time of silent listening gives time for thinking and forming an opinion, too.

If one finds that the patient operates in decisive life situations on the basis of the mechanism of orality, the diagnosis is simple—we are confronted with an oral case. If not, the generally acknowledged analytic rules are pertinent.

I believe that oral patients are incapable of *starting* analysis according to the classical technique.[2] To begin with, the analytic technique of free associations is the first handicap. To "give" association comes immediately in conflict with the *main defense mechanism* of these neurotics who unconsciously live on the basis of *pseudo-aggression.* Constantly bothered by their superego reproaching them because of their wish to be refused, they defend themselves with pseudo-aggressive refusal. Asked to *give* associations, they *refuse*. If the analyst uses the classical technique, he is confronted even in the first days with an unsurmountable resistance, either of silence, or fury, or the patient's tendency to run away. Or, if the patient remains in analysis, an amazing degree of hatred and suspicion comes to the fore: he makes out of the analyst the "bad mother" in the transference. Long experience with these neurotics taught me that the only way of coping with this difficulty at

[1] I believe that every patient should be given, before analysis starts, a short and simplified introduction of what an analysis is. I have seen too many disagreeable results when an analysis started with the simple advice of producing free associations. The analyst's avoidance of any explanation at the start is taken by intelligent patients as an insult to their intelligence. It is, of course, true that analysis is an affective process—the trouble is that the patient does not know it. Neither is he familiar with resistance; he cannot be warned early enough.

[2] Summary in "Specific Types of Resistance in Orally Regressed Neurotics." The Psa. Rev., *34*:1, 1947.

the beginning is to change the technique for them: one has to give, give and give *words.* The tiring result is that one has to talk much more with these neurotics than is usual in classical analysis. I described this fact first in 1932 in my paper "Problems of Pseudo-Imbecility." [3] It is clear that by confronting the patient with a "giving mother," one does not escape his transference of a "refusing mother." But—and this but weighs heavily—one gets the possibility of creating an atmosphere in which one can analyze all.

For analysis two people are necessary; these patients, however, are present—so to speak—only in an "infinitesimal dosis." The part of the ego capable of discernment and some kind of cooperation can be artificially increased by the device of "giving words."

The patient with whom that idea first occurred to me presented this: He started analysis with a woman analyst who interrupted treatment after a few months because of the patient's agitation, especially his pathologic jealousy of her baby. The patient became suicidal and attacked his mother. When he came to me, he evaded any correction and even understanding of his attitude by shutting his ears and shouting for hours "Don't understand, don't understand. . . ." I tried to "circumvent" his attitude by talking for many hours. Every time I interrupted my "tale" for a second, the patient started his stereotyped "Don't understand." The analysis was, as it were, conducted in a vacuum: the patient seemed to take no part in it. It was like telling a child fairy-tales. Only after "contact" was established in that way, analysis could be started. It was amazing, by the way, to what degree the patient remembered later the contents of my "stories," as he called them. I had the impression that the contents of my talk was immaterial; I gave hundreds of clinical examples. Talking about the weather would have had the same effect: the decisive point was my *giving* of words (= milk, love, attention).

Here is another example of what hopeless conflicts the analyst railroads himself into if he adheres to the classical technique with orally regressed patients: Mr. X., a patient with psychogenic aspermia entered trial-analysis with a colleague in another country. The patient was advised to adhere to the basic rule; the result was that he became agitated, depressed and "suffered hell." The analyst did not open his mouth

[3] Int. Z. f. Psa., *18*:528–538, 1932. Abstract in Int. J. of Psa., *14*:408–10, 1933.

during four weeks and broke the silence of a Sphinx for the first time after twenty appointments to announce that he believed that the patient was a case for analysis. The patient left in a fury. He could not explain what made him so angry since he had spoken all the time about business matters. Some time latter, he entered analysis with me. Said the man: "Should you, too, tell me that I have to use the couch and talk, talk and talk, I am leaving immediately." The answer was that neither was necessary in his case, he merely had to listen. For weeks I talked; an atmosphere favorable for analysis had to be created artificially. Classical analysis can start with these people only *after* that—in my opinion—necessary pre-stage.

The most *typical* resistance in oral cases is the constant projection of the "bad mother" upon the analyst with resultant craving for "injustices," and reactive pseudo-aggression. These patients are really "*injustice collectors*" of imaginary wrongs. Every word, every gesture of the analyst is misconstrued as deliberate malice. Here are a few examples:

Mr. Y., a man of 35, was a musician and composer in the realm of his own fantasy. Practically, he devoted his life to the "proof" that his family prevented his success in becoming a composer simply by refusing to finance his studies. The idea of earning money himself did not enter his head seriously, though he made a few attempts only to reduce them to absurdity. After complicated conflicts with his family lasting for fifteen years, his fiancee convinced the parents that the young man needed psychiatric treatment. The question arose how to find an analyst. The patient and the girl decided that the usual method of procuring the name of an analyst—recommendation—was not to be trusted. Therefore, they decided to read the issues of psychiatric-psychoanalytic journals of the last two years and to make up their minds on the basis of the "quality of publications." Since the young man did not have "enough energy" to finish the job, the young lady took over marking the papers. In this queer "scientific" contest I came out on top of the list; therefore I was consulted. After a trial-treatment of one month I was able to convince the family that the most reasonable attempt at solution of the patient's conflict was: conceding analysis, allowance *and* music lessons. Reluctantly the family accepted the proposal. The patient was pleased only to accuse me immediately that I "sold him out." He suspected that I had suggested to his parents the following deal: "Let me treat him and I shall convince him to give up music and become a good business-man." In other words, he immediately projected upon me—in spite of clear evidence to the contrary—the "bad" pre-oedipal mother-image. After having established that fantasy, he could fight me in righteous indignation with pseudo-aggression. It was exceedingly difficult to convince the schizoid patient that his "basic fallacy" [4] was a—fallacy.

The next step in his "injustice-collecting" was his assumption that even if I were helping him in his music in good faith, I was interested in him only for the duration of treatment. Since his musical education needed five years, the analysis, however, only a particle of that time (more precisely: his parents would pay only for approximately one year), I would drop him after one year. Therefore, he concluded, there was no point in starting his studies.

To follow up the patient's "arguments" for continuation of inactivity: even if his studies would make sense, analysis would occupy too much time. He was compelled to think about analytic interpretations, which disturbed him. Therefore, I was responsible that he could not work.

My next "crime" in his projections pertained to his "colds." After a few weeks of treatment in the fall, he wanted to take "a rest" for a while. Since I advised him to continue treatment instead, I was responsible for his not feeling well with his "resultant" colds.

In my attempts to show him that he wasted time and inwardly did not want success in music and life, but continuation of his fallacy "Everybody but myself is responsible," I pointed out one day: "It is amazing that a man of your intelligence is taken in by every nonsense which the unconscious sends as ingenious 'red herring' into your consciousness." This explanation of his resistance was parried by the patient the next day: "I am furious with you since you attacked my intelligence." When I proved to him that I had paid him a compliment and did not attack nor doubt his intelligence, he remained unconvinced.

When it was proved that he wasted time and did not study, he replied that "organizing" his studies took time. Besides, constant "interruptions" prevented his studies. Asked what these interruptions

[4] See the writer's "The Danger Neurotics Dread Most: Loss of the Basic Fallacy." The Psa. Rev., *33*:2, 1946.

consisted of, he stated that he had to visit auctions since he hoped to earn money one day by becoming an expert in Chinese art. When it was pointed out to him that the "interruptions" were self-created, he smiled and complained: "It is hard to talk to you." And so on, and so on.

Dr. Z., a physician, 28 years old, consulted me because of premature ejaculation two weeks after publication of my monograph on psychic impotence, in 1937. He stated that he had great confidence in me since he had studied my book thoroughly. He told me in an excited tone that he considered it a great injustice that he should wait till he could afford analysis and asked in no uncertain terms to be treated on credit. He knew that this was unusual, he knew also from reading Freud's works that—in contradistinction to general usage that physicians do not pay for medical services—such an arrangement is impossible in psychoanalysis since every patient takes up 1/8 or 1/7 of the analyst's working day.[5] And still he asked to be treated free of charge. He admitted that his father could pay for his treatment but he did not want to divulge his troubles with his potency to his family. He admitted further that his wife's family had some means, but the same secrecy had to be applied there. He revealed also that he had saved some money, but that he needed it for furnishing his future apartment; he still lived with his family. He refused to apply for treatment in our clinic; he did not want to be treated by young and—as he believed—inexperienced analysts. He even made fun of himself that he consulted a specialist in that field, telling the joke of a man who consulted a specialist without being capable of paying the fee. Asked by the indignant physician how he dared consult him without having the necessary funds, the man answered: "Well, nothing is too expensive where my health is concerned. . . ."

It was obvious that the young doctor started to act the "mechanism of orality" with me even before he saw me the first time: he just wanted to be refused. I was at that time interested in the psychologic problem embedded in gratitude [6] and decided (though, of course, without telling

[5] *Ges. Schr.*, VI, p. 95 Freud states that two simultaneous analyses of physicians would deprive the analyst of one-fourth or one-third of his earning capacity "which is identical with the results of a severe traumatic accident."

[6] Later published in "Psychopathology of Ingratitude," Diseases of the Nervous System, VI, 7, 1945.

the real reason to the patient) to treat him for some months on his conditions. I explained to him that I was expecting a Swiss patient in several months and had to keep an appointment free; in the meantime he could get that appointment. There was a chance that he could be helped during that time; if not I would continue treatment though on a reduced schedule.

It was really amusing to observe the contortions of the patient in order to maintain his "basic fallacy": that I (projection of mother) was "unjust" towards him. Consciously, he was very grateful and pleased to be in "good hands" as he called it. He solved his seemingly hopeless problem—to transform a kind act on my part into a malicious one—by assuming that I wanted to use him as a "guinea-pig" for my theories. He had to admit that in the monograph on impotence hundreds of cases were described, so that my interest in discovering something new in his specific disease could not be too great.

The next objection was that I was speculating on his gratitude should he once become famous. He admitted that there was not much hope on that score.

The next step was the patient's assumption that I had made a vow to the effect that the first patient who wanted to be analyzed after reading the monograph, should be treated without fee. I assured him that I used different methods to straighten out my accounts with fate.

The patient had—after that bubble collapsed—another idea. He suspected that I felt guilty that physicians reading my book could be disturbed. "Look at me," said the patient, "I knew that I had my difficulties in potency but I never took it tragically. After reading your book I became jumpy." In other words, he construed a fantasy according to which I owed him something. . . .

It took a few months to show him the irrationality of his behavior. He had a hard time to keep up his fallacy.

Miss A. M.,[7] a young girl of 17, with "personality"-difficulties manifesting themselves in constant conflicts at home and in attaching herself to "wrong" men who constantly disappointed her, was always shabbily dressed. Since her parents were well-to-do people who cared for the

[7] I am running out of initials. The case A.M. has no connection with previously described cases A. and M.

children this fact was unexplainable. Asked why she was poorly dressed, the girl answered: "I have nothing to wear." Conferences with her parents showed the following clinical picture. The girl had literally dozens of dresses; she just did not wear them. If she did, she either tore them to pieces, made them dirty, or "forgot" about their existence only to complain that her mother did not care. In other words, the girl worked the "mechanism of orality" overtime. How strong this defensive "putting-the-parents-into-the-wrong" was, is visible in the fact that her neurotic attitude even overshadowed her vanity; she just played self-created masochistic Cinderella with a pseudo-aggressive defense. In analysis she constantly tried to get masochistic gain through injustices allegedly experienced with the analyst.[8] The simple fact that her parents recommended him, made him in her eyes into a paid executive organ of the parents, in the other words, "unjust." [9]

Another difficulty which oral patients present is a strange faculty of "sucking out," draining and wearing down the analyst. Abraham was the first to mention the "sucking out"-trait in the oral make-up,[10] attributing it, however, to a direct continuation of the original, oral-aggressive wish to get. Further clinical experience taught that the *historically* explainable wish to get and the *clinically* observable one, are by no means identical. Interpolated is the masochistic elaboration of aggression and guilt, as stressed repeatedly in this book. The practical conclusion is that every time we see *aggression* in an orally regressed *neurotic*, we have to classify it as *pseudo-aggression*, covering a masochistic aim. *Nothing is more dangerous and at the same time futile than to interpret in analysis to an oral neurotic his "oral greed" and "oral aggression" per se.* In doing so, one plays the game of the patient's unconscious and can never cure him if one takes his pseudo-aggression at its face value. Only by *de-bunking his pseudo-aggression as covering cloak for the deeper repressed masochistic wish to be refused,* can one achieve success with these patients.

The specific technique of these patients consists of constant "elimina-

[8] It infuriated her that the analyst did not accept her excuse to the effect that all her "disappointments" with men were based on inexperience.

[9] She admitted, though, that were he not recommended, she would not have "confidence". A good example that the psychic masochist "cannot lose".

[10] "Psychoanalytic Studies to Character Formation," Int. Psa. Verlag, 1925, p. 44.

tion" of everything they learn in analysis. These patients are confronted with the following—truly tragicomic—conflict. They have to keep up the "basic fallacy" that the analyst, representing in the transference the "bad, refusing" mother, is bad and refusing. When the analyst adheres to classical analysis with these patients the "proof" is simply established: the analyst's silence is equaled to refusal. When, however, the analyst behaves differently—as I suggested—and *gives* constantly, the patient's conflict is more complicated: First he misconstrues everything as malice; this helps for some time. If the analyst, moreover, explains the resistance correctly and continues to "give," the precarious neurotic balance, based on the basic fallacy, is endangered. Here the strange technique of "sucking out" sets in with these patients. *They nullify every voluntary "giving" on the analyst's part by aggressively "taking away."* They maintain therefore the basic fallacy with the unconscious trick: "He does not give because he is nice and generous, I take it against his will." *Therefore* the "sucking out"-attitude.

The basic fallacy of the refusing monster of a mother (projected upon the innocent analyst) can thus be maintained—for some time. This does not lead anywhere, however, since the patient must reinforce his alibi: though nullified as "giving" person, his own superego constantly reproaches the patient: "Mother gives." Therefore, the patient cannot even use the "aggressively taking away" of information, since he must immediately "eliminate" everything achieved in that way.[11] This leads to constant "forgetting" of interpretations and to confusion.

These patients ask a hundred questions, wear the analyst down. If he treats these questions as rhetorical ones and does not answer directly but tries to analyze the reason for that "draining" attitude—the patient has once more the proof positive that the analyst is refusing. If he—avoiding that Scylla—answers with angelic patience, he comes into the Charybdis of human endurance, since he becomes a speaking machine trying in vain to straighten out the patient's confusion. These patients provoke so long till an impatient remark of the analyst or even the tone of his voice gives them the badly needed alibi: "Mother is refusing after all."

What is the solution for the poor analyst? My advice is this:

[11] An example of this type is described in Part I of the paper "Further Contributions to the Psychoanalysis of Writers." The Psa. Rev., *3*: 1947, and *1*: 1948.

Arrange your schedule in such a way that two oral patients never follow each other. Do not take oral patients at all if you do not have the angelic patience coupled with the needed inner strength to cope with such cases.

Orally regressed neurotics are often wrongly diagnosed as hysteric cases. The reason is obvious: the superficial impression of these people is often misleading. An orally regressed man often impresses one as one fixated on the negative Oedipus; an oral woman as "typical" hysteric. If the mistake in the diagnosis is not corrected, such an analysis must end with failure.[12]

One can distinguish three types in orally regressed neurotics:

All oral neurotics are under constant pressure of inner guilt pertaining to the accusation that their only aim in life is the psychic-masochistic wish to collect injustices. Their only inner defense is: "Not I am masochistic, the outer world is unjust." To establish that alleged but always self-created injustice is their main job which absorbs all their energies.

Oral people are totally uniform as far as their *unconscious* tendencies and defense mechanisms are concerned. Phenomenologically they represent differences so great that the untrained observer would doubt their genetic classification. For instance, the *garrulous* and *silent* types are seemingly opposites. And still, both elaborate the same conflict with different means: both use pseudo-aggression as defense against their wish to be refused. The silent type in directly visible pseudo-aggression, the logorrhoic type under the disguise of *giving*. What he gives, however, is—concentrated malice. It is clear that both types make difficulties in analysis: they either "kill" you through silence or thousands of words uttered in a minimum of time.

The "*draining*" variety, is somewhere in between the two. He is insistent in squeezing you out and waits silently till you exhaust yourself. He is logorrhoic in proving to you his legitimate right of draining you. Of some clinical importance is the fact that the "draining" type not only "takes aggressively" to prove that the "giving mother" is not

[12] An example of this type in a male patient is contained in my paper, "Further Contributions to the Clinical Picture of Psychogenic Oral Aspermia," Case A., Int. J. of Psa., London, *18*:196–234, 1937. In a female patient: "On a Predictable Mechanism," Case 4, The Psa. Rev., *30*:19-32, 1943.

good and never gives voluntarily but is deprived against her will, as stressed before, but also for another reason. It is simply the counteraction against the eternal superego reproach: You want *passively* to be disappointed. The defense is established: On the contrary, I want to drain him *actively*. . . .

Closely connected with these problems are complexities arising from the patient's complaints about "*lack of progress*" in analysis.[13]

"I don't see any progress," is the most typical objection of patients and their relatives (especially of those who pay for treatment) which is uttered during the course of analytical treatment. The layman's idea of progress during analysis is based on a direct proportion of checks and time consumed; after three months the progress should be greater than after two months, and so on, in direct arithmetical and even geometrical progression. In other words, a direct increase of progress at an ever increasing pace is expected and asked for. We know that nothing of that kind happens in psychoanalysis; after six months the patient might feel subjectively worse than he did at the very beginning of the treatment. The simple reason being that after all that time, the patient may perhaps begin to understand, *affectively*, what he has to give up; the most cherished wishes and resultant defenses of his unconscious. At this point, we are once more confronted with the outcry: "I don't see any progress."

How can we avoid these misunderstandings? The answer is simple: we cannot. We can try to explain in a preventive manner, at the beginning of the treatment, how analysis typically works. As long as the underlying unconscious wishes and defense mechanisms are not destroyed, modified or changed, the neurosis will manifest itself in symptoms, signs, ego limitations and depressions. Furthermore, we can ask the naive patient every time he complains about lack of progress, "Do you use the word progress in the layman's meaning, or in the analytical connotation?" Thus, with never ending patience, we have to make the patient understand that, analytically, progress during the first phases of the treatment does not mean the immediate disappearance of the symptoms, but understanding. That understanding is first intellectual and after much time is spent in repetition in the transference and

[13] First published in Medical Record, March 1947 under the title "Progress During Psychoanalytic Treatment."

after a long "working through" of the resistance, an affective one. The result is the typical discussion in the first months of the analysis: "Do you deny that you now understand your problem better than you did before?" asks the analyst. "I did not come to you to become a professor of psychology, I came only to be cured," answers the indignant patient.

Our problem starts with three question marks:

1. Is our general opinion correct, that for quite some time we have no reason to expect therapeutic changes during analysis?

2. What about cases where the symptoms disappear without recurrance but without an analytic destruction of the underlying reasons?

3. What is the typical sequence of events: Do the symptoms disappear first, and then the personality changes, or *vice versa?*

Therapeutic Changes in the First Phases of Psychoanalysis

Let us start with the first question. It is analytically obvious that without changing the basic structure of a neurosis, no basic change in the patient can occur; but, and that but weighs heavily, during analysis the feeling of guilt is mobilized and results in an increased pressure against the specific defense mechanism used by the patient. Consequently, very often, the changes of the defense mechanism, in the first weeks of treatment, are quite striking and give the patient and the environment the mirage of normalcy. Some typical examples follow:

Case I—Mr. A. N., a schizoid, aged thirty-six, entered analysis because of an unsolved transference to his former analyst, who, in another country, had treated him ten years ago. After being brought to understand his inner passivity as the basis and his paranoic projections as the defense, the man rapidly changed in one respect; he became a good businessman, whereas previously he just, to quote him, "trotted along." This change, the mobilization of a stronger defense mechanism under the pressure of guilt, analytically activated his defense and gave him the mirage of a "cure."

Case II.—Mr. A. O., aged forty-two, was to an amazing degree, under the thumb of his aggressive wife. Asked what the conflicts with his wife consisted of, he answered angrily that "his allowance was too small." He and his wife had the strange arrangement that he delivered all the money he earned in a free profession, about twenty thousand dollars a year, to his wife (he signed blank checks!) and she graciously gave him five dollars per week as his allowance. This patient, horrified at the extent of his self-damaging tendencies, changed in a few weeks. The man who characterized his behavior as "nice, kind and full of the milk of human kindness", became, after a few weeks of treatment, "harsh and overbearing" toward his clients. In other words, by using the defense mechanism of pseudo-aggression, he proved to himself that he was not a "sissy" any more; overlooking, of course, that he also damaged himself with his new ways.

Case III.—Mrs. A. P., a nymphomaniac, who lived the life of a half-prostitute, became very penitent after a few weeks of treatment. She claimed that, while she had previously been the "life of every party", she was now rather shy and had completely "lost her grip on men." This provoked her fury, and she claimed that "she came into analysis to lose her frigidity and not to become a nun."

It is of advantage if the analyst is prepared for these eventualities and warns the patient beforehand. These transitory pseudo-successes (they are but defense mechanisms) are dangerous, because they give the patient either the illusion of a cure, (Mr. A. N.); or, damage the patient professionally or socially, (Mr. A. O.); or they may be the signal for running away from analysis, (Mrs. A. P.). One can avoid these dangers, to a certain degree at least, by preventively explaining to the patient why he will try to assume the other extreme, and also ask him not to be too naive when confronted with a new trick of the unconscious.

At first, the unconscious ego reacts to the analytical "danger" in the same way as to any other difficulty threatening the neurotic balance; [13a] it tries to counteract the difficulty in a routine manner. This routine consists, first, of increasing the strength of the already established defense-mechanism, and secondly, if that is not sufficient, the exchange of the defense mechanism; thereby keeping the neurotic balance. However, the quickly established, new defenses, visible in the early stages of analysis, have nothing whatsoever to do with a real cure, but accomplish exactly the opposite: the maintenance of the neurosis with new devices. Sometimes the establishment of new defense mechanisms is preceded by a period of depression and confusion. The patient

[13a] See the writer's paper "The Danger Neurotics Dread Most: Loss of the Basic Fallacy," Psa. Rev., *33*:2, 1946.

bitterly complains of both, using them for the purposes of his resistance. Only the fact that analysis goes after these new defense mechanisms too, convinces the unconscious ego that "routine" handling of the situation does not suffice and that more drastic measures are necessary. It then basically depends on the amount of the "free floating" feeling of unconscious guilt, whether the patient chooses the desparate measure of running away from analysis altogether, or allows further attacks against his neurosis, with the ultimate prospect of cure. This phase teaches us, however, never to underestimate the elasticity of the unconscious ego, which is very cunning in devising ever new defenses to keep the neurotic balance.

Another type of pseudo-progress, which is too well-known to be discussed at length, is the positive transference mirage. The moment the negative transference comes into play, the bubble collapses. There are no short-cuts to an honest, psychoanalytically achieved cure.

To put the matter bluntly, we want the patient to feel as good as he can, even in analysis; but focusing our attention to the end-result, we are not too much interested in his transitory well-being, provided that he makes progress in *our* meaning of the word. Our situation is comparable to that of a surgeon, who is bothered by the patient with questions as to whether he should read detective stories, or serious novels during his period of suspension in a surgical position, after a complicated multiple fracture.

It is theoretically an interesting problem whether or not the conclusion as to the probable end-result, can be drawn from the initial, newly installed, defense mechanisms. The answer is, paradoxically, yes and no. Since we see that the patient's feeling of guilt can be mobilized, the analytically initiated defense mechanisms are a favorable sign.[14] Should one, however, draw too far reaching conclusions from these quickly established defense mechanisms toward the surety and acceleration of an ultimate cure, one will be disappointed. Nothing will prevent the patient from playing the whole repertoire of his "use and misuse of interpretations."[15]

[14] See the writer's: "Working Through in Psychoanalysis," The Psa. Rev., *32*:4, 1945.

[15] See the paper: "Use and Misuse of Analytic Interpretations by the Patient," Psa. Rev., *33*:4, 1946.

Sometimes the initial, newly created defense mechanisms are dangerous, since the patient misjudges them completely and furiously decides to leave analysis. Here is an example: A writer, a female aged forty, reported that from the age of five until she was ten, she was as she put it, "selling her looks" to an old man across the street, for fifty cents per exhibitionistic performance. This action could be reconstructed as her first desperate, unconscious attempt to cope with her own voyeuristic conflict; not she, but the old man (father-image) committed the crime of peeping. The mechanism used was first, projection; second, an exchange of one part of scopophilia for the other (voyeurism into exhibitionism); third, an unconscious identification with the old man's voyeuristic pleasure. The child exhibited twofold; in the performance given and in confessing it to her sister, who was horrified. She thus preferred to take the blame for the defense mechanism (exhibitionism), only to cover up something more important,—peeping.[16] Why did she, however, accept money? At that time, her father was beating her mercilessly, and every beating was administered with a specific ceremony, including undressing and an official appeal for punishment. The child, at an early age, suspected that her father's motives were not of an entirely punitive nature. In taking money from the old man across the street, she unconsciously directed irony toward her father: "He enjoys it and should pay me for the pleasure, as does the other man." Secondarily, unconscious ideas of self-degradation were included: "This is what father makes out of me."

As previously stated, the patient was a writer and her voyeuristic tendencies were quantitatively increased. In her private life, she behaved in an extremely exhibitionistic fashion. As usual, she used exhibitionism as a defense for her deeper repressed voyeurism. Interesting were the rationalizations of this patient when she was asked why she had not done something about her father's cruelty. She claimed that she was "ashamed of her bruises" and of the possibility that the neighbors would have considered her father "crazy." What the child really was afraid of, was that people might understand her masochistic pleasure in this paternal torture. That it was not modesty which pre-

[16] For details pertaining to the problem of voyeurism versus exhibitionism see "A Clinical Approach to the Psychoanalysis of Writers," Psa. Rev., *31*:1, 1944; and "Further Contributions to Psychoanalysis of Writers, Ibid., *3*: 1947 and *1*: 1948..

vented her from the exhibitionistically conceived complaints and exposing her father, was apparent in the transference. She projected upon the analyst the "bad mother-father" attachment and misconstrued everything as "mistreatment." Without understanding what she was repeating, she started to mobilize outsiders against analysis. The reason was a newly established defense mechanism; since her feeling of guilt was increased because of the analysis of her masochistic wishes, she *now* did what she had *not* done as a child, namely, complain about "mistreatment." Thus denying masochistic pleasure, she even produced suicidal ideas and, completely oblivious of the fact that she had attempted suicide three times previously, (the first time at the age of seven!) she started to accuse the analysis of driving her toward death. Every attempt to make the patient understand what she was doing, was futile. In her mobilization of outsiders against analysis, an ironic twist, a quasi-moral alibi was discernible: "You ask why I didn't complain; well, I do now." Thus, analysis was "punished" for disturbing her masochistic pleasure via a newly created defense mechanism.

The Disappearance of Neurotic Symptoms Without the Destruction of Their Unconscious Basis

Let us compare the three following cases:

Case I—Mr. A. R., aged thirty, consulted the author on a Friday, because of a potency disturbance. Each time he attempted intercourse, the erection collapsed. The description and the case history gave the impression of a hysteric individual, so upon the advice of the author, he decided to start treatment on Monday. Sunday night the prospective patient called the author to inform him that the treatment would not be necessary, since he had just had successful intercourse for the first time in his life. His "inflationary potency," as he later called this episode in his troubled life, lasted three months, only to collapse as suddenly as it had appeared.

Case II—Mr. A. S. started treatment because of severe premature ejaculation. He was in great despair, due to the fact that his wife had left him because he could not satisfy her sexually. During analysis, he behaved like a school boy making fun of the teacher. The interpretations of the oral and anal contributaries of his sexual difficulties were, for him, a never ending source of irony and scorn, and he constantly criticized the author. The fact that the furniture of the author's office was "modern," was a constant object for merry making. He refused to analyze his senseless objections, especially his constant praise of his own antique furniture, with the excuse that axiomatic statements do not have to be proven. Every attempt to show him that his objections pertaining to problems of tastes, covered something else (e.g., sexual comparisons in the transference repetition), since there was no necessity to agree on that score, was futile. One day, after seven weeks of treatment, the patient informed the author that he could no longer afford analysis, since he had invested the money reserved for that purpose in remodeling his apartment with modern furniture. "A guy has the constitutional right to change his opinion," he stated, and furthermore, "he was cured anyhow," since during the last few days, he had acquired a girl friend and had repeatedly had normal intercourse. He left analysis despite the writer's objections and *remained potent.* His unresolved psychic masochism found an even more dangerous depository; by hiding political literature for his so-called friends of different political parties in his country, he railroaded himself in later years into a position where he was repeatedly arrested and had to serve jail sentences, although he himself was indifferent to all kinds of politics.

Mr. A. T. entered analysis because of premature ejaculation. He was a typical case [17] and was *cured* after twenty-one months of analysis.

What is the difference between these three cases? From the standpoint of naive description, they were all "cured" and a cynic could even say that Messrs. A. R. and A. S. saved time and money. If we look at the cases analytically we can state: Mr. A. R. was unconsciously so frightened of analysis, that he preferred to temporarily give up his symptom for the purpose of escaping analysis with a good conscience. His *success because of unconscious fear,* lasted only three months. His subsequent analysis revealed that the element which unconsciously frightened him most, was his repressed oedipal attachment to his mother. His unconscious ego temporarily preferred to sacrifice the symptom instead of sacrificing the whole neurosis. Mr. A. S. achieved the same result after seven weeks of analysis. As his later life proved,

[17] "Short Genetic Survey of Psychogenic Potency Disturbances," Psychiat. Quart., *19*:3 and 4, 1945.

he shifted the guilt pertaining to his pregenital libido and aggression to provoking jail sentences. The fact that he was really innocent, as far as politics were concerned, was a part of his inner alibi; "I am innocent of the other crime, too." The amazing fact was that he remained potent; general experience with "*success because of unconscious fear*" prove conclusively that they collapse after some time. This is one of the pathognomic features of these pseudo-successes; the other being that no direct connection is visible between the material worked through in the transference neurosis, and the disappearance of the symptoms.[18] There is only one exception to that empirical rule; cases of potency disturbances. Had the man had any other neurotic symptom, i.e., agoraphobia, erythrophobia, insomnia, neurotic headaches, or what not, the symptoms would have recurred. Why exactly, do some cases, not all by far,—as visible in the case of Mr. A. R.—show no recurrence? It is a matter of conjecture. I believe that the narcissistic defeat, the most painful possible for a man, embedded in a disturbance of potency, has something to do with it.

There are no miracles in the psychic economy; quantities of libido and aggression may be shifted to other points, the sum total remains the same. From a practical angle, Mr. A. S. did not improve his situation. Jail is even more painful and objectively damaging than is a potency disturbance. There are no bargains to be had from a neurotic superego.

Closely connected with the aforementioned facts is the problem as to why *incorrect interpretations often "help"* The problem is best explained by reproducing parts of a discussion with an intelligent and belligerent paranoiac patient. A colleague wanted the author's opinion in a case which first started with the symptom of blushing (erythrophobia), whereas paranoia was the real trouble. After a few appointments, the patient went into a hypomaniac mood, accompanied by great excitation, complete insomnia and ideas of grandeur. The colleague discontinued his analysis and gave superficial psychotherapy for some time. Fully agreeing with the colleague, the author suggested to the patient that he continue psychotherapy with the colleague, with the modification that the psycho-

[18] Problems of "successes because of unconscious fear" are discussed in the paper "Eight Prerequisites of Psychoanalytical Treatment of Homosexuality," Psa. Rev., Vol. 32, 1945.

therapy should be somewhat deeper, i.e., that his projections should be explained. The patient objected furiously; "According to your statement I am an incurable case. Analysis is impossible in my case, superficial psychotherapy did not work, what else is there to do?" It was explained to him that there is something in between psychoanalysis and superficial psychotherapy; psychotherapy using analytical knowledge. The patient remained angry and skeptical: "If you don't shoot in the center, how can you get a bull's eye?" He was given the following example, "Imagine you have an employee who regularly steals from the cash register but you, the boss, are completely unaware of it. One day, the young man appears very pale to you. You want to make a joke about his too extensive night-life and remark, 'You look very pale to me.' The man misunderstands your remark, believing because of his guilty conscience, that you refer to his thefts. *Don't you think that on the basis of this wrong conclusion, the man could stop stealing for some time?*"

There is only one reasonable surety against a recurrence of neurotic symptoms and signs; destruction brought through psychoanalysis of the basis on which these symptoms rest. This is the honest and solid way. Besides this there are many spurious ways to make a symptom disappear; in neurotic cases, however, strange as it may sound, honesty is the best policy.

Neurotic Symptom vs. Neurotic Personality

The general conception of a neurotic symptom versus a neurotic personality is this; the neurotic "character" is the basis, the neurotic "symptom," the apex of the pyramid. It is like an island emerging from the sea; only the superficial layers are visible. Neurotic difficulties are first absorbed by the personality; only after the "sponge" is oversaturated do the neurotic symptoms and signs make their appearance. The "queer" personality precedes the "queer" symptom.

It is obvious from that conception that it is easier to change neurotic symptoms than the personality. A good percentage of our patients leave analysis after their symptoms disappear, and they refuse to give us the opportunity to change their personality. True, every analysis is from the very beginning, an analysis of the whole personality; still, our patients make a precise distinction between both—only symptoms are acknowledged by them as sickness. The old saying, "You have to take me as I am" is still used to a great degree.

We are therefore not surprised when, even in most favorable cases, symptoms change first, the personality later. This sequence of events is observable in approximately ninety percent of all analyses. In ten per cent, the sequence of events is reversed and here the confusion begins.

The most simple answer is that it just depends on the neurotic deposition of *libido* and *destrudo*. If the main deposition is in the neurotic personality, the symptom changes first. If, however, the opposite is the case, and the main deposition is in the neurotic symptom, the personality changes first. This is sound reasoning, although, unfortunately, a totally unproductive one, since there is no possibility of finding out in advance where the respective deposition is, nor do we understand why the main deposition is not in all cases, first in the personality and only later in the symptoms.

The next possibility is an investigation of different types of analytically treated neurosis. In overlooking the results of phallic, anal and orally regressed cases, we could determine whether any rule in the sequence of changes (symptom vs. personality) is discernible. One could theoretically imagine that, in hysteric cases, it is easier to change symptoms and personality, than the personality in oral cases. Nothing of that regularity is visible. There are hysteric cases in which the personality changes remarkably, while the "simple" symptom persists for a long period of time. On the other hand, there are oral cases in which the symptoms disappear quickly and the personality is more difficult to change. To turn the tables; there are hysteric cases in which the symptoms change quickly, although the personality is resistant; whereas, in some oral cases, the personality changes and the symptoms persist. In other words, the problem is not to be solved only on the basis of stating the level of regression.

A third approach could resign itself to the empirical rule that symptoms change quicker than the personality. The rather exceptional cases in which the opposite happens, could be registered as unexplainable.

A fourth theory could claim that one should always take into account that the nonchangeable part, be it symptom or personality, was incorrectly interpreted. Such cases do exist; we exclude them because we speak of typical cases in which we assume that the analyst knows what he is talking about.

A fifth possibility is this: one could doubt whether the changes observable in the personality are not pseudo-changes in the first place.

I am personally not satisfied with these solutions and am rather surprised that our literature does not contain even the simple statement of the problem itself. I believe that every patient, unconsciously, does not want to make more compromises than *the minimum of the minimum of the minimum.* Forced out of his position, he gives in more and more, only to find one decisive resting place for the remnants of his neurosis. I believe, furthermore, that the subdivision in symptomatic and characterological neurosis, although practically useful, is much too schematized. The borderlines are flimsy and rather artificial; they remind one of the wooden signs erected on a plain, stating, "You are entering the state of . . ." The plain is the same, before and after the sign.

Basically, what is at stake for the neurotic is this: analysis forces him to give up the decisive parts of his neurosis. His unconscious trio wants to avoid that danger and finds in the end one point of refuge. Whether this point is called "symptom," or "character" is immaterial; basically, it is the "*buen retiro*" of his neurosis.

Let us take two clinical examples; Mrs. A. U., a hysteric, entered analysis because of frigidity and constant conflicts with her husband. She caused the greatest difficulties to the analyst and for a long time, projected upon him the hatred toward her father (mother). She "fought like a wild animal" (her own words in retrospect) against male prerogatives, her penis-envy was overdimensional. After some time, it was possible to discard this hatred as having been a fear of being seduced by her father. Upon longer "working through", she "came to terms" with analysis; the conflicts with her husband, the scenes and threats of leaving home and the danger of suicide disappeared. She even became a successful businesswoman, and learned to adapt herself to a difficult reality. Sex, which she previously hated became "fun," but no orgasm was forthcoming. Here we have an example of remarkable personality changes with the retention of the neurotic symptom.

What was at the bottom of her frigidity? The superficial layers were a hysteric penis-envy and an oedipal rape fantasy. After long "working through," sex became "fun" without achieving an orgasm. It turned out that her conception of sex was that of "being blasted to pieces," being killed. She concentrated all her masochistic fantasies at that point, and her frigidity was a defense against that imaginary danger. In a dream she represented the intercourse of two snakes; the male snake whirled the female snake in the air for so long a time that the latter died. The patient's holding on to her frigidity simply meant that this part of her neurosis was untouchable, therefore the defense, too, was indestructible.

In contradistinction to this case, Mr. A. V. went into analysis because of paranoiac jealousy. After long working out of the negative Oedipus and the voyeuristic components,[19] his symptom subsided. His personality was, however, imbued with psychic masochism patterned after the formula "nobody loves me." He cleverly constructed situations of that type, and for a very long time was holding on to that depository of his sexualized passivity.

Comparing both cases, we have to state that though the sequence of changes was exactly opposite, (Mrs. A. U., a personality change first; Mr. A. V., a symptom change first), they had one point in common; *the most conspicuous deposition of the neurosis was changed first.* In the case of Mrs. A. U., the conflicts with her husband and her inability to earn money were in the foreground; in the case of Mr. A. V., the "great man" was offended that he was ridiculously conspicuous in his jealousy. In other words: the deposition of remnants must be first, *inconspicuous* to the outsider, second, *give an alibi* that "so much has changed already," third, *the narcissism must not be hurt too much.* It is possible that these three points give the clue for the choice of the deposition of neurotic remnants.

Symptom or personality; both are used as a depository of the remnants of neurosis—even in well conducted analyses. It can be admitted, however, that some confusion remains concerning the specific choice. Why steal the show from future generations of scientifically interested psychoanalysts?

19 See the writer's: "Contributions to The Problem of Jealousy," Int. Z. f. Psa., und Imago, *24*:4, 1939.

8

Prognosis of Orally Regressed Neurotics and a Glance at the Shape of Things to Come in Psychopathology

WORKING with my definition and clinic of orality I can state that the prognosis in orally regressed cases is excellent, provided they are "exposed" to the correctly applied "mechanism of orality." A series of neurotic difficulties became thus for the first time curable, for instance psychogenic oral aspermia, oral frigidity, writer's block, retirement neurosis, pseudo mental debility,—others, with a traditionally poor prognosis, such as perversion homosexuality, premature ejaculation of the severest variety, erythrophobia, alcohol addiction, gambling, impostor-like features, etc.—accessible to successful therapy.

Freud once maintained that the study and exploration of neurosis is far more important than therapeutic successes and therapeutic furor. That was quite proper for the first decade of analysis, but it gave—unfortunately—every poor therapist a convenient excuse. Freud never meant his statement to be misinterpreted in this way, but it was. In any case, the golden age of excuses is past. Confronted with a patient, we have to tell him after six weeks of exploratory analysis, whether or not we subjectively believe that he has a *fair chance* of being cured. If he doesn't, we have to send him away. Only one exception is justified: if the patient, fully informed about our doubts of being capable of helping him, takes the chance of spending one to two years of his time and the adequate amount of money in an attempt to reverse the pessimistic prognosis. These cases are of two kinds: in exceptional instances, the patient's intuition is better than the physician's knowledge—these cases are helped. The majority of the "insisters" misuse the hopeless situation for masochistic purposes exclusively and have to be dismissed.

The tragicomedy of ignorance of, or, "non-acceptance" of, the "mechanism of orality," consists in the fact that many colleagues give an optimistic prognosis in oral cases in good faith, and are afterwards disappointed with the results, not to mention the patient's negative propagandistic wrath. The good faith is based on confusing these cases with hysteric ones.

I believe in the correctness of an observation, made by the late Hanns Sachs, to the effect that analytic psychiatry so far has merely scratched the surface of the psychic apparatus. This is no doubt true: what we already know is but an infinitesimal part of what we still have to learn. Future generations of analysts will smile condescendingly at our relative ignorance but, perhaps, benevolently give us credit that we did the most with the tools at our disposal. Perhaps they will react with the same smiling respect with which our generation of analysts regards Freud's report of a detail in the first published dream analyzed with his method. This report, published in "Interpretation of Dreams" in 1899, describes Freud's "Dream of Irma's Injection," dreamt in 1895. In the dream, the creator of analysis defends himself against the inner reproach that he did not fully cure a specific patient (Irma), using among others the argument that Irma did not accept his interpretations and therefore could not have been cured in the first place. Freud had not yet discovered the tremendous importance of unconscious "resistance," and believed at that time, fifty some years ago, that two types of patients existed, those who accepted and those who did not accept analytic interpretations. He believed furthermore that only patients of the first type could be cured. In the light of his later discoveries, this viewpoint lost its validity, but it serves as illustration how every step in analysis had to be discovered and tested gradually, on the basis of bitter clinical experience. We have to console ourselves: knowledge of the workings of the different parts of the unconscious personality did not spring like Pallas Athene from Zeus' head—at once, beautiful and complete. This is the difference between mythology and science.

Of course, the statement that the prognosis of orally regressed neurotics is excellent, if treated on the basis of the correctly applied "mechanism of orality," needs some amplification. Not every neurotic wishes to give up his neurosis in toto. Quite the contrary, he wishes unconsciously to rescue as much of his neurosis as possible and to make only the most minimal amount of compromises. Hence it is easier to change his symptom than his personality. Frequently, the patient declares himself cured prematurely and leaves analysis against the analyst's protest. These one-half or three-quarters "cured" patients are full of *gratitude: for the rescued part of the neurosis.* Consciously, the reason for gratitude is only stated in different terms.

The statement that oral neurotics have an excellent prognosis is therefore restricted to cases in which the analyst has sufficient time and coöperation.

It is also to be acknowledged that not every case is curable. Exactly the incurable patients and those who run away from analysis during a resistance-phase, are the loudest propagandists against us; they need confirmation from the ignorant environment how "stupid" and "dangerous" analysis is. The cured impotent man or frigid woman keeps the secret of the artificially acquired potency—that is understandable; not less than the silence of the cured drinker or homosexual. The uncured or runaway patient, however, talks—and loudly, for that matter.

Other cases with not too "secret" a symptom—i.e., writing block, blushing, divorce-mania, etc.,—are less reticent in acknowledging analytic cure. Still, personally, I don't believe in grateful cured patients.[1] The inner resentment remains. "Not even the analyst can with impunity lay hands on the infantile elements in the human psyche."

An especially dangerous pitfall in analytic therapy of orally repressed neurotics is the fact that some patients "cannot take it" when their psychic masochism is correctly analyzed and their aggression discarded as pseudo-aggression. The result is that the pseudo-aggression is reinforced to a degree which makes analysis impossible. Especially typical is the situation in which one has to show the patient that his (especially her) lack of effective complaints in early infancy against the "cruelty" of educators had not been based on reticence and modesty, but on masochistic enjoyment. These patients whose guilt is mobilized, frequently start a whole propaganda campaign against the analyst, mobilizing naive outsiders (sometimes even analysts), stating that the

[1] See my contribution to the Symposium on the Theory of the Therapeutic Results in Psychoanalysis, held at the XIVth International Psychoanalytic Congress, Marienbad 1936. Published in Int. J. of Psa. (London), XVIII, pp. 146–60, 1937.

analyst is cruel. Instead of understanding their nearly paranoiac projections, they act out: "You asked why I didn't complain? Well, I'm complaining *now*."

The danger of confusing hysterical and orally regressed cases is very acute. *Every* human being harbors an Oedipus complex. Hence it can be found and analyzed in every patient. The problem is: is the trouble seated there (as it is in hysterical cases) or is it used as a blind to cover up pre-oedipal conflicts? In oral regression the latter is the case.

The decisive point in an analytic interpretation is the *emphasis* and consistency with which the specific point is stressed. It is not sufficient to show that a patient damages himself *too* in adhering to his neurotic difficulties. Every patient is comparable to a reader of a book who remembers but one phrase. It is of decisive importance whether he remembers enjoyment of "psychic masochism" or "aggression." Both lead to guilt: the latter is defense against the former.

I believe that a classification of aims of psychiatric therapy and ways of achieving that aim, should be firmly established in the mind of the therapist. The real situation is far from satisfactory on that score. Here is a short summary of my personal views.[2]

Every psychotherapist—whatever his method of treatment of neuroses might be—is confronted with a suffering human being, *consciously* and in good faith frantically calling for help. *Unconsciously*, the situation is quite different, and exactly at that point the real difficulty starts.

Fifty years of psychoanalysis have proven conclusively that every neurotic enjoys *unconsciously* repressed fantasies in his various symptoms. He pays an exorbitant price for these symbolically materialized unconscious wishes, a price visible in his depressions, feeling of guilt, self-damaging tendencies.

In my opinion the subjective suffering which every neurosis produces is *not* the real reason why a neurotic consults the psychotherapist. Only if the inner balance between inner wishes and inner punishment for exactly these wishes is disturbed does the neurotic seek help.

[2] "Prognosis in Psychotherapy" in the Framework of Symposium on Psychotherapy held in the New York Society for Psychotherapy and Psychopathology on December 19, 1946.

This assumption explains why not all neurotics who have enough money, knowledge of existence of psychotherapy, and the necessary time and opportunity, do consult us. This, by the way, sheds a strange light on the problem of statistics in our specialty of medicine: they are always too favorable. Even if we are absolutely truthful about our successes and failures, we must give a distorted picture: our figures are too optimistic. This is simply the result of the material of our observation; we deal only with relatively favorable and selected cases. The simple fact that a patient consults us at all means that his inner balance is disturbed and, therefore, amenable to therapy. To express it differently: let's assume that a statistic of successes and failures in cases of psychogenic potency disturbance would be compiled by ten analysts for a series of ten years. The results would give a clue ábout cases who consulted us and would say little about curability of that specific neurotic symptom in general.

The disturbed balance between unconscious wishes and unconscious punishment—the prerequisite for consulting the psychotherapist—results in shaky defense-mechanisms. What the patient wants *consciously* is obvious: removal of suffering. What he wants *unconsciously* is—to put it paradoxically—maintenance and even improvement of neurosis. *An improvement, to be sure, which leaves his unconscious pleasures intact and removes his guilt. In other words, an impossible task.*

Since the patient's defenses are at the moment he consults us weak and his inner guilt unsatiated, he is inwardly scared that his whole neurosis will be taken away from him, the same neurosis which provides him unconsciously with such deep pleasure.

At that point the roads part. One type of psychotherapy—let's call it a *psychotherapy aiming at destruction of neurosis*—attempts to attack the unconscious wishes and defenses. Other types of psychotherapy—let's call it a *psychotherapy aiming at temporary conscious improvement of the patient's suffering*—will leave the edifice of the neurosis intact, though it may improve the patient's conscious well-being—temporarily. Therefore, the patient's behavior will be quite different during both precedures, whatever labels you attach to these two types of therapy. I was repeatedly struck by statements of patients who, before entering analysis, were treated by adherents of different schools of the second type of psychotherapy. They reported with friendly and amazing benevolence about their therapists, giving them credit for trying to do their best, acknowledging short-lived improvements, etc. When, however, one of these patients was even a short time in analysis which he did not finish, mostly terminating it by running away, nothing of the described kindness and benevolence was discernible. With anger and contempt, these patients were mercilessly attacking the analysts. The question arose: why the benevolence and malice, respectively.

I was forced to conclude that the benevolence and gratitude pertained to the fact that the neurosis was not even touched. That is less paradoxical than it sounds in the first moment. The patient who enters psychotherapeutic treatment expects unconsciously a *day of judgment*. Therefore, if nothing of that tragic expectation materializes, the patients feel unconsciously grateful. This does not cure him, but the feeling of benevolence is thus explainable.

It is customary to subdivide psychotherapies into suggestion and analysis. I believe that the term "suggestive therapy" should be defined more precisely. These types of therapy do not work with simple suggestion at all.

First, they reassure unconsciously the patient by not touching his basic conflicts, giving them different rationalizations as crutch.

Second, the therapist offers himself—though the patient does not know that—as artificial and transitory weapon against the patient's inner punitive conscience. The establishment of that new authority was stressed by a series of authors, starting with Ferenczi.

The inner "district attorney" (superego) accuses the unconscious ego of specific unconscious wishes. The ego uses unconsciously the therapist's rationalizations—whether they blame social, economic, cultural, environmental, or some other causes—as inner shield against these accusations. Thus, by establishing a new "protective" temporary, external authority, to be played off against the old, "accusing," internal authority, a temporary respite is achieved, manifesting itself in temporary "improvement." The accent is on "temporary", since the inner guilt proves itself to be stronger despite the new "protector."

The third and decisive reason is achievement of "*success because of unconscious fear.*" The latter term needs some elaboration.

The patient's psychic situation at the time of entering treatment is unconsciously that of a child "scared to death" of being found out in some forbidden doing. Imagine a child afraid of the discovery that it masturbates. Apply the simile to the unconscious, with a different "crime" and with exclusion of conscious awareness, and the situation is approximately described.

Well, the therapist may or may not conform to the patient's inner fears. Amusingly enough, the patient is inwardly more convinced of the psychotherapist's omniscience and psychologic x-ray-eyes than reality warrants. Still, on the basis of that unconscious misunderstanding, temporary improvements can take place. The situation is reminiscent of the following situation. Imagine an employee who steals regularly from the cash register; the boss, however, is completely unaware of it. One morning the young man looks very pale. The boss wants to tease him about his too extensive night life and remarks, "You look very pale to me." The guilty one misunderstands the harmless remark, because of his guilty conscience believing that the boss refers to the theft. It is quite possible that on the basis of the wrong conclusion the young man stops stealing—for a couple of weeks.

This trend of thoughts explains why even incorrect interpretations help—temporarily. The same holds true for *maintaining inner guilt on a sidetrack*. Let's take the example of a patient with impotence based on unconscious feminine identification, who claims that what disturbs him most is the fact that he cannot satisfy his wife sexually, hence is "cruel" toward her. If the therapist bolsters his pseudo-aggressive defense by explaining that aggression is the cause of the patient's difficulty, without analyzing his passivity—well, the neurosis is strengthened because unconscious wish and unconscious defense are confused.

Let us compare three cases: the previously mentioned Messrs. A. R., A. S. and A. T.,[3] the patients with "inflationary potency," "success because of unconscious fear," and the cured impotent man, respectively. If we look at these cases analytically we can state: Mr. A. R. was so scared *unconsciously* of analysis that he preferred to give up temporarily for the purpose of escaping analysis with good conscience. His "*success*

[3] See p. 325 ff.

because of unconscious fear" lasted only three months. His unconscious ego preferred temporarily to *sacrifice the symptom instead of sacrificing the whole neurosis.* Mr. A. S. achieved the same result after seven weeks of analysis, using via identification "borrowed strength." He shifted, as his later life proved, the guilt and psychic masochism pertaining to his pregenital libido and aggression to provoking jail sentences. The fact that he was really innocent, as far as politics were concerned, was a part of his inner alibi: "I am innocent of the other crime, too." The amazing fact was that he remained potent. General experience with "successes because of unconscious fear" prove conclusively that they collapse after some time. This is one of the pathognomic features of these pseudo-successes; the other being that no direct connection is visible between the material worked through in the transference neurosis and the disappearance of symptoms.

As stated, there are no miracles in the psychic economy: quantities of libido and aggression may be shifted to other points, the sum total remains the same. Symptoms may be exchanged—that's the maximum. From a practical angle, Mr. A. S. did not improve his situation. Jail is even more painful and objectively damaging than is potency disturbance. There are no bargains to be had from a neurotic superego.

So far we have stressed only one prognostic factor: what the psychotherapist does with the patient. It would be, of course, erroneous to assume that the prognosis depends exclusively on the physician's actions or omissions of actions. Every prognosis in the therapy of a neurosis rests on two pillars: one is the physician, the other the patient's unconscious. More specifically: *the patient's unconscious feeling of guilt.* I am of the opinion—stressed in a series of papers [4]—that the unconscious feeling of guilt is the decisive part in therapy of neurotics. Basically it is the *static or dynamic deposition* of that unconscious guilt. Every neurotic has, of course, a superabundance of guilt. This feeling is deposited in neurotic symptom, signs, personality difficulties, sense of depression, ego limitations, etc. The whole problem of prognosis depends on the therapist's ability to "*mobilize*" that inner guilt. This presupposes, however, an at least potentially fluctuating,

[4] Summary in the writer's contribution to the Symposium "Theory of Therapeutic Results," held at the XIVth Int. Psa. Convention, 1936 (publ. Int. J. of Psa., 1937) and "Working Through" in The Psa Rev., 1945.

dynamic deposition. When the vicious circle between neurotic wish and neurotic punishment is frozen, so to speak, the deepest psychotherapy is powerless.

A witty patient characterized every psychotherapy as eternal fight between the couch and the door. The question is in what state the patient decides that fight. He can run away; he can achieve a success because of unconscious fear; he can establish a new defense mechanism, or—even be cured.

It has been already stressed in previous chapters that the unconscious ego reacts at first to the *analytic "danger"* in the same way as to any other difficulty threatening the neurotic balance: [5] it tries to *counteract it in a "routine" manner.* This routine consists, first, of increasing the strength of the already established defense mechanism, and, if not sufficient, to exchange, secondly, the defense mechanism, only to keep the neurotic balance. From this fact follows that the quickly established new defenses visible in the early stages of analysis, have nothing whatsoever to do with a real cure, but exactly the opposite: *maintenance of neurosis with new devices.* Only the fact that analysis goes after these new defense mechanisms, too, convinces the unconscious ego that "routine" handling of the situation does not suffice and more drastic measures are necessary. It depends, then, basically on the amount of "free floating" feeling of unconscious guilt, whether the patient chooses the desperate measure of running away from analysis altogether, or allows further attacks against his neurosis—with the ultimate prospect of cure. This phase teaches us, however, never to underestimate the *elasticity* of the unconscious ego which is very cunning in devising ever new defenses only to keep the neurotic balance.

It is analytically obvious that without changing the basic structure of a neurosis, no basic change in the patient can occur. But, and that but weighs heavily, during analysis the feeling of guilt is mobilized and results in increased pressure against the specific defense mechanism used by the specific patient. Consequently, very often in a well-conducted analysis the *changes of the defense mechanism,* which means substitution through another one, are striking in the first weeks of treatment, giving the patient and the environment the mirage of normalcy.

[5] See the writer's paper: "The Danger Neurotics Dread Most: Loss of the Basic Fallacy," The Psa. Rev., 33:1, 1946.

To sum up: Prognosis in psychotherapy depends on the type of psychotherapy used *and* the potentially dynamic part of unconscious guilt which can be mobilized. The patient asks of psychotherapy something unachievable: improvement of unconscious pleasures with elimination of inner guilt. The patient tries unconsciously to make the minimum of compromises, mainly giving up temporarily a symptom or establishing new defense mechanisms—always trying to hold on to his basic neurosis. "Successes because of unconscious fear"—encountered in every type of psychotherapy—are a mirage. It depends on the type of psychotherapy whether one stops at that point—with or without some illusions—or "goes after" these pseudo-successes, too. Only if these attempts at maintaining the neurosis are fully analyzed, can real success be achieved.

Confronted with the all-important problem of psychic masochism we would like to know where that "tendency" comes from. "Chemically," psychic masochism is misplaced baby aggression, based on the triad: inadequately expressed (or inexpressible) aggression—guilt—libidinization of guilt. Exactly because psychic masochism is not a drive but an unconscious defense mechanism, we are able to change it in psychoanalysis. In other words, we are *therapeutically* well advanced.

Theoretically, our progress is poorer. True enough, we can explain the genesis, but we are, so far, incapable of stating why one child, confronted with identical external factors, chooses the "solution" of psychic masochism more extensively than the other. That has been the great X in psychopathology. That X is not solved by playing around with words like "strong" and "weak" ego.

There is, of course, always the biological and quantitative recourse. Both are admission of ignorance in psychology—if applied to a psychological problem. We can say that—according to the Eros-Thanatos theory—there is a biological tendency to direct aggression against oneself; more, that all aggression is originally but self-aggression, only secondarily shifted outside, towards objects, through Eros' counteractions. We can also assume that since the quantity of biological endowment of aggression varies in different individuals, children have to cope with quantitatively different conflicts arising from handling these quantities. Finally, we can suspect that infantile megalomania, the offense against which starts the ball of aggression rolling, is different in different children, hence the ability of "taking" and "absorbing" the offense varies, too.[6]

All these (and similar) excuses can be used; the fact remains that we don't know. We can console ourselves that therapy is more important than theoretical speculation—for the patient. In the meantime, an undisguised admission of "we don't know *yet*", seems indicated.

Finally, we can venture a guess as to why every person considers psychic masochism in his unconscious ego as the greatest inner danger. The reason seems to be that it endangers life: one step further and suicide or extinction of life is the result. Newer studies of the psychology of suicide seem to point in this direction.[7]

Does the psychic masochist "learn" something from his bad experiences? No. Since he lives on the basis of his conscious illusions, mainly that of being an innocent victim of other people's cruelty and malice, he gets more and more bitter. Even the minimum of life experience, unavoidable and given as gift and taxfree to everyone, is lost on him. Paraphrasing Coleridge, one could say that the psychic masochist without treatment becomes progressively a "*sadder and not a wiser man.*" Elderly neurotics prove that point conclusively.[8]

[6] One can also adduce the different "libidinous types" which, according to Freud, constitute a biological fact (statement of Anna Freud, in a discussion in the Vienna Psychoanalytic Society, interpreting her father's opinion). As a matter of fact, the suggestion has been put forward for the use of a double yardstick in the genesis of different neuroses: the level of regression *and* the libidinous type (L. Eidelberg). The idea is usable, but does not explain too much. First of all, it seems doubtful to me whether the libidinous type is really a biological fact; I rather subscribe to the assumption that the "type" represents one of the later results of inner conflicts. Secondly, it leaves us still where we started: with the quantitative factor. One can say e.g., that the homosexual is "so narcissistic" that he runs after the "duplication of his own defense mechanism," the penis as breast substitute in the other fellow. One can further state that the writer is "so highly narcissistic" that he "eliminates" the masochistic attachment to the refusing mother by acting *on himself* the "corrected" picture of giving mother and receiving baby. That may be so and the quantity of narcissism may account for the *duality* and *unity*-situation. However, since we cannot measure these quantities, theoretically it helps us little. Obviously there are many undiscovered subdivisions in the framework of "libidinous types."

[7] See the author's "Problems of Suicide," The Psychiatric Quarterly, 1947.

[8] First printed under the title "Elderly Neurotics" in Diseases of the Nervous System, VIII, 2, 1947.

Neurosis is a progressive, not a self-limiting disease. Ample proof of this statement is the simple observation that untreated neuroses deteriorate as time passes. Symptoms and signs may be exchanged but the sum total increases.

The question is raised: Why do neuroses progress? There are two interrelated reasons: First, is the fact that unconscious wishes, previously satisfied in symbolic innuendos, want more substantial realization. Second, the inner conscience increases its lust for punishment. The whole neurotic structure is based on appeasing and buying off the inner conscience with depression, unhappiness and suffering. Every neurosis is based on deep self-damaging tendencies. The neurotic may be compared to the man who offers a thousand dollars for a 65 cent motion picture admission ticket. An outsider would consider that man either "crazy" or drunk, or, if he cares to attribute to him rational motives at all, will think that something in the picture attracts him "magically," so that the money spent corresponds to the pleasure he expects. The amount of conscious unhappiness which every neurosis produces, is so overdimensional that the neurotic "deal" is impossible without the presence of that self-damaging tendency. Since every neurosis represents, as Freud proved fifty years ago, a compromise between unconscious repressed wishes and unconscious repressed inhibitions, the infantile pleasure must be out of proportion. Neurotics are not fools, in the popular meaning of the word. They do, however pay a ridiculous price for the camouflaged "pleasures" imbedded in their particular neurosis. But the pleasure is real enough for them, of course, only in unconscious reality.

Both *parties constituentes* want to get more out of the "deal." The unconscious wish desires materialization, in a panic of "Time runs short," the unconscious part of conscience seeks more punishment. I have, however, the impression that at that late stage of the game, the inner conscience is the real malefactor. While we may have little respect for the policeman who allows himself to be bribed for years, the officer himself, on the other hand, becomes more demanding. He has to assert himself. His "trick" is to lure the victim into an "impossible situation" and then to increase his demands. That explains why the forties and the fifties are so frequently the neurotic danger spot.

Other facts also point in the direction of increased power of inner conscience: the very fallacy on which every neurosis rests, is too often confronted with reality and "debunked." Every collapse of that fallacy is used by the inner conscience "to increase the rent." Assuming that the basic fallacy of a specific neurotic consists of the fantasy that not he is a glutton for punishment, but the "bad" mother or father treated the child "badly." The neurotic repetitiveness will result in reincarnation of the same situation in marriage and social-professional life. Such a neurotic will marry a shrew, be mistreated by her, his friends will take advantage of him, his competitors get the better of him. The masochistic neurotic will see to it that the proper people for that purpose are chosen. Consciously, of course, he will consider himself the innocent victim. He will not fool his inner conscience, though. The "hell within," to use a Miltonic phrase, will ironically point out that he himself, the alleged victim, is the manufacturer of his own defeats. To counteract that inner voice, the next "mistake" must be greater and the resultant "injustice" increased. Thus a veritable race is instituted with increasing stakes.

Maintaining the "basic fallacy," becomes an indispensable prerequisite to the continuation of the neurosis. Since the inner conscience objects more and more, the alibi before one's own reasoning power must be stronger. This leads to greater external troubles. How else can the neurotic convince himself that the outer world is cruel? Only by unconsciously provoking a greater injustice. The increased difficulties encountered by the aging neurotic in the pursuit of his specific brand of unhappiness, produce a strange mechanism, that of *pseudo-naiveté*. The neurotic can fool himself about his motives less and less. Therefore, he must produce before himself a new mirage. That mirage of expected success is counteracted by the "voice of experience." It is the skepticism of the experience which warns even a neurotic. To silence that objection, a greater amount of self-deception is discharged. That naiveté is *pseudo-naiveté,* because the obvious facts are overlooked. "Experience," said Oscar Wilde, "is the name everybody gives to his mistakes." That additional deterrent must be overcome—and the technique is—*pseudo-naiveté.*

This explains why the "mistakes" committed by the elderly neurotic are more irrational than identical "mistakes" made twenty years earlier. The outer world sees in this only precocious senility. But it is nothing of the kind; the poor neurotic has simply greater inner obstacles to overcome.

Interestingly enough, when the neurotic tries escape into a "narcissistic retreat," his inner conscience objects. The last escapade, representing once more a neurotic repetition, leaves the aging neurotic a little more despondent. The thwarted neurotic tries to retire from disappointing objects and for a short time he appears to learn from past experience. Unpleasant encounters with friends contribute to that retreat: "I want only acquaintances." But here again the power of the inner conscience obstructs that way out. The narcissistic retreat is paid for with inner guilt. The inner conscience favors object-relations. From early youth, education, and later, inner conscience, have objected to concentration on one's self, which is identified with selfishness, and in a deeper layer, with infantile masturbation. That old prohibitive pattern is inwardly mobilized and used to push the disillusioned neurotic once more into object-relationship. His *buen retiro,* paid for with pessimism and a "nobody-loves-me" attitude, becomes untenable. Then if the neurotic resumes the old patterns of neurotic repetitiveness, the inner conscience clamps down once more. Which all goes to show that one cannot "do business" with the inner conscience.

A merciful fate helps in the end; the elderly neurotic acquires some organic disease. A clever psychiatrist once stated: "Punishment is one of life's natural therapies." That punishment in form of organic disease absorbs, especially if sugarcoated with a good dose of hypochondria and self-reproach over missed opportunities, so much of the neurotic's need for punishment that even the elderly neurotic sometimes makes a resigned and rather calm impression. People even wonder about stoicism.

Neurosis being a progressive disease, the old repressed infantile wishes ask for more substantial satisfaction, the inner conscience claims more punishment. Different techniques are used, showing how the inner conscience lures the aging ego into more dangerous escapades. The natural solution is in the end an independently arising organic disease which saturates the neurotic wish for punishment. *From the cradle to the grave, the neurotic is an insatiable glutton for punishment.*

I believe that the future of analysis will bring in addition to overcoming the usual children's diseases, reorientation on genetic principles, greater than the minimum *practically* used today, though in *principle* fully admitted. I believe that the present thinking from the top of the psychic pyramid downwards, will be replaced by thinking from the base of the pyramid upward. This will automatically increase the importance of orality. This "*dies certus an incertus quando*," the day which will surely come, the only uncertainty being the little question of when, will place the "mechanism of orality" in its proper perspective.

The decisive obstacle in understanding the rôle of orality, is the painful fact of having to accept the universality of the problem, including the scientific rejector. Psychic masochism, imbedded in the neurotic wish to be refused, will play an integral part in the didactic analysis of the future analyst.

Nosologic entities, as treasured today, will be seen in the place where they belong: as rescue stations from the deeper oral danger. Nobody denies their clinical existence. Their present lack of interconnection with the basic problem in the human psyche—with orality—is however questioned.

A socially-minded patient predicted to me—after understanding with horror the tragic importance of orally based psychic masochism—that in high schools of the future an obligatory course on self-damaging tendencies will be taught. The pupil will be indoctrinated with the technique of not provoking inner disappointments, and coping with unavoidable external ones; the motto being: "The world owes you exactly nothing, not even a kick in the jaw."

The reformer-tendencies of the patient even let him believe that that school-subject would diminish the great army of psychic masochists.

I cannot share his optimism. Even if the school-system taught the subject-matter of "psychic masochism," the pupil would not recognize it in himself. He would, pushed by others, enter—perhaps—treatment earlier, if at all.

Should, however, an optimist expect that the duration of psychoanalytic treatment of orally regressed neuroses, will be shortened, he will be sorely disappointed: one and a half to two and a half years of regular treatment, at least three full appointments per week, are unavoidable.

Future generations will undoubtedly see the emergence of psychiatric out-patient departments on a mass scale. It is a fair guess that psychic masochists will—statistically—be the most typically encountered type of help-seeking individual, though he himself will not know it.

Whether or not, the psychic masochism of humanity will prematurely "solve" the problem of masochism via an atomic deluge, before proper safeguards can be established against the *psychic cancer* of the human race—her strange *unconscious wish to suffer*—is a matter of hope and conjecture.

Index

3
4
5
6
7
8 f
9 g
0 h
1 i
8 2 j